Literatim

Literatim

Essays at the Intersections of Medicine and Culture

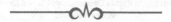

Howard Markel

OXFORD
UNIVERSITY PRESS

OXFORD
UNIVERSITY PRESS

Oxford University Press is a department of the University of Oxford. It furthers
the University's objective of excellence in research, scholarship, and education
by publishing worldwide. Oxford is a registered trade mark of Oxford University
Press in the UK and certain other countries.

Published in the United States of America by Oxford University Press
198 Madison Avenue, New York, NY 10016, United States of America.

Library of Congress Cataloging-in-Publication Data
Names: Markel, Howard, author.
Title: Literatim : essays at the intersections of medicine and culture /
Howard Markel.
Description: New York, NY : Oxford University Press, [2020] |
Includes bibliographical references and index.
Identifiers: LCCN 2019033686 (print) | LCCN 2019033687 (ebook) |
ISBN 9780190070007 (hbk) | ISBN 9780190070021 (epub) |
ISBN 9780190070014 (updf)
Subjects: MESH: Medicine in Literature | Medicine in the Arts |
Motion Pictures | Famous Persons | History of Medicine | Collected Work
Classification: LCC R733 (print) | LCC R733 (ebook) | NLM WZ 7 |
DDC 610—dc23
LC record available at https://lccn.loc.gov/2019033686
LC ebook record available at https://lccn.loc.gov

9 8 7 6 5 4 3 2 1
Printed by Integrated Books International, United States of America

For Catherine D. DeAngelis, MD, MPH,

with gratitude and affection

CONTENTS

Literatim

Introduction

In 1959, shortly before his death, legendary Hollywood film director Preston Sturges (who I write about more fully later in this book) remarked, "The only amazing thing about my career . . . is that I ever had one at all."[1] The same might be said about my career as a professor, physician, and historian of medicine.

As a young boy, some of my best companions were the characters I met on the pages of novels, theatrical scripts, and screenplays. Fascinated by human stories, conflicts and contradictions, both moral and physical, and worlds so vastly different from my middle-class, suburban Detroit upbringing, I was inspired to try my hand at writing. As an active participant in my high school's theater program (thankfully, in an era when taxpayers still supported the arts as a critical part of the public school curriculum), I attempted to write a series of incredibly bad plays. Soon enough, I was confronted by the difficult time I had (and have) in coming up with believable plots, a serious handicap for any budding fabulist.

To compensate for that failing, I finished high school with the idea of becoming a physician who found his stories in the care of his patients and the drama of the hospital. As Dr. William Carlos Williams wrote, such clinical encounters afforded glimpses into the

> . . . underground stream [of humanity] . . . it is then we see, by this constant feeling for a meaning, from the unselected nature of the material, just as it comes in over the phone or the office door, that there is no better way to get an intimation of what is going on in the world.[2]

Soon after matriculating into the University of Michigan in the fall of 1978, I stumbled upon what turned out to be the best first step in navigating the thorny thickets of medicine, academia, and writing. It was then a professor convinced me that a student determined on medicine could also study English literature. The

Literatim: Essays at the Intersections of Medicine and Culture. Howard Markel, Oxford University Press (2020).
© Oxford University Press.
DOI: 10.1093/oso/9780190087647.001.0001

lengthy Western canon was still rigidly adhered to and almost exclusively taught in those days. And because so many of our discussions centered on the conflicts and dilemmas these writers explored, I often looked at my reading lists as an intensive course in moral philosophy, but with far better and more enjoyable texts.

Studying English literature also served as a welcome respite from the rigors of the rote memorization and smelly laboratory work I encountered in my "pre-medical" classes. I was especially partial to the Victorian novelists Charles Dickens, Anthony Trollope, Thomas Hardy, the Brontë sisters, and George Eliot. Thanks to a scholarship from my college and encouragement from my parents, in 1981 I was able to make a life-changing journey to the British Isles, where I explored the Victorians in their native habitat and, later, roamed the streets of Dublin with a copy of the modernist James Joyce's *Ulysses* in hand. A bona fide prose man, I struggled with and learned to appreciate the poetry of Milton, Keats, Yeats, Byron, Eliot, Seamus Heaney, and William Carlos Williams's college roommate, Ezra Pound. Less rigorously taught at the time but no less important were a slew of other American litterateurs I came to cherish, including F. Scott Fitzgerald, H.L. Mencken, Mark Twain, Sinclair Lewis, Theodore Dreiser, Richard Wright, Herman Wouk, and Philip Roth.

To feed my love of drama, I devoured the plays and comedies of Shakespeare, of course, but also the theatrical gems by Oscar Wilde, Ben Jonson, Christopher Marlowe, George Bernard Shaw, Eugene O'Neill, George S. Kaufman and Moss Hart, Sean O'Casey, J.M. Synge, and Arthur Miller (a Michigan graduate, class of 1938, who frequently visited the Ann Arbor campus to lecture to budding writers).

Every night but Mondays, five different cinema guilds or cooperatives took over the various auditoria on the Ann Arbor campus and screened the spun gold of the Hollywood film factories. All through my undergraduate and medical school years, I watched two or three of these classic movies a week, all for the admission of a dollar or two, a rare privilege in those pre-video, DVD, and streaming days. The raucous antics of the Marx Brothers, anything starring Humphrey Bogart, James Stewart, Cary Grant, or James Cagney, the screwball comedies of Preston Sturges, Frank Capra's all-American "Capra-corn," the glorious MGM musicals, the holy trinity of silent comedy—Chaplin, Lloyd, and Keaton—and the tense dramas of Alfred Hitchcock, Elia Kazan, and Budd Schulberg, to name but a few of the offerings, essentially served as my fifth, uncredited course each term.

Even though English majors during the early 1980s had one of the highest acceptance rates into medical school, mine was a rarely taken path in Ann Arbor. When my class of more than 250 medical students matriculated at the University of Michigan Medical School in 1982, I was the only English major of the lot. Today, most of my medical students would handily agree on such a duality and, indeed, many of them are drawn from departments of English, history, comparative literature, music, art history, and many other fields not all that scientific. Back in the dark ages of the 1980s, however, this track was still considered to be heresy and (almost) every good medical student came armed with a baccalaureate in biology, chemistry, or molecular biology.

It was as a first-year medical student when I discovered the allure of narrative history. Divining and telling stories of the lives of doctors, diseases, and patients from the past appealed to the left side of my brain; the rigor required in terms of documenting every statement made with a text or piece of evidence never failed to tickle the right side of my frontal cortex. It was a *Eureka!*-like moment that I have yet to recover from. Angels sang, harps strummed, and a warm, fuzzy feeling energized my body. At last, I had found my literary quarry. I now knew what I wanted to write about and explore. And with due respect to all who love or create fiction, I have always found that real-life events are typically far better than anything any human could ever contrive.

In 1986, with the ink on my medical diploma barely dried, I drove an overstuffed Honda Civic south to the Johns Hopkins Hospital in Baltimore to begin my training as a pediatrician. On call, every third night for three years, I honed my writing skills composing careful histories of the patients I admitted to the Hopkins and, because I often found myself wide awake in the early morning hours, writing a book about baby care advice ghostwritten by the famed Baltimore journalist H. L. Mencken in 1910 and edited by Theodore Dreiser, who was then in between novels and serving as the editor for a woman's magazine published by the Butterick Dress Pattern Company.[3]

After internship and residency, I crossed Monument Street, the potholed byway separating the Johns Hopkins Hospital and the Johns Hopkins Institute of the History of Medicine. Narrow in physical distance, it represented the widest intellectual difference of my career. The doctors I had studied under at the Hospital were chiefly interested in disease, cures, scientific discovery, and, most of all, action; my professors at the Institute were more drawn to long, garrulous arguments over social and national contexts, clever cultural fantasies that rarely adhered to reality, and history "from the ground up," meaning the lives of patients as well as great doctors. I took the best offerings from both fields and have always believed I was a better physician because I was a historian of medicine and that I was a better medical historian because I was a physician.

In retrospect, it was a youthful, if not outright naive, belief that I could succeed as a doctor who studied the humanities and actually make a living at it. When I told my father, upon completing my residency training in pediatrics, that instead of joining a lucrative private practice on New York City's Park Avenue, I was matriculating into the Johns Hopkins Ph.D. program in the history of medicine, he shook his head and wearily replied, "Howard, you find new ways of making less money each year."

Similarly, on the last day of my pediatrics residency, a rather prominent immunologist came up to the floor I was supervising. He was arrogant, self-assured, and confident that he would someday win the Nobel Prize—an achievement he has still not been accorded, by the way. As I scribbled my last notes, the doctor asked me what I was going to be doing the following morning. I proudly told him of my graduate school plans and he looked at me, incredulously, as if I had just told him I planned on flying to Jupiter on the back of a Hershey bar. "Why do you want to study medical history," he asked, "when you can make it?" I came up with an answer but in the interest of full disclosure, it was not until a few weeks later, while shaving and still stewing in resentment: "Oh yeah?" I thought as I imagined another meeting with him, "Just you wait. I'm going to write the history of medicine and guess what? You're not going to be in it!"

In the years since, I have been blessed to occupy my work life reading, re-reading, and thinking about literary and historical works as well as extracting complex—and sometimes confusing—stories of illness from ailing patients and myriad other sources. As a physician, I have always found this approach to be helpful in figuring out a great many medical problems. As a writer, this worldview has enabled my understanding and explanation of the human condition, which is, after all, the purview of both physicians and authors. Although writers and physicians use markedly different tools and approaches, both are recording and interpreting narratives. Patients, too, I have found, are eager to tell their stories of physical and psychological illness.

From the distance of nearly three decades, my career looks like a rather direct path, but in reality it was somewhat circuitous and represented a significant gambling of resources. There were no guarantees I would be able to find such a position in a medical school, and there were relatively few role models with which to compare or model my career goals. I was, as they used to say in the days of early aviation, flying by the seat of my pants.

A serious and rather sad interruption was occasioned by the early years of the AIDS epidemic in the United States, during the 1980s and early 1990s. My training in pediatrics and adolescent medicine afforded me significant expertise treating sexually transmitted diseases, and when a colleague asked me to help out in a Baltimore AIDS clinic, I could hardly say no. It turned out to be one of the most gratifying, albeit often heartbreaking, experiences of my career, both in becoming (I hope) a compassionate and caring clinician and, intellectually, as a historian of epidemics, quarantines, and public health.

Recently, a student asked me if when I was writing my doctoral thesis and, later, books about late 19th-and early-20th century epidemics, did I ever think that work would be put to use a decade later in my collaborative work with the U.S. Centers for Disease Control and Prevention to help develop federal and international policies of pandemic preparedness planning. I told her that I may have briefly held such hopes—all authors hope that their work makes a difference—but I soon gave those notions up as a long shot at best. In reality, I think I always had a goal of playing a role in the public conversation about serious and important matters. I just didn't broadcast it, in case it failed to come true. I might add that there were many days when this goal seemed quite distant.

Around this same time period, 2000–2011, I began writing and reporting regularly for the *New York Times*. There, I learned from some of the best editors in the world how to tell a story accurately, quickly, and with far fewer words than the excess verbiage too often employed by the professoriate. Similarly, between 2010 and 2012, I took up writing and broadcasting short pieces called "Science Diction," in which I discussed the origins of scientific and medical terms on the National Public Radio show *Science Friday*. One of my favorite career coincidences, however, occurred in 2011 when a literary critic, in an otherwise favorable review of my best-selling book, *An Anatomy of Addiction*, snidely complained that there was, in my writing style, "a certain *PBS*-ness of the soul."[4] The next day, a producer for the *PBS NewsHour* who had laughed at the review in the morning paper invited me to consider writing a monthly column for that show's website, a joyful chore I have performed since 2012.

Many of the essays comprising this volume first appeared in two of the world's premier medical journals, the *New England Journal of Medicine* and the *Journal of the American Medical Association*, but there are a few other essays I wrote for some other superb publications, including *The Lancet, The American Journal of Medicine, Public Health Reports*, and *Archives of Pediatrics and Adolescent Medicine*. Completing the volume are dozens of the more informal essays I have written for the *PBS NewsHour*. The conceit of my monthly column for the *NewsHour* is to highlight the anniversary of a momentous event (or person's work) that continues to shape modern medicine. Given that these shorter pieces were written for a public *broadcasting* network, they are aimed at a far larger and more diverse audience and, as a result, do not include citations or references. In every instance, I worked with talented editors who enabled and expanded my peculiar passion for historicizing great events, works of literature, films, plays, and even musical comedies that touch upon the practice of medicine and the experience of illness. Most important, they allowed me to explore sundry topics as traditional as the Hippocratic Oath and the invention of the stethoscope to popular cultural tales of Rodgers and Hammerstein's medical musical, *Allegro*, and the painful life of Cole Porter, along with a shelf of other books, plays, and films that have helped me to better understand the human condition.

Herewith, collected into one volume, are a stack of essays for your consideration. They are arbitrarily divided into four parts: I. Medical Literature; II. Medical Texts; III. Medical Performances; and IV. "A Certain *PBS*-ness of the Soul." You can read these essays *in seriatim* or by way of occasional visits as time allows. I hope your enjoyment of them is equal to a tiny percentage of the joy I experienced in the wonderful hours spent writing them.

Positano, Italy
February 20, 2019

REFERENCES

1. Howard Markel. Not So Great Moments: The "Discovery" of Ether Anesthesia and Its "Re-Discovery" by Hollywood. *JAMA*. 2008; 300(18): 2188–2190.
2. William Carlos Williams. *The Autobiography of William Carlos Williams*. (New York: Random House, 1951), pp. 358–360.
3. Howard Markel, Frank A. Oski. *The H. L. Mencken Baby Book*. (Philadelphia: Hanley & Belfus, 1989).
4. Dwight Garner. The Lure of Cocaine, Once Hailed as Cure-All. *The New York Times*. July 19, 2011, p. C1.

PART I

Medical Literature

CHAPTER 1

∾

"I Swear by Apollo"

The Hippocratic Oath

E very spring for almost 30 years, I have happily donned a rented robe, hood, and
mortarboard to attend medical school commencement exercises. The purpose
of this annual foray into pomp and circumstance goes well beyond applauding the
achievements of graduates who are about to enter the medical profession. For me,
commencement is the perfect opportunity to renew my vows, as it were, standing
shoulder to shoulder with both newly minted doctors and like-minded colleagues
as we take the Hippocratic Oath.

Although many scholars dispute the exact authorship of the writings ascribed to
the ancient physician Hippocrates, who probably lived sometime between 460 and
380 B.C.E., the oath named for him is simultaneously one of the most revered, pro-
tean, and misunderstood documents in the history of medicine.[1] To begin with, it is
often misquoted. For example, many people mistakenly ascribe our mantra of "First,
do no harm" (a phrase translated into Latin as *"Primum non nocere"*) to the Oath, although it appears nowhere in that venerable pledge. (See Below) Hippocrates came
closest to issuing this directive in his treatise *Epidemics,* in an axiom that reads, "As
to diseases, make a habit of two things—to help, or at least, to do no harm."

Most doctors practicing today are surprised to learn that the first recorded
administration of the Hippocratic Oath in a medical school setting was at the
University of Wittenberg in Germany in 1508 and that it did not become a standard
part of a formal medical school graduation ceremony until 1804, when it was incorporated into the commencement exercises at Montpellier, France.[2] The custom
spread in fits and starts on both sides of the Atlantic during the 19th century, but
even well into the 20th century relatively few American physicians formally took
the oath. According to a survey conducted for the Association of American Medical

Literatim: Essays at the Intersections of Medicine and Culture. Howard Markel, Oxford University Press (2020).
© Oxford University Press.
DOI: 10.1093/oso/9780190087647.001.0001

Colleges in 1928, for example, only 19 percent of the medical schools in North America included the oath in their commencement exercises.[3] With the discovery of the atrocities that were committed in the name of medicine during World War II and the growing interest in bioethics in the succeeding decades, oath taking began playing an increasing part in graduation ceremonies.[4]

This spring, nearly every U.S. medical school will administer some type of professional oath to its share of about 16,000 men and women who are eager to take possession of their medical degrees. Yet it is doubtful that Hippocrates would recognize most of the pledges that are anachronistically ascribed to him. Such revisionism is hardly unique to our era. Indeed, the tinkering with Hippocrates' oath began soon after its first utterance and generally reflected the changing values, customs, and beliefs associated with the ethical practice of medicine.

Consequently, there are stark differences between the promises made in the original version and the oaths sworn today. To take the most obvious example, few if any of us now believe in the ancient Greek gods Apollo, Asclepius, Hygieia, and Panaceia, and we therefore no longer pledge allegiance to them. Textual and documentary evidence indicates that religion in general—regardless of its form—now has a distant relationship with medical science: a "content analysis" of the oaths administered at 147 U.S. and Canadian medical schools in 1993 showed that only 11 percent of the versions invoked a deity.[5]

In Hippocrates' day, the student made a binding vow to honor his teacher as he would his parents and to share financial and intellectual resources with his mentor and the mentor's family. Unfortunately for those of us engaged in medical education today, this pledge has long since passed into disfavor.

There are two highly controversial vows in the original Hippocratic Oath that we continue to ponder and struggle with as a profession: the pledges never to participate in euthanasia and abortion.[1] These prohibitions applied primarily to those identified as Hippocratic physicians, a medical sect that represented only a small minority of all self-proclaimed healers. The Hippocratics' reasons for refusing to participate in euthanasia may have been based on a philosophical or moral belief in preserving the sanctity of life or simply their wish to avoid involvement in any act of assisted suicide, murder, or manslaughter. We have fairly reliable historical documentation, however, that many ancient Greeks and Romans who were confronted with terminal illness preferred a quick, painless death by means of poison to letting nature take its course. Moreover, there were no laws in the ancient world against suicide, and it was not uncommon for physicians to recommend this option to a patient with an incurable disease. Similarly, abortion, typically effected by means of a pessary that induced premature labor, was practiced in both ancient Greece and the Roman Empire. Many Christian revisions of the Hippocratic Oath, especially those written during the Middle Ages, prohibited all abortive procedures. Not surprisingly, the contentious debate over both of these issues continues today, although the relevant sections are simply omitted in most oaths administered by U.S. medical schools. As of 1993, only 14 percent of such oaths prohibited euthanasia, and only 8 percent prohibited abortion.[5]

Another discarded relic is the vow never to "use the knife, not even on sufferers from the stone." In an era before antiseptic and aseptic surgery, anesthesia, and the scientific management of fluids, blood loss, and surgical shock, it was wise indeed to refer sufferers of these painful concretions to persons who specialized in removing them. Many healers in the ancient world focused their work specifically on kidney and bladder stones, others on cataract removal, and still others on the treatment of external injuries such as wounds. But as recently as the end of the 19th century, most surgical operations were treacherous affairs that carried a high risk of death. Consequently, the passage about "the knife" remains difficult to interpret. Historians have debated for centuries whether this vow bans all surgical procedures by the Hippocratics because of their inherent danger, reflects the fact that these physicians considered surgery beneath their dignity, or represents a promise not to practice outside the bounds of one's abilities.

The Hippocratic physicians understood the importance of avoiding any type of sexual relationship with their patients, yet only 3 percent of the oaths administered by U.S. medical schools at the end of the 20th century specifically prohibited such contact.[5] On the other hand, virtually all the oaths administered today include the assurances that Hippocrates insisted were touchstones of the successful patient–doctor relationship: the promises of acting in the best interest of the patient and of confidentiality.

Often, the additions made to the Hippocratic Oath are as historically interesting as the deletions. Many of the oaths taken this spring will include vows not to alter one's practice on the basis of the patient's race, nationality, religion, gender, socioeconomic standing, or sexual orientation. Others include assurances of the physician's accountability to his or her patients, protection of patients' autonomy, and informed consent or assistance with decision making. In a very real sense, all these changes help to make the act of oath taking eternal, a process that constantly changes to accommodate and articulate changing views of medicine and society.

But regardless of the language or provenance of the hundreds of texts collectively classified as Hippocratic, on commencement day the historian in me invariably takes a back seat to the physician. Whether I am reciting from bowdlerized or amended versions or the original Greek text, as I rise to take the oath with my peers, my heart grows full with reverence for the profession I have chosen.

Despite occasional complaints questioning the relevance or purity of the oath taking, this symbolic act is a tradition that is unlikely to become superannuated. It serves as a powerful reminder and declaration that we are all a part of something infinitely larger, older, and more important than a particular specialty or institution. Given the myriad challenges facing almost every aspect of medicine in the 21st century, the need for physicians to make a formal warrant of diligent, moral, and ethical conduct in the service of their patients may be stronger than ever.

As every experienced doctor knows, the few minutes we spend giving voice to a professional oath are far easier than the years we must devote to its faithful execution. As Hippocrates famously said, "Life is short, the art long, opportunity fleeting, experience perilous, and the crisis difficult," but the legacy of medicine suggests that we are capable of fulfilling this noble charge.

HIPPOCRATIC OATH

[Translation from the Greek by Ludwig Edelstein. From *The Hippocratic Oath: Text, Translation, and Interpretation*, by Ludwig Edelstein. Baltimore: Johns Hopkins Press, 1943].

I swear by Apollo Physician and Asclepius and Hygieia and Panaceia and all the gods and goddesses, making them my witnesses, that I will fulfill according to my ability and judgment this oath and this covenant:

> To hold him who has taught me this art as equal to my parents and to live my life in partnership with him, and if he is in need of money to give him a share of mine, and to regard his offspring as equal to my brothers in male lineage and to teach them this art—if they desire to learn it—without fee and covenant; to give a share of precepts and oral instruction and all the other learning to my sons and to the sons of him who has instructed me and to pupils who have signed the covenant and have taken an oath according to the medical law, but no one else.

I will apply dietetic measures for the benefit of the sick according to my ability and judgment; I will keep them from harm and injustice.

I will neither give a deadly drug to anybody who asked for it, nor will I make a suggestion to this effect. Similarly I will not give to a woman an abortive remedy. In purity and holiness I will guard my life and my art.

I will not use the knife, not even on sufferers from stone, but will withdraw in favor of such men as are engaged in this work.

Whatever houses I may visit, I will come for the benefit of the sick, remaining free of all intentional injustice, of all mischief and in particular of sexual relations with both female and male persons, be they free or slaves.

What I may see or hear in the course of the treatment or even outside of the treatment in regard to the life of men, which on no account one must spread abroad, I will keep to myself, holding such things shameful to be spoken about.

If I fulfill this oath and do not violate it, may it be granted to me to enjoy life and art, being honored with fame among all men for all time to come; if I transgress it and swear falsely, may the opposite of all this be my lot.

[*This essay originally appeared as: Markel, H.: Becoming a Physician: "I Swear By Apollo"—On Taking the Hippocratic Oath. New England Journal of Medicine 2004; 350:2026-2029.*]

REFERENCES

1. Edelstein L. The Hippocratic Oath: text, translation and interpretation. In: Temkin O, Temkin CL, eds. *Ancient Medicine: Selected Papers of Ludwig Edelstein.* (Baltimore: Johns Hopkins University Press, 1967), pp. 3–64).
2. Nutton V. What's in an oath? *Journal of Royal College of Physicians* (London). 1995; 29: 518–524.
3. Carey EJ. The formal use of the Hippocratic Oath for medical students at commencement exercises. *Bulletin of the Association of American Medical College.* 1928; 3: 159–166.
4. Smith DC. The Hippocratic Oath and modern medicine. *Journal of the History of Medicine and Allied Sciences.* 1996; 51: 484–500.
5. Orr RD, Pang N, Pellegrino ED, Siegler M. Use of the Hippocratic Oath: a review of twentieth century practice and a content analysis of oaths administered in medical schools in the U.S. and Canada in 1993. *Journal of Clinical Ethics.* 1997; 8: 377–388.

CHAPTER 2

⚭

The Death of Dr. Samuel Johnson

A Historical Spoof on
the Clinicopathologic Conference

The lexicographer, essayist, and social philosopher Samuel Johnson was one of Britain's greatest men of letters. Johnson was born in Lichfield in Staffordshire, Great Britain, on September 18, 1709. The son of a struggling bookseller, Samuel was educated at Pembroke College, University of Oxford. He was forced to leave after three years without a degree, due to his father's insolvency. Young Sam Johnson worked as a schoolmaster (the famed actor David Garrick was among his pupils) before leaving Lichfield for London in 1737 to make his way as a writer. Beginning in 1738, Johnson became a regular contributor to the periodical *Gentleman's Magazine,* and published a series on physicians, including Boerhaave and Sydenham, reflecting an interest and love of "physick and chymistry which never forsook him."[1] Also, Johnson assisted his former schoolfellow Robert James, M.D. (1705 to 1766), in preparing *The Medicinal Dictionary.*

Johnson's first taste of fame was experienced in 1738 with the publication of *London,* a satiric imitation of Juvenal, followed by *The Life of Savage* (1744), *The Vanity of Human Wishes* (1749), and his tragedy *Irene* (1749). It was in 1747, however, that Johnson began his most important work, *The Dictionary of the English Language,* which first appeared in two volumes in 1755. Further, Johnson distinguished himself as a brilliant moralist by creating almost every issue of the periodicals *Rambler* (1750 to 1752) and the *Idler* (1758 to 1760). Other important works from the pen of Samuel Johnson included *The History of Rasselas, Prince of Abissinia,* which he composed during the evenings of one week to pay off his mother's funeral expenses in 1759, an eight-volume edition of Shakespeare's work

Literatim: Essays at the Intersections of Medicine and Culture. Howard Markel, Oxford University Press (2020).
© Oxford University Press.
DOI: 10.1093/oso/9780190087647.001.0001

he edited in 1765, and the ten-volume critical and biographic opus, *Lives of the Poets* (1779 to 1781).

Physicians and medical scholars are doubly fortunate in being able to appreciate not only Samuel Johnson's prodigious literary work, but his medical history and postmortem examination results as well. For example, he represents one of the first recorded cases of emphysema in the medical literature.[2] Morgagni described an autopsy in 1742 in which "the cavity of the thorax was almost wholly filled by the lungs being very turgid, and heavy; but still less heavy than turgid; for they contained a great quantity of air and not much serum . . .".[3] But it was the British physician and anatomist Matthew Baille (1761 to 1823), studying the lungs of Samuel Johnson, who first specifically referred to the anatomic abnormality of emphysema in his 1793 text, *Morbid Anatomy of the Most Important Parts of the Human Body.* "The air cells are seen much enlarged beyond their natural size, so as to resemble the air cells of the lungs in amphibious animals."[4] Laënnec would not begin his brilliant delineation of emphysema, based upon auscultation, percussion, and postmortem examinations, until 1819.[5]

Biographers and medical historians have long been fascinated with the many ailments and diseases of Samuel Johnson.[6-13] Indeed, Johnson's medical history is replete with episodes of cardiac, respiratory, infectious, and neuropsychiatric disorders. Further, the physicians who attended Johnson, particularly during the last years of his life, included such prominent medical figures as William Heberden, who first described angina pectoris in 1772, the surgeons Perceval Pott, who described Pott's disease or tuberculosis of the spine, and William Cruikshank of the Royal Academy of Medicine, and Thomas Lawrence, who was president of the Royal College of Physicians, London, from 1767 to 1775. Although Richard Cabot is given credit for developing the clinicopathologic conference to an art form in medical education in 1910 and which were famously published for decades in the *New England Journal of Medicine* as "Case Records of the Massachusetts General Hospital,[14] one can only fantasize what a brilliant exercise a clinicopathologic conference based upon Samuel Johnson's death would have been. This highly fictional but historically based thought experiment describes such a conference as it might have occurred at the Royal College of Physicians in London, sometime in early 1785.

PRESENTATION OF CASE

Dr. Richard Brocklesby (general practitioner, the patient's neighbor): This patient was a 75-year- old white man who presented to my office with chief complaints of weakness that had grown progressively worse over the past two years, frequent spasmodic episodes resulting in a constriction of the breast and severe shortness of breath upon minimal exertion, and irretractable dropsy of the lower extremities and abdomen. The patient, a well-known man of letters and conversationalist, lamented his inability to perform his daily work or even to read in bed: "I used formerly, when sleepless in bed, to read like a Turk."[15]

The patient first noted respiratory difficulties seven years ago when he began experiencing shortness of breath brought on by walking up a long flight of steps. In January 1777, he had an attack of influenza that developed into spasmodic asthma. He was treated with the modality of phlebotomy, and 36 ounces of blood were removed over the course of two days, 10 to 12 ounces at a time. Although this procedure gave the patient some respite from the respiratory embarrassment, the dyspnea on exertion soon returned.

The patient consulted Dr. Thomas Lawrence for his asthmatic condition in late 1777, and a trial of the emetic ipecacuanha was instituted. Little relief was found and the drug was discontinued. From 1777 to 1783, shortness of breath gradually worsened to a point where he could sleep only in an upright position, and a catarrhous cough that was productive in nature developed. Over this period of time, repeated phlebotomies were performed that were more than likely detrimental to the patient's general constitution, and were finally discontinued in 1781. At this time, tincture of opium was prescribed as a means of relief. Although the patient continued to complain of spasmodic asthma and its gradual worsening in nature and frequency, he was still able to attend to his daily activities, which were largely sedentary in nature.

In June 1783, he had a minor paralytic stroke that caused a slight drooping of the left side of the face, aphasia, and agraphia; treatment consisted of ammonia blisters behind the ears and over the head and a nutritive diet supplemented with wine and brandy. The stroke resolved within a week without any further sequelae, and the patient resumed his work.

Spasmodic asthma continued to plague him, and, from December of that year to February 1784, he was confined to his bed. Severe dropsy of the legs and thighs with accumulation of fluid in the abdomen also developed. By mid-February 1784, a course of vinegar of squills was prescribed in an attempt to alleviate some of the patient's dropsy. He complained of nausea and dyspepsia upon taking the squills, but obtained minor relief from the worsening dropsy. By March 1784, however, upon the least amount of cold exposure or labor, he would experience a constriction of the breast accompanied by a catarrhous cough that seriously impaired his ability to breathe when in a recumbent position and that obliged him to sit up all night. His only rest and occasional sleep were by means of laudanum and syrup of poppies.

By the summer of 1784, the patient's condition improved somewhat with laudanum and restricted activity combined with a remarkable spirit, and he embarked upon a tour of Staffordshire and Derbyshire with visits to Lichfield, Birmingham, and Oxford. He noted that he was too dyspneic to "scale the Library steps" at Oxford, and, at Ashbourne, the patient observed that his dropsy advanced so far that he "could not without great difficulty button . . . [his trousers] at the knees."[16] He returned to London in November in a condition that could only be described as critical.

The patient expressed a desire to remain in his home to recuperate. Physical examination revealed a weak, markedly obese man lying in bed on several pillows. The peripheral pulses were poor and felt best at the neck. The pulse was rapid with a galloping rhythm. The jugular veins were distended. Chest examination was remarkable for tachypnea, markedly reduced diaphragmatic excursion, and audible expiratory wheezes. The abdomen was protuberant with a demonstrable fluid wave and pitting of the lower half of the abdominal wall. The liver edge was tender and firm, and palpable at least four inches below the right costal margin. Dropsy with marked pitting of the feet, ankles, legs, and presacral area was present.

On November 10, 1784, a consultation of his physicians was held, including myself, Dr. William Heberden, and Mr. William Cruikshank. It was then decided to scarify his legs in an attempt to give him some relief from the severe state of anasarca. Scarification was repeated by Mr. Cruikshank on December 8th, when the patient urged "cut deeper; you are afraid of giving me pain, whilst I am anxious for life."[17]

The patient, who publicly advocated that physicians give their patients a complete and accurate prognosis of their illnesses, was informed that it was doubtful he would recover without a miracle. He then resolved to "take no more physick, not even my opiates; for I have prayed that I may render up my soul to God unclouded."[18] On December 13, he asked for a case of lancets that he had stored in a drawer, and, before he could be stopped, he made a deep incision in the calf of one of his edematous legs, which resulted in a blood loss so great that he quickly fell into a stupor. By 7 P.M., the "Great Cham of English Literature" died.

I should also mention that the past medical history was significant for scrofula at infancy, which he contracted from a wet nurse, and which resulted in numerous suppurating scrofulous glands permanently scarring his face. Despite being taken to London as a child to receive the royal and purportedly healing touch of Queen Anne, he had subsequent development of corneal leukomas of the left eye secondary to tuberculous keratitis, rendering him blind in that eye. Beginning in childhood and lasting throughout his life, the patient also exhibited a wide and complex variety of nervous tics in which "his mouth [was] almost constantly opening and shutting as if he were chewing. He [had] a strange method of frequently twirling his fingers and twisting his hands. His body [was] in constant agitation, see-sawing up and down; his feet are never a moment quiet and in short, his whole person is in perpetual motion."[19] The patient's psychiatric history was significant for recurring episodes of mental depression beginning at age 20, when a physician stated that his melancholy would probably terminate in madness. He understandably had a lifelong fear of insanity and frequently suffered from hypochondriasis. The patient also had several episodes of gout beginning in 1773, and chronic dyspepsia and flatulence since 1737; he was a late riser, an extremely large eater, almost exclusively sedentary, and although he stopped drinking completely at age 57, he had a long history of consuming vast quantities of port wine and tea.

DIFFERENTIAL DIAGNOSIS

Dr. William Heberden (Fellow, Royal College of Physicians; Member, Royal Society of Medicine; Associate, Royal Society of Medicine, Paris; and formerly lecturer in *Materia medica*, University of Cambridge): It is with distinct pleasure, and not without some sorrow, that I discuss this case. The patient, when calling for me during his fatal illness, referred to me as "*Ultimus Romanorum*, the last of our learned physicians." Alas, I was not able to utilize that knowledge to undo the damage of what Dr. Johnson diagnosed as the incurable disease of being 75. To summarize Dr. Brocklesby's fine case presentation, the patient was a 75-year-old man with a history of scrofula, blindness of the left eye, gout, chronic dyspepsia and flatulence, gesticulations, and nervous tics and episodes of mental depression, who had an interesting form of spasmodic asthma eight years ago that rarely abated, a mild paralytic stroke from which he recovered completely in 1763, dropsy, and congestive heart failure of at least two years' duration.

I shall focus on the patient's lung and circulatory disorders, particularly his asthma, orthopnea, and catarrhous cough, since these were his major medical complaints, and most likely what lead to his death. The entity asthma is, unfortunately, poorly differentiated, and I fear what we call asthma, based solely on the symptoms of shortness of breath, may indeed be several respiratory disorders covered by the same blanket of terminology. I think this is particularly the case with the patient under discussion. The Greek physician Aretaeus of Cappadocia (c. 120 to 200 C.E.) produced one of the first descriptions of asthma: "If from running, gymnastic exercises, or any other work, the breathing becomes difficult, it is called asthma; and the disease orthopnea is also called asthma, for in the paroxysms the patients also pant for breath. The disease is called orthopnea, because it is only when in an erect position that they breathe freely; for when reclined there is a sense of suffocation. From the confinement in the breathing, the name orthopnea is derived. For the patient sits erect on account of breathing; and, if reclined, there is danger of being suffocated."[20] It is important to note, however, that although positional difficulty with breathing, or orthopnea, can be associated with the paroxysms of asthma, it is probably a more common clinical manifestation of severe left ventricular failure and is seen in advanced cases of dropsy. I suspect that most episodes of our patient's orthopnea, in his last few years, were secondary to such heart failure.

Dr. Thomas Willis (1621 to 1675), the British physician, was more successful in differentiating the various forms of asthma that formerly tended to be incorporated as one entity.[21] Willis described a form caused by an obstruction of the bronchi, such as thick humors, viscous or purulent matter, or extravasated blood-patients with such a disorder often complain of catarrhous or productive cough. This type of "asthma," if you will, is more properly classified as a chronic inflammation of the airways, which our patient indeed had for at least eight years. A second type categorized by Willis was called convulsive asthma: here, no great compression or obstruction of the bronchi exists; instead, we believe that a cramping of either the smooth muscular fibers of the airways, both small and large, or the peripheral nerves servicing the breast and lungs results in convulsive episodes of an understandably distressing shortness of breath. Such patients experience orthopnea like that seen in patients with severe dropsy, but, unlike subjects with heart failure, only have this condition during their attacks. Willis did note, however, hypertrophy or enlargement of the heart muscle (particularly the right ventricle) upon postmortem examination in patients with long-standing asthma of both types. A final form of asthma is a mixed-disease entity consisting of both the obstructive and convulsive components I just described.

The patient we are discussing complained of dyspnea for more than eight years. Further, it appears from the history that he had asthma several years before dropsy and congestive heart failure developed. It may be that his chronic respiratory problems of a catarrhal cough, spasmodic episodes of "constriction of the breast," and gradual loss of energy and increasing shortness of breath led to his heart failure, severe dropsy, and orthopnea, which made it impossible for him to lie completely flat without having great difficulties in breathing. A vicious cycle is therefore created by this form of mixed obstructive-spasmodic asthma (also known as a chronic inflammation of the airways), causing heart failure and resulting in more breathing problems and fatigue, and so on. It is possible to theorize that this mixed obstructive-spasmodic asthma pathologically impedes the outflow of the right side of the heart in some yet unexplained fashion. In order for the right side of the heart to pump against a greater head of pressure, it must hypertrophy or become stronger, leading to eventual heart failure. The exact mechanism of this failure, however, remains to be completely understood.

At this point, I would like to pause and discuss the somewhat effective course of therapy for dropsy tried in early 1784, vinegar of squills, which was discontinued because of the severe side effect of nausea. I have asked Dr. William Withering of Birmingham, a recently elected Fellow to the Royal College, to describe his experience with this therapeutic and others like it.

Dr. William Withering (Fellow, Royal College of Medicine, practitioner in Birmingham, author of *A Botanical Arrangement of All the Vegetables Naturally Growing in Great Britain*, 1776; in 1785, he provided the first description of the congestive heart failure drug now known as digitalis, in *An Account of Foxglove*): Vinegar of squills is an extract of the bulbous root of *Urginea scilla* in a solution of vinegar. For this drug to be effective as a diuretic, it must be prescribed in large amounts, often causing severe nausea, anorexia, and emesis as was seen in this patient. A much more potent diuretic and therapeutic for severe dropsy is extract of foxglove or *Digitalis purpurea*. I was first introduced to foxglove by an old woman in Shropshire in 1775, who had sometimes cured dropsy after regular practicum had failed; I am currently preparing for publication an account of my experience with it. The extract must be carefully administered or nausea, indistinct vision and anorexia will result, but I have never yet found any permanent bad effects from it. I use foxglove in the ascites, anasarca, and hydrops pectoris; and so far as the removal of the water will contribute to cure the patient, so far may be expected from this medicine; but I wish it not to be tried in ascites of female patients believing that many of these cases are dropsies of the ovara; and no sensible man will ever expect to see these encysted fluids removed by any medicine.[22] Parenthetically, I might add that my maternal grandfather, Dr. George Hector, delivered this patient in 1709 at Lichfield.

Dr. Heberden: In passing, it is interesting to note that this patient, whose paralytic stroke of June 1783 resulted in temporary aphasia and agraphia, regained his ability to speak and write within 48 hours, and also had recovery of his muscular power. I suspect that this stroke was caused by an embolus, which dissipated quickly, or may even have been a localized spasm of the cerebral arteries in the area of the cortical motor speech center at the base of the inferior frontal convolution of the left hemisphere.

Dr. George Fordyce (Fellow of the Royal Society; Fellow of the Royal College of Physicians; and physician to St. Thomas's Hospital): Dr. Heberden, what was the diagnosis of the medical students?

Dr. Heberden: The students reviewed the multiple possible causes of progressive shortness of breath and heart failure. They believed the disease to be a chronic obstructive and destructive one of the lung tissue that has not yet been described in the literature.

Clinical diagnosis: Spasmodic asthma, dropsy, heart failure. *Dr. Heberden's diagnosis:* Mixed obstructive-spasmodic asthma leading to congestive heart failure.

PATHOLOGIC DISCUSSION

Dr. James Wilson (Lecturer in anatomy, Hunterian School of Medicine, Great Windmill Street, London): On opening into the cavity of the chest, the lungs did not collapse as they usually do when air is admitted, but remained distended, as if they lost the power of contraction; the air cells on the surface of the lungs were also very much enlarged; the right lobe adhered very strongly to the diaphragm; the internal surface of the trachea was somewhat inflamed; no water was found in the cavity of the thorax. The heart was exceedingly large and strong, the valves of the aorta were beginning to ossify; no more fluid than was common was contained in the pericardium. In the abdomen seemed to be incipient peritoneal inflammation and ascites; the liver and spleen were firm and hard; the spleen had almost the feel of cartilage. A gallstone about the size of a pigeon's egg was taken out of the gall bladder; the omentum was exceedingly fat; nothing remarkable was found in the stomach; the folds of the jejunum adhered in several places to one another; there was also a strong adhesion by a long slip between the colon and bladder; the pancreas was remarkably enlarged; the kidney of the left side tolerably good, hyatids beginning to form on its surface; that of the right side was almost entirely destroyed and two large hyatids formed in its place. Dr. Johnson never complained of any pain in this part; the left testicle was perfectly sound in structure, but also had a number of hyatids on its surface, containing a fatty gelatinous fluid; the right testicle had hyatids likewise, but the spermatic vein belonging to it was exceedingly enlarged and varicose. The cranium was not opened. Mr. White, assisting me to sew up the body, pricked his finger with the needle; next morning he had red lines running up the arm, and a slight attack of fever.[23]

To begin with, the immediate cause of this patient's death was congestive heart failure, as evidenced by the hypertrophy of the heart muscle, the enlarged pancreas, and the liver, which was firm and beginning to show signs of cardiac sclerosis; the firmness of the spleen is also pertinent. The patient had, in addition, dropsy of the lower extremities and gross ascites. It is possible to theorize that the patient had high blood pressure, which led to the cystic changes in his kidneys, particularly the right kidney, and may have been a factor in the paralytic stroke that occurred two years ago. The patient's chronic dyspepsia and flatulence may have been caused by the large gallstone found in the gallbladder; the adhesions noted in the folds of the jejunum and between the colon and bladder may also have been contributing factors.

Most interesting was, undoubtedly, the nature of the patient's lungs on gross examination. Air vesicles of an extremely rare type were found on the lung surfaces. Dr. Heberden noted that he had never seen such a condition, and Mr. Cruikshank professed to have observed only two instances of such air vesicles.

Dr. Baille, would you comment on the morbid anatomy of these lungs?

Dr. Matthew Baille (Assistant, and nephew, to Dr. William Hunter, of the Royal College of Physicians and Hunterian School of Medicine, Great Windmill Street, currently working on a textbook of morbid anatomy): The most impressive feature was the formation of large cells on the surface and within the parenchyma of the lungs, resembling those of an amphibian's. Dr. Wilson has already mentioned the gross distension of these lungs as well as their diminished compliance. The enlargement of the air cells, which explains these findings, cannot well be supposed to arise from any other cause than the air not being allowed common free egress from the lungs, and therefore accumulating in them. It is not improbable also that this accumulation may sometimes break down two or three contiguous cells into one, thereby forming a very large cell. These morphologic changes could certainly explain the patient's breathing difficulties and probably led to his right-sided heart failure, although he clinically showed signs of the mixed asthmatic process described by Dr. Heberden.[24]

Anatomic diagnosis: Enlargement of the air cells of the lungs (a new clinical entity); congestive heart failure.

THE FINAL WORD

As epilogue to this fictional post mortem, it is worthwhile noting that Matthew Baille's description of emphysema, or as he called it, "enlargement of the air cells of the lungs," appeared in 1793 and was based on the postmortem examination of Samuel Johnson's lungs. It was one of the earliest descriptions of emphysema in the medical literature.[24] Although this hypothetical clinicopathologic conference is an exercise of creative medical history rather than a documented report, it should serve as further evidence of a statement made by James Boswell in 1791:

Such was Samuel Johnson, a man whose talents, acquirements, and virtues were so extraordinary, that the more his character is considered, the more he will be regarded by the present age, and by posterity, with admiration and reverence.[25]

[This essay originally appeared as: Markel, H.: The Death of Samuel Johnson, L.L.D. A Clinicopathologic Conference. American Journal of Medicine 1987; 82:1203-1207.]

REFERENCES

1. Boswell, J. *The Life of Samuel Johnson.* (New York: Modern Library, 1952), pp. 39, 45.
2. Major R.H.: *Classic Descriptions of Disease,* 3rd Edition. (Springfield, Illinois: C.C. Thomas, 1945), pp. 582–583.
3. Morgagni J.B.: *The Seats and Causes of Diseases, Integrated by Anatomy,* Vol I (abridged and translated by Cooke, W.); (Boston: Wells and Lily, 1824), pp. 368–370.
4. Rodin, A.E. *The Influences of Matthew Baille's Morbid Anatomy.* (Springfield, IL: C.C. Thomas, 1973), pp. 29–30.
5. Laennec, R.T.H.: *A translation of selected passages from De L'Auscultation Mediate* (translated by Hale-White W). (London: John Bale, Sons and Danielsson, 1923), pp. 101–111.
6. Squibb, G.J.: Last illness and post-mortem-examination of Samuel Johnson the lexicographer and oralist, with remarks. *London Medical Journal.* 1849; 1: 615–623.
7. Cahill, W.C.: The medical history of Dr. Samuel Johnson. *American Medicine.* 1901; 2: 338–338.
8. Packard, F.R.: The medical history of Samuel Johnson. *New York Medical Journal.* 1902; 75: 441–445.
9. Rolleston, H.: Medical aspects of Samuel Johnson. *Glasgow Medical Journal.* 1924; 110: 173–191.
10. Rolleston, H.: Samuel Johnson's medical experiences. *Annals of Medical History.* 1929; 1: 540–552.
11. Hutchison, R.: Dr. Samuel Johnson and medicine. *Edinburgh Medical Journal.* 1925; 32: 389–406.
12. Chase, P.P.: The ailments and physicians of Dr. Johnson. *Yale J Biol Med.* 1925; 23: 370–379.
13. McHenry L.G.: Samuel Johnson's tics and gesticulations. *J Hist Med.* 1967; 22: 152–168.
14. White P.D.: Richard Cabot, 1669-1939. *N Engl J Med.* 1939; 220: 1049–1052.
15. Boswell, J. *The Life of Samuel Johnson.* (New York: Modern Library, 1952), p. 540.
16. Ibid, p. 229.
17. Ibid, p. 537.
18. Ibid, p. 54.
19. Rolleston, H.: Medical aspects of Samuel Johnson. *Glasgow Medical Journal.* 1924; 110: 173–191.
20. Adams F., ed.: *The extant works of Aretaeus the Cappadocian.* (London: The Sydenham Society Publications, 1856), p. 316.
21. Willis, T.: *Pharmaceutical Rationalis,* Volume II. (London: Dring, Harper, and Leigh, 1679), p. 82.

22. Withering W.: *An account of the foxglove and some of its medical uses with practical remarks on dropsy and other diseases.* (London: C.G.J. and J. Robinson, 1785).
23. Rolleston, H.: Medical aspects of Samuel Johnson. *Glasgow Medical Journal.* 1924; 110: 173–191.
24. Baille M.: *The morbid anatomy of some of the most important parts of the human body,* 1st ed. (London: Johnson and Nicol, 1793).
25. Boswell J.: *The Life of Samuel Johnson.* (New York: Modern Library, 1952), p. 546.

CHAPTER 3

cℳっ

Charles Dickens' Work to Help
Establish the Great Ormond Street
Children's Hospital in London

When contemplating the medical ramifications of poverty and the importance of child advocacy, we can hardly do better than to point in the direction of Charles Dickens, England's celebrated novelist and social reformer. The
reading of just a few of his novels, or the biting essays he composed for his weekly
magazines, *Household Words* (1850–58) and *All the Year Round* (1859–70), shows
that rarely have children had a more eloquent or effective proponent. A brilliant
example of Dickens' broad-based activism on behalf of children was the establishment of London's Great Ormond Street Children's Hospital.[1] His philanthropic
acts of kindness in developing this famous center of children's health and healing
exemplifies so well his deep sense of civic responsibility, his great concern for
youngsters of all kinds and classes, and his keen understanding of the need for a
special place to care for sick children.

Dickens' intense interest in the plight of abandoned, orphaned, and impoverished
children began, not surprisingly, with his own abject childhood. His father John
was arrested for debt in 1824 and imprisoned first in the King's Bench Prison
and, subsequently, the Marshalsea Debtor's Prison. Although John and Elizabeth
Dickens and most of their children were imprisoned in the Marshalsea, the 12-year-
old Charles was removed from school and sent to work at the rat-infested Warren's
Blacking (shoeshine) Warehouse for 5 months. During this time, the young
Dickens had vague episodes of illness that may have been more closely related to his
emotional distress than to organic causes. Dickens' humiliation and psychological
scars from the experience were carried long into his adulthood. Although he never
spoke of this period during his lifetime, he did leave behind an autobiographical

Literatim: Essays at the Intersections of Medicine and Culture. Howard Markel, Oxford University Press (2020).
© Oxford University Press.
DOI: 10.1093/oso/9780190087647.001.0001

snippet documenting his tenure at the warehouse to his friend and biographer John Forester.[2,3] In 1850, Dickens incorporated these troubled times into his semiautobiographical novel, *David Copperfield*. He depicted his father as the insolvent Mr. Micawber. Early in the book, young David Copperfield (Dickens' literary alter-ego) is orphaned and sent by his malevolent step-father as "a labouring hind in the service of Murdstone and Grinby," a wine factory with striking similarities to Warren's Blacking Warehouse.[4,5]

Dickens recreated his traumatic childhood and those of other unfortunate youths in all his novels; indeed, his works teem with the tribulations and travails of rejected or orphaned children.[6] Given Dickens' intense fascination with the plights of abandoned children, it is not surprising that he was also interested in their diseases (both physical and psychological), which often developed as a result of living in squalid conditions.[7] The descriptions of illness that appear in Dickens' novels are accurate and based upon real disorders rather than invented maladies with inconsistent symptoms, as was the more common practice among many Victorian novelists.[8] But this careful attention to detail was not merely gained by the occasional skimming of a medical textbook or by occasional conversations with one of the many physicians with whom he was friendly. Dickens was a regular reader of *The Lancet* and subscribed to the sanitarian doctrine of disease. The novelist also made frequent visits to hospitals in the greater London area where he had the opportunity to meet and observe the sick.[9,10]

Despite London's reputation as one of the great capitals of Europe, it still had no children's hospital within its metropolitan borders until Great Ormond Street opened in 1852. In fact, there was no such facility in all of England, even though there were long-established children's hospitals across Europe, from Paris to St Petersburg, that not only flourished but also were maintained typically at government expense. This striking deficit was not lost to the medical profession in general and, more specifically, to Charles West, a doctor who threw his entire energies into the founding and establishment of a British children's hospital. Working with the physician-reformer Thomas Southwood Smith, Edwin Chadwick (who authored the landmark *Report from the Poor Law Commissioners on an Enquiry into the Sanitary Condition of the Labouring Population of Great Britain*), and the physician-chemist, Henry Bence Jones, West convened a Provisional Committee and took out a series of advertisements soliciting contributions and support in the *London Times*, the *London Morning Post*, and the *London Standard* in mid-February, 1850. It was not until February 6, 1852, however, that a 31-bed hospital opened in a house at 49 Great Ormond Street in London's Bloomsbury area.[11]

During this period, Dickens was hard at work writing *Bleak House* and launching his successful weekly journal *Household Words*. But it seems very likely that he was aware of West's work. Long an avid supporter of a multitude of causes concerning the poor and their children, especially those pertaining to health and living conditions, Dickens was friends with both Chadwick and Smith. Another original board member of the Children's Hospital, architect Henry Austin, was Dickens' brother-in-law. Moreover, one of the first financial contributions to the cause was Baroness Angela Georgina Burdett-Coutts, who was a close friend of Dickens, an ally of many of his social-reform activities, and godmother to Dickens' eldest son, Charles, Jr.[12,13]

With his editorial assistant Henry Morley, Dickens first visited the Children's Hospital, Great Ormond Street, during its initial weeks of operation. Together they composed a moving essay entitled "Drooping Buds", which appeared as the lead article in the April 3, 1852, issue of *Household Words*. Although literary scholars have argued over which collaborator penned which phrase, the essay does have a distinctly Dickensian quality in its style and outrage.[14] Dickens and Morley explained the unnecessary tragedy of the alarming infant and childhood mortality rates in Victorian England:

> Our children perish out of our homes: not because there is in them an inherent dangerous sickness (except in the few cases where they are born of parents who communicate to children heritable maladies), but because there is, in respect to their tender lives, a want of sanitary discipline and a want of knowledge. What should we say of a rose-tree in which one bud out of every three dropped to the soil dead? We should not say that this was natural to roses; neither is it natural to men and women that they should see the glaze of death upon so many of the bright eyes that come to laugh and love among them . . .[15]

Perhaps more intriguing to the modern-day reader is the authors' understanding of the distinction between diseases of childhood and infancy and those of adulthood. This, of course, is a concept the modern-day medical practitioner takes as an accepted truth, but in 1852, long before the specialty of pediatrics was formally established, it was one bordering on the vanguard:

> It does not at all follow that the intelligent physician who has learnt how to treat successfully the illnesses of adults, has only to modify his plans a little, to diminish the proportions of his doses, for the application of his knowledge to our little sons and daughters. Some of their diseases are peculiar to themselves; other diseases, common to us all, take a form in children varying as much from their familiar form with us as a child varies from a man . . .[16]

The article also included a pen portrait of the hospital with its wide array of toys and the spacious "airy and gay" rooms that were richly decorated with murals depicting "rosy nymphs and children." Six children (five girls, one boy) were inpatients at the time of the visit.[17] "Drooping Buds" had a far wider circulation than the 40,000 readers who regularly subscribed to *Household Words*. Dickens gave the Children's Hospital permission to reprint the essay as a pamphlet for potential donors, and, although this helped to publicize the hospital, it only went so far. Indeed, 6 years later, in 1858, the hospital still only had 31 beds despite a childhood death rate in London of more than 21,000 per year (out of a total of 50,000 deaths per year). To remedy the Children's Hospital's stunted growth, Dickens proposed to chair a benefit festival on February 9, 1858, at the Freemason's Tavern, Great Queen Street, Lincoln's Inn Fields. Queen Victoria agreed to be the patron, and a panoply of distinguished and concerned Londoners signed on as stewards for the evening's festivities. It was culminated, of course, by a vigorous speech by Dickens on the plight of England's impoverished children.[18,19] The journalist T. A. Reed described the event as one of Dickens' greatest triumphs as an orator: "I never heard him, or reported him, with so much pleasure . . . His speech was magnificent . . .".[20] A brief excerpt of his oration fits nicely with what became his signature "Dickensian pathos":

> Some years ago, being in Scotland, I went with one of the most humane members of the humane medical profession, on a morning tour among some of the worst lodged inhabitants of the old town of Edinburgh . . . In a room in one of these places, where there was an empty porridge-pot on the cold hearth, with a ragged woman and some ragged children crouching on the bare ground near it—where, I remember as I speak, that the very light, refracted from a high damp-stained and time-stained house-wall, came trembling in, as if the fever which had shaken everything else there had shaken even it—there lay, in an old egg-box which the mother had begged from a shop, a little feeble, wasted, wan, sick child. With his little wasted face, and his little hot, worn hands folded over his breast, and his little bright, attentive eyes, I can see him now, as I have seen him for several years, look in steadily at us . . . Many a poor child, sick and neglected, I have seen since that time in this London; many a poor sick child I have seen most affectionately and kindly tended by poor people, in an unwholesome house and under untoward circumstances, wherein its recovery was quite impossible; but at all such times I have seen my poor little drooping friend in his egg-box, and he has always addressed his dumb speech to me, and I have always found him wondering what it meant, and why, in the name of a gracious God, such things should be![21]

The speech, and a subsequent benefit reading by Dickens of *A Christmas Carol*, raised over £3,000 for the hospital. The funds were used both to increase patient bed space and to support medical staff. Dickens returned to the topic of the Great Ormond Street Hospital several times, such as his essay "A Smaller Star in the East", which appeared in his 1860 essay collection *The Uncommercial Traveller*[22] and, with Morley, in a progress note on the "good and wholesome work" of the hospital entitled "Between the Cradle and the Grave" in the February 1, 1862, issue of his magazine *All the Year Round*.[23] Perhaps best known, however, is Dickens' glowing tribute to the Children's Hospital in his last completed novel, *Our Mutual Friend* (1865).[24] In 1867, West, the founder of the hospital, best assessed how vital Dickens' support was to the institution: "Dickens, the children's friend, first set [the hospital] on her legs and helped her to run alone."[25] Dickens created a world of characters and events that leapt from the page for his millions of readers. He is as captivating a writer and entertainer today as he was during his lifetime in the 19th century. Less well known, especially among the medical community, is Dickens' tireless work as a social activist for public health and children's causes. His work to establish the Great Ormond Street Children's Hospital represents only a small part of this aspect of his career. Dickens' love and advocacy for children may have emerged from his own traumatic childhood. That he could create something so positive out of such a negative experience speaks to his character and resilience. His life, words, and deeds are superb lessons in humanity from which all of us engaged in the medical profession can profit. Dickens expressed this philosophy of life himself in a letter he wrote to his friend and fellow writer Wilkie Collins in 1858:

> Everything that happens shows beyond mistake that you can't shut out the world; that you are in it, to be of it; that you get yourself into a false position the moment you try to sever yourself from it; and that you must mingle with it, and make the best of it; and make the best of yourself into the bargain.[26]

[This originally appeared as: Markel, H.: Charles Dickens' Work to Help Establish the Great Ormond Street Children's Hospital of London. The Lancet. 1999; 354:673–675.]

REFERENCES

1. Kosky J. *Mutual Friends. Charles Dickens and the Great Ormond Street Children's Hospital.* (New York: St. Martin's Press, 1989).
2. Forster J. *The Life of Charles Dickens*, Vol I. (London: Dent, Everyman's Library, 1966), p. 21.
3. Ackroyd P. *Dickens*. (New York: Harper Collins, 1990), pp. 56–99
4. Johnson E. *Charles Dickens. His Tragedy and Triumph*, Vol I. (New York: Simon and Schuster, 1952), pp. 27–46.
5. Dickens C. *David Copperfield*. (London: Chapman and Hall, 1850), p. 183.
6. Johnson E. *Charles Dickens. His Tragedy and Triumph*, Vol I. (New York: Simon and Schuster, 1952), pp. 684–685.
7. Markel H. The Childhood Suffering of Charles Dickens and his Literary Children. *The Pharos*. 1985; 48: 5–8.
8. Markel H. Charles Dickens and the Art of Medicine. *Annals of Internal Medicine*. 1984; 101: 408–411.
9. Poynter F.N.L. Thomas Southwood Smith—The man. *Proceedings of the Royal Society of Medicine*. 1962; 55: 381–392.
10. Fielding K.J. *The Speeches of Charles Dickens*. Clarendon Press of Oxford University Press, 1960), pp. 40–43, 222–25, 246–53.
11. Kosky J. *Mutual Friends. Charles Dickens and the Great Ormond Street Children's Hospital.* (New York: St. Martin's Press, 1989), pp. 143–167.
12. Ibid, pp. 117–141.
13. Ackroyd, P. *Dickens*. (New York: Harper Collins, 1999), pp. 380–383, 393–94; 532–33.
14. Stone H. *The Uncollected Writings of Charles Dickens*, Vol II. (London: Allen Lane/The Penguin Press, 1969), p. 401.
15. Dickens C, Morley H. Drooping Buds. *Household Words*, April 3 1852, No. 106, p. 45–48. (quote is from p. 45).
16. Ibid, p. 45

17. Kosky J. *Mutual Friends. Charles Dickens and the Great Ormond Street Children's Hospital.* (New York: St. Martin's Press, 1989), pp. 163–165.

18. Dickens C, Morley H. Drooping buds. *Household Words*, April 3, 1852, No. 106, p. 47.

19. Ackroyd P. *Dickens.* (New York: Harper Collins, 1999), p. 801.

20. Kitton F.G. *Charles Dickens by Pen and Pencil.* (London: Sabin, Dexter, 1890), p. 46.

21. Fielding K.J. *The Speeches of Charles Dickens.* (Oxford, UK: Clarendon Press of Oxford University Press, 1960), pp. 250–251.

22. Dickens C. *The Uncommercial Traveller.* (London: Chapman and Hall, 1860).

23. Dickens C., Morley H. Between the Cradle and the Grave. *All the Year Round*, February 1, 1862, No. 145, pp. 454–456.

24. Dickens C. *Our Mutual Friend.* (London: Chapman and Hall, 1865), pp. 246–251.

25. Kosky J. *Mutual Friends. Charles Dickens and the Great Ormond Street Children's Hospital.* (New York: St. Martin's Press, 1989), p. vi.

26. Letter from Charles Dickens to Wilkie Collins. Sept 6, 1858. IN: Storey G., Tillotson K. (eds.), *The Letters of Charles Dickens 1856–58*, Vol 8. (Oxford, UK: Clarendon Press, 1995), pp. 649–651.

CHAPTER 4

⌯⌲

The Medical Detectives

Sir Arthur Conan Doyle and the Case
of Robert Koch's Lymph

O n a hot and steamy summer day in Berlin—August 4, 1890, to be precise—
the 10th International Medical Congress opened with a flair and fanfare that
few conference-weary doctors of the 21st century would recognize. At the invitation of Kaiser Wilhelm II, almost 6,000 physicians from around the globe flocked to
the city that represented the modernity and optimism of medical progress. Perhaps
even more enticing was the jam-packed program of lectures delivered by a veritable who's who of medical greats, including Joseph Lister, Rudolf Virchow, and
James Paget.

Topping the bill two days later, on the afternoon of August 6, was none other
than Dr. Robert Koch, perhaps the greatest medical detective who ever lived.
During the preceding 14 years, the distinguished professor of hygiene and bacteriology at the University of Berlin had become a household name as he successively
discovered the microbial causes of anthrax (in 1876), tuberculosis (in 1882), and
cholera (in 1883). Although Koch was never a commanding speaker (he reputedly
had a thin, reedy voice and tended to infuse his sentences with a distracting number
of "umms" and "errs"), his colleagues had long since learned to pay closer attention
to his words than to his style of presentation, knowing that still another demonstration of something spectacular was likely to transpire.

The eager physicians filling the seats of the stifling-hot auditorium were not dis-
appointed. Within moments after beginning his speech, Dr. Koch announced that
he had discovered a "remedy for tuberculosis." As expected in a world connected by
telegraphs and multiple editions of newspapers and magazines—and one in which

Literatim: Essays at the Intersections of Medicine and Culture. Howard Markel, Oxford University Press (2020).
© Oxford University Press.
DOI: 10.1093/oso/9780190087647.001.0001

tuberculosis was a leading cause of death and illness—Koch's discovery made news around the world. Hours after the lecture, physicians began to clamor for supplies of what was then called "Koch's lymph" to treat their desperate patients. The excitement only intensified when the lecture was formally published in the November 13, 1890, issue of *Deutsche Medizinische Wochenschrift* and reprinted, in English translation, in the November 15, 1890, issue of the *British Medical Journal*.[1] The following day, the front page of the *New York Times* heralded the remedy as "Koch's Great Triumph. The Discovery Called a Greater One Than Jenner's."

Koch was careful never to state explicitly that he had discovered a "cure." Instead, he reported that his "remedy" destroyed the tissue in which the tuberculosis germs had settled, so that the entire diseased area would simply be sloughed off and then expelled through coughing. Moreover, Koch was careful to state that the remedy worked best in cases that were "not too far advanced," although he theorized that it might be of some benefit in patients with large pulmonary cavities.

One of the millions of people reading about this incredible discovery was a young general practitioner who was struggling to build a practice in Southsea, Great Britain. During the long stretches of time between appointments with his patients, the doctor took up his fountain pen and wrote beautiful essays, stories, and even novels. In 1887, only a few years before Koch's announcement, the young doctor had published a novel entitled *A Study in Scarlet* in *Beeton's Christmas Annual*. It was a compelling tale that introduced the world to a character destined to become the most famous detective ever to grace the written page. The sleuth's name was Sherlock Holmes, and he employed a method he called "deductive reasoning," which was actually based on the diagnostic approach of a doctor. The physician author, of course, was Arthur Conan Doyle.

In his 1924 autobiography, Conan Doyle described the Koch announcement and the events that followed as "life transforming." Only a few hours after reading the translation of Koch's paper in the *British Medical Journal*, which was accompanied by the notice of a demonstration of the tuberculosis remedy that was to take place in Berlin later that week, Conan Doyle dashed out of his house and boarded a train for London with the intention of getting to Germany as soon as possible. He later recollected, "I could give no clear reason for doing this, but it was an irresistible impulse and I at once determined to go. Had I been a well-known doctor or a specialist in consumption it would have been more intelligible, but I had, as a matter of fact, no great interest in the more recent developments of my own profession."[1]

Once he reached London, the doctor's pragmatic side intervened, and Conan Doyle stopped by the offices of W.T. Snead, the editor of the magazine *Review of Reviews*. Securing letters of introduction from Snead to prominent Berliners and, even more important, a green light to write about the event, Conan Doyle then hopped a boat across the English Channel. Once in France, he secured a seat on the Continental Express to Berlin and arrived on November 16. Almost as soon as he stepped off the train in Berlin, Conan Doyle set out for the university building where Koch's colleague, Dr. Ernst von Bergmann, was scheduled to demonstrate the miraculous tuberculosis remedy the following morning. Alas, Conan Doyle's trip appeared to be for naught when he learned that tickets to von Bergmann's clinical demonstration were "simply not to be had and neither money nor interest could procure them."[2]

At this point, the intrepid Conan Doyle decided to seek out Koch at his home, but he was told by a butler that the professor was unavailable. As Conan Doyle later recounted, "To the Englishman in Berlin, and indeed to the German also, it is at present very much easier to see the bacillus of Koch than to catch even the most fleeting glimpse of its discoverer."[3] The closest Conan Doyle got to Koch was witnessing the upended sacks of mail emptied on the professor's doorstep and the thousands of letters from around the world containing desperate pleas regarding "the sad broken lives and wearied hearts which were turning in hope to Berlin."[3]

Bright and early on the morning of November 17, Conan Doyle went back to the medical auditorium at the University of Berlin. But neither bribes nor his clumsy attempts at slipping by the ticket taker secured him entry. Realizing that his magazine story was evaporating into thin air, Conan Doyle patiently waited for von Bergmann and literally threw himself in the path of the formidable physician, causing a pileup of the younger doctors who made up the professor's faithful retinue and academic rear guard.

"I have come a thousand miles. May I not come in?" begged the British medical journalist. The query prompted the senior physician to stop, glare through his pince-nez spectacles, and haughtily reply: "Perhaps you would like to take my place? That is the only one vacant!" Humiliated by the laughs and jeers of those who did possess the necessary coupons for entry, Conan Doyle began to turn around and leave the hospital. Fortunately, a tuberculosis specialist from Detroit named Henry J. Hartz was appalled by von Bergmann's display of bad behavior and lack of professional collegiality. Hartz promised to meet with Conan Doyle later that afternoon and share his notes on the demonstration. Even better, the following morning, Hartz quietly escorted Conan Doyle into von Bergmann's clinical wards to examine the patients who had received Koch's lymph.

Within a day after analyzing the mass of clinical data, however, Conan Doyle came to a startling conclusion: "The whole thing was experimental and premature." What is more, he had the temerity to make this statement publicly, first in a letter to the editor, published in the London *Daily Telegraph* on November 20, 1890,[4] and then, more definitively, in his article in the *Review of Reviews*, which ran in December of that year. While the rest of the world rejoiced over the reported conquest of tuberculosis, Conan Doyle argued that "Koch's lymph" might remove traces of the enemy, but it left deadly germs "deep in the invaded country." Its real value, Conan Doyle asserted, was as "an admirable aid to diagnosis," in that a "single injection" would help doctors decide definitively whether a patient was "in any way tubercular."

Conan Doyle was right. Koch's lymph, or what we now refer to as tuberculin, was essentially a glycerin extract of a pure culture of tuberculosis germs. In the decades before the development of the much safer purified-protein-derivative test for tuberculosis, it became an essential diagnostic tool. A few months later, in early 1891, after several highly publicized treatment failures, many exacerbated cases of tuberculosis, and not a few deaths closely associated with the administration of the so-called curative medication, Koch publicly retracted his even-tempered announcement of a remedy for tuberculosis and announced that although Koch's lymph was an excellent means of diagnosing tuberculosis, the actual cure was nowhere in sight.[5]

One cannot help but be impressed by the way in which the young Conan Doyle, the creator of the greatest detective in English literature, figured out what took Koch, one of the most illustrious medical detectives in history, and his accomplished colleagues many more months to realize. Sadly, the paper trail ends before we can definitively ascertain how Conan Doyle cracked "The Case of Koch's Lymph."

[*This essay originally appeared as: Markel, H.: The Medical Detectives. New England Journal of Medicine 2005; 353:2426–2428.*]

REFERENCES

1. Koch, R. A further communication on a remedy for tuberculosis. *British Medical Journal* 1890; 4: 1193–1201.
2. Conan Doyle, A. *Memories and Adventures*. (London: Hodder and Stroughton, 1924), pp. 82–93.
3. Dr. Koch and his cure. *Review of Reviews*. 1890; 2: 552–556.
4. The Consumption Cure. *London Daily Telegraph*. November 20, 1890:3.
5. Koch, R. Professor Koch's remedy for tuberculosis. *British Medical Journal*. 1891; 1: 125–127.

CHAPTER 5

∽

The Last Alcoholic Days
of F. Scott Fitzgerald

F. Scott Fitzgerald dropped dead after eating a chocolate bar and reading the *Princeton Alumni Weekly* magazine. A little after 2:00 in the afternoon of December 21, 1940, he erupted from his chair, clutched the mantelpiece of the nearby fireplace for support, and fell to the carpet with a resounding thud. A badly recovering alcoholic whose relapses were legendary, Fitzgerald drank and smoked himself into a terminal spiral of cardiomyopathy, coronary artery disease, angina, dyspnea, and syncopal spells. He had already sustained a mild heart attack in October 1940, outside Schwab's Drug Store on Sunset Boulevard. On December 21, that last Sunday of his life, Scott was hoping for some rest and, perhaps, a bit of inspiration for *The Love of the Last Tycoon,* the novel he was composing about Hollywood but would never complete.[1]

The evening before, Fitzgerald had attended the premier of the screwball comedy *This Thing Called Love*, starring Rosalind Russell and Melvyn Douglas, at the Pantages Theatre. After taking a seat next to his devoted companion, the popular and pretty Hollywood gossip columnist Sheila Graham, Scott experienced severe chest pain. By the closing credits, he needed Graham's help getting out of the theater and home to bed. Ever the manipulative addict, Scott convinced her to delay consulting his physician until the following day.[2]

Two decades earlier, Fitzgerald was the toast of the literary world and a living legend of the Roaring Twenties, the era he called "the most expensive orgy in history."[3(p.21)] Even now, the mention of his name instantly conjures up vivid images of flappers with bobbed hair and collegians wearing raccoon coats. But on the afternoon he took one last, labored breath in his tiny and sparsely furnished apartment, Scott's meteoric fame was irrevocably lost to him. He was 44 years old.

Literatim: Essays at the Intersections of Medicine and Culture. Howard Markel, Oxford University Press (2020).
© Oxford University Press.
DOI: 10.1093/oso/9780190087647.001.0001

There are many ways to teach patients and students about the ravages of alcoholism, but few case histories can match Fitzgerald's alcoholic avalanche. A progressive and relapsing disease, alcoholism often requires an unlucky spin of at least 3 wheels of misfortune: nature, nurture, and emotional trauma. With his strong family history for alcoholism; a personality marked by excessive risk taking, reckless behavior, and what he called "a two cylinder inferiority complex"; and a dizzying series of emotional traumas—most notably his wife Zelda's descent into madness—Scott came up short all 3 times.[4]

Fitzgerald was drinking to excess by the time he matriculated into Princeton in 1916. As with all active alcoholics, his problem only grew worse with each passing year and every empty bottle of his favorite spirit, gin. Scott often exaggerated his inebriation so that he could shed his inhibitions and become the life of the party. Throughout his life, he made a fool out of himself at parties and public venues, spewing insults, throwing punches, and hurling ashtrays—behaviors followed by blackouts and memory loss. From cavorting in public fountains to engaging in bloody barroom brawls, Scott's antics were widely reported on two continents. The fool became a pariah in the social settings in which he most craved acceptance, but his consumption of liquor never really stopped.[4] Predictably, his excessive drinking sapped his health and creative energy. As he told his editor, Max Perkins, in 1935:

> It has become increasingly plain to me that the very excellent organization of a long book or the finest perceptions and judgment in time of revision do not go well with liquor. A short story can be written on a bottle, but for a novel you need the mental speed that enables you to keep the whole pattern in your head and ruthlessly sacrifice the sideshows. . . .[5]

Between 1933 and 1937, Scott was hospitalized for alcoholism 8 times and thrown in jail on many more occasions. Most famously, in February, March, and April 1936, Scott confessed the details about his breakdown on the high-profile pages of *Esquire* magazine. He called his *De Profundis* "The Crack-Up." Guilt-ridden, hauntingly sad, and occasionally petulant, Scott admitted to a mass audience that he had "prematurely cracked" and that his alcoholism was destroying him. In an era when such an admission was still considered a weakness of character or a moral failing, Scott's public *mea culpa* was more than an act of candor or bravery; it was tantamount to professional suicide.[3(pp.69-84)] In the months that followed, Scott's incapacitation was widely reported in a number of publications, including the front page of the *New York Post*. The headline on the morning of September 25, 1936, screamed, "The Other Side of Paradise: Scott Fitzgerald, 40, Engulfed in Despair."[6]

In 1937, Fitzgerald somehow managed to convince his agent, Harold Ober, to wrangle him a job as a contract writer for the fabled Metro-Goldwyn-Mayer (MGM) studios. He had flirted with Hollywood before, but this job represented his best chance at success in writing screenplays. He was paid a comfortable, but hardly staggering by Hollywood standards, $1,250 a week. Although he briefly offered his services for such films as *Gone With the Wind, A Yank at Oxford,* and *Madame Curie,* one of the few screenwriting credits he did manage to capture was for the 1938 MGM film *Three Comrades,* a motion picture Scott reviled because he felt that producer Joseph Mankiewicz had mangled his perfect script.[7]

Chain smoking and stuffing himself with fudge, chocolate bars, and bottles of Coca Cola, an alcohol-starved Scott simply could not master the art of screenwriting by assembly line or committee. He rebelled against the system by getting drunk.

Scott's MGM contract was not renewed, and he tried freelancing at some of the other studios for brief and not terribly lucrative stints. Too many times, he did what chronic alcoholics often do: he relapsed. On the mornings after, his young secretary, Frances Kroll, discretely disposed of the empty gin bottles.[8] Most intriguing, he attempted to adapt one of his most famous short stories, *Babylon Revisited,* for producer Lester Cowan. Cowan paid Scott a paltry $2,300 for both the story and the screen adaptation but never made the film. Years later, Cowan sold the script to MGM for $100,000, a transaction that resulted in a 1954 movie called *The Last Time I Saw Paris,* starring Elizabeth Taylor and Van Johnson.[9]

During Zelda Fitzgerald's long confinement to a series of insane asylums, Scott remained true to her in his own fashion. But near the end of his life, the lonely and ailing writer fell in love with Sheila Graham. Struggling to abstain from liquor, he worried intensely about finances, his precarious health, and the education of his daughter Scottie. More than once, Sheila recommended that Scott join a sobriety support group that had been founded by a stockbroker named Bill Wilson and a physician named Bob Smith in 1935. It was called Alcoholics Anonymous. Scott's response was contemptuous: "I was never a joiner. AA can only help weak people because their ego is strengthened by the group. The group offers them the strength they lack on their own."[10,11]

Instead, Scott chose to go it by himself, hoping that willpower alone would free him of his addiction. Despite periods of weeks to months "on the wagon," the binges never really stopped, and each one took a greater toll on Scott's battered brain and body. One time, he boasted of tapering his gin consumption but was still drinking 37 beers a day. In late October 1939, a few weeks after a disastrous and prolonged drunken spree, Fitzgerald wrote his daughter Scottie a eulogy of sorts for himself:

> Anyhow I am alive again—getting by that October did something—with all its strains
> and necessities and humiliations and struggles. I don't drink. I am not a great man, but
> sometimes, I think the impersonal and objective quality of my talent, and the sacrifices
> of it, in pieces, to preserve its essential value has some sort of epic grandeur. Anyhow
> after hours I nurse myself with delusions of that sort.[12]

Fourteen months later, before his formal interment in the family plot in Rockville, Maryland, F. Scott Fitzgerald's body was placed on view in the William Wordsworth Room of the Pierce Brothers Mortuary in Los Angeles. One of the few mourners to pay her respects was the Algonquin Round Table wit, poet, screenwriter, and raging alcoholic Dorothy Parker. The undertakers dedicated their most artistic abilities to expertly coloring Scott's gray hair back to its golden brown and disguising the wrinkles marring the profile admired by millions. Scott's hands, however, told a more accurate tale of too much alcohol and unhealthy living; they were as withered and frail as those belonging to an old man.

Parker alternately praised Scott as the era's greatest novelist and roundly criticized him as a "horse's ass." Softly, under her breath, the bereaved and tipsy poet whispered, "The poor son-of-a-bitch."[13] Those who subsequently heard about the remark assumed Parker was making one of her famously inappropriate, sharp comments. In fact, she was quoting a line Scott wrote near the end of *The Great Gatsby*. It was first uttered by the character "Owl-Eyes," as he stood over the coffin of Jay Gatsby.[14(p.154)]

One cannot read the wonderful prose of F. Scott Fitzgerald without realizing that he was filled with hope and humanity or without gaining an understanding of alcoholism as a physical, mental, and spiritual disease. Every morning during the last, sad years of his life, Scott awoke with the hope that he could tell his alcoholic demons to scram. Some days he enjoyed a modicum of success in that task; there were still many more, however, when he reached for a drink, and then another, sliding closer and closer to his grave. Fitzgerald, after all, was the man who famously observed, "The test of a first-rate intelligence is the ability to hold two opposing ideas in mind at the same time and still retain the ability to function."[3(p.69)]

In retrospect, a far better passage for Parker to have recited while standing over Scott's silent body would be the last luminous lines of his Long Island literary masterpiece:

> Gatsby believed in the green light, the orgiastic future that year by year recedes before us. It eluded us then, but that's no matter—tomorrow we will run faster, stretch out our arms further. . . . And one fine morning—So we beat on, boats against the current, borne back ceaselessly into the past.[14(p.159)]

[This essay originally appeared as: Markel, H.: The Last Alcoholic Days of F. Scott Fitzgerald. Journal of the American Medical Association. 2009; 301 (18):1939–1940.]

REFERENCES

1. Fitzgerald FS. *The Love of the Last Tycoon: The Authorized Text.* Bruccoli MJ, ed. (New York, NY: Scribner, 1993).
2. Graham S, Frank G. *Beloved Infidel: The Education of a Woman.* (New York, NY: Henry Holt & Co, 1958), pp. 330–335.
3. Fitzgerald FS. *The Crack-Up.* (New York, NY: New Directions, 1993), p. 21.
4. Bruccoli MJ. *Some Sort of Epic Grandeur: The Life of F. Scott Fitzgerald.* (New York, NY: Carol & Graf, 1981).

5. Fitzgerald FS. Letter from Fitzgerald to Max Perkins, March 11, 1935. In: Kuehl J, Bryer JR, eds. *Dear Scott/Dear Max: The Fitzgerald-Perkins Correspondence*. (New York, NY: Charles Scribner's Sons, 1971), pp. 218–219.
6. Mok M. The other side of paradise: Scott Fitzgerald, 40, engulfed in despair. *New York Post*. September 25, 1936:1.
7. Latham A. *Crazy Sundays: F. Scott Fitzgerald in Hollywood*. (New York, NY: The Viking Press, 1970), pp. 120–149.
8. Ring FK. *Against the Current: As I Remember F. Scott Fitzgerald*. (Berkeley, CA: Donald S. Ellis/Creative Arts Book Co, 1985).
9. Fitzgerald FS. *Babylon Revisited: The Screenplay*. (New York, NY: Carroll & Graf, 1993), pp. 7–14.
10. Graham S. *The Real F. Scott Fitzgerald: 35 Years Later*. (New York, NY: Grosset & Dunlap, 1976), p. 113.
11. Kurtz E. *Not-God: A History of Alcoholics Anonymous*. (Center City, MN: Hazelden, 1979).
12. Fitzgerald FS. Letter from F. Scott Fitzgerald to Scottie Fitzgerald, October 31, 1939. In: Bruccoli MJ, ed. *F. Scott Fitzgerald: A Life in Letters*. (New York, NY: Touchstone Books, 1994), pp. 419–420.
13. Meade M. *Dorothy Parker: What Fresh Hell Is This?* (New York, NY: Villard Books, 1988), pp. 298–299.
14. Fitzgerald FS. *The Great Gatsby*. (New York, NY: Charles Scribner's Sons, 1925).

CHAPTER 6

∽

Blowing the Whistle

The Internship of William Carlos Williams, M.D., and His Abrupt Resignation From the New York Nursery and Child's Hospital

I t is fitting that it was a pathology professor, William Henry Welch, who best described what constituted a complete and successful career in medicine: "the almost perfect adaptation of [one's] talent and temperament to the accidents and circumstances of his life"[1](p. xi) (Welch WH, review of *The Life of Sir William Osler*, Harvey Cushing Papers, Yale University Manuscript Collections, Microfilm 124, p. 39). Although Welch was writing about the exemplary life of Sir William Osler, the axiom could be equally applied to the poet-physician William Carlos Williams. Dr. Williams' pediatrics internship at the New York Nursery and Child's Hospital between 1908 and 1909 makes for a lovely example of Welch's observation; it was an intriguing period in William's life that both tested his character and demonstrates how chance or circumstance can have remarkable consequences in life. During the year of his internship, Williams engaged in a protracted battle with the hospital's administration over an order that he endorse a report of hospital bills to be sent to the State of New York. Williams objected because the hospital would not provide him with the appropriate documentation that the listed services were actually rendered. Although many of Williams' senior physicians told him to simply sign the billing report and be done with the matter, the young pediatrician's moral convictions resulted in his abrupt resignation from his post many months before he completed his internship. To the historian's delight, Williams' papers and letters easily allow a reconstruction of this chain of events that not only drastically altered

Literatim: Essays at the Intersections of Medicine and Culture. Howard Markel, Oxford University Press (2020).
© Oxford University Press.
DOI: 10.1093/oso/9780190087647.001.0001

the course of Williams' medical career but also had a lasting impact on American literature. For the pediatrician of the 21st century, the episode affords a parable about the importance of honesty in medical reporting and the uncomfortable role of "whistle-blower."

In 1902, shortly after receiving his high school diploma from the Horace Mann School in New York City, Williams matriculated into the University of Pennsylvania Medical School, which did not yet require a baccalaureate degree for entrance. As a homesick student, Willie wrote his mother in the fall of 1904 about the frustrations of having to sit and observe his professors practice medicine when he was so clearly destined for medical greatness: "I will be much happier when I can really do something. When I can work to do somebody good besides myself. All my worrying comes from being impatient to really do something. I want to get with the world and work for some definite end" (W. C. Williams, letter to R. H. Williams, October 25, 1904, Yale University, Beinicke Rare Book Library).

Williams soon recognized during his medical studies that he had a passion for both reading and creating literature. He gained the artistic sustenance he required by dabbling at writing poetry. These early attempts, which Williams subsequently lost or destroyed, were by his own admission bad imitations of poet-physician John Keats. He also embarked on lifelong friendships with several Penn Literary College undergraduates who were destined for great careers in the arts and letters, including the artist Charles DeMuth and the poets Ezra Pound and Hilda Doolittle (who wrote under the pen name, H.D.). After graduation from medical school in 1906, Williams wished his more artistically minded friends *bon voyage* as they set sail for the all-but-mandatory trip of self-discovery in Europe. Williams remained behind and moved to New York, NY, where he was to embark on a general internship at the French Hospital of the French Benevolent Society on West 34th Street. Almost 50 years later, on April 11, 1950, when preparing a biographical sketch for the U.S. Information Service, Washington, DC, Williams explained the pragmatism behind his decision to temporarily put his literary aspirations on hold:

> Writing has been a lifelong occupation for me—at the same time I have practiced medicine. For I knew as a young man that to write as I wanted to write there would be very little money in it for me. And being an American I was born with the practical sense, which told me there was nothing to be gained by dying for art. Rather, I wanted to live for it . . .

Among his many patients at the French Hospital were impoverished New Yorkers in varying states of neglected health, and laborers injured while building the once-glorious Pennsylvania Railroad Station designed by the firm of McKim, Mead, and White. In addition to emergency cases, he also treated a great variety of general medical and surgical maladies, ranging from acute heart attacks and malignant neoplasms to performing appendectomies and other surgical procedures (annual report, Societe Francais de Bienfaisance de New York, October 1907). At the close of his 18-month stint at the French Hospital, the young Dr. Williams applied for and received a coveted position as a pediatrics intern at the Nursery and Child's Hospital (annual report, New York Nursery and Child's Hospital, 1910-1911, 1911).[2]

The field of pediatrics was essentially in its infancy during the first decade of the 20th century. Although Williams was preceded by the first generation of American pediatricians, a group of men who devoted at least 50 percent or more of their professional interests to the diseases of infancy and children, few of these physicians undertook a formal pediatrics residency. Indeed, most of the leading American pediatricians of the early 20th century learned their specialty by working at community dispensaries and orphanages in large cities that catered to the needs of impoverished children. Furthermore, in 1908, there were only a handful of hospitals in the United States devoted solely to the illnesses of children, in which a young physician could learn the intricacies of pediatric medicine, and most of these institutions were situated in the large Atlantic seaboard cities of Boston, Mass, Philadelphia, Pa, and New York. Williams was actually part of a cohort of pediatricians that marks the beginning of formally trained, children's health care physicians.[3-5]

The New York Nursery and Child's Hospital was founded in 1854, making it one of the first hospitals devoted to children in the United States. It had a dual mission, in that it was an obstetrics hospital that catered largely to unwed or destitute mothers and, given the socioeconomic status of many of its patients, also attended to the needs of the children born there. As the years progressed, it offered excellent maternity, general pediatrics, and quarantine or isolation ward services, in addition to foster care programs for those infants who had no parents. Located in Manhattan on Amsterdam Avenue and 61st Street, the hospital was situated on the northern reaches of New York City's notorious Hell's Kitchen neighborhood and adjacent to an African American neighborhood called San Juan Hill. As Williams reminisced about the neighborhood where he learned pediatrics some 40 years later: "We didn't go out much after dark unaccompanied. There were shootings and near riots and worse practically every weekend."[6](p. 93)

He did not have to worry too much about having much free time to wander about any neighborhood of New York. From his first day, on July 1, 1908, Williams was busy morning until night—and oftentimes around the clock—delivering babies, attending to the acute medical needs of desperately ill youngsters, and advising unwed mothers. In those days, Williams envisioned a prominent career as a New York City pediatrician with a huge practice and an even larger income. In 1908, there were fewer than 200 pediatricians practicing in the United States. Those physicians who did manage to carve out comfortable professional niches were typically affiliated as clinical professors with the leading U.S. medical schools and the authors of numerous articles and books. Competition was especially fierce in New York, in which many of the most widely respected pediatricians practiced, including Abraham Jacobi, M.D., who is acclaimed as the father of American pediatrics[7]; L. Emmett Holt, M.D., who wrote the best-selling baby-care book, *The Care and Feeding of Children*, and was, in terms of annual sales and public influence, the "Dr. Spock" of the early 20th century[8,9]; and Henry Koplik, M.D., a developer of free milk distribution programs for impoverished infants and the describer of the pathognomic sign of measles, still referred to as "Koplik's spots."[10] More impressive to a young physician embarking on a career in pediatrics, these professionals all maintained luxurious salaries from the fees generated by attending to the wealthiest children of their community.

Williams was in the early phases of such a career path when a senior physician at the hospital, Charles Gilmore Kerley, M.D., invited him to join his private practice for a year or two as an associate. This was no mere indentured servitude. Kerley, too, was a nationally known pediatrician and author of several best-selling books for both physicians and parents, including a popular baby-care book, *What Every Mother Should Know*, which went through 8 editions, and a novel, *Where Is My Mother?* based on his experiences as a resident physician in an orphanage.[11,12] In 1912, Kerley was elected president of the American Pediatric Society, the elite academic society of his field. The senior physician's office was on West 81st Street, just a few doors from Central Park, and the practice was heavily populated with the children of well-heeled parents residing in the palatial apartment houses along Central Park West.[13] If Williams succeeded in Kerley's office, he was likely to be offered a permanent spot as a partner—an incredible opportunity in the competitive and not always lucrative medical marketplace of New York City of the early 20th century.

Williams' career aspirations dimmed when he was appointed senior resident at the Child's inpatient pediatric service in late December of 1908. One of his responsibilities was to review and sign the monthly reports documenting the hospital's admissions, discharges, and medical services, which were then sent to the state authorities in Albany, NY, for reimbursement. Although the medical care provided at the hospital was excellent, the administration was, in Williams' words, "riddled with corruption." Therefore, when asked by the hospital superintendent, a "dark, sweaty-looking creature" named Miss Malzacher, to sign the monthly report, Dr. Williams appropriately asked to review the medical records of that month's patients to make sure the services listed were correct. Malzacher refused his request explaining, "This is a business matter, not a medical matter."[6](p.102)

After a few days of pointless face-offs, Miss Malzacher sent the report to Albany, NY, without Williams' endorsement. The New York State Department of Charities promptly returned the billing report with the request that the senior resident physician actually sign the form to attest to its veracity. Again, Williams refused to sign it, despite urgent pleas from Malzacher, his patron-to-be Kerley, and several other attending physicians, who found Williams' behavior eccentric, to say the least. To one of his superiors, the Fifth Avenue obstetrician J. Milton Mabbott, M.D., whom the house staff nicknamed "Maggoty" Mabbott because of his predilection for lingering over attractive women when performing pelvic examinations, Williams pointedly asked: "If someone handed you some scribbled figures and told you to copy them into an official report, figures which you had no way of verifying, could you as a self-respecting person put your name to those figures and would you do it?" Mabbott was reported to have exited the conversation muttering, "No, I'll be damned if I would."[6](p. 103)

When it mattered most, however, Williams enjoyed little support from Kerley, Mabbott, or the other staff physicians, and the board of trustees suspended him from the hospital for two weeks. The most likely reason Williams was not given supportive documents for the billing report was that they did not exist. To make matters more complicated, Superintendent Malzacher was involved in a passionate affair with the president of the hospital's board of trustees, who was unwilling to support a righteous young physician over his corrupt but beloved mistress. Williams' code of ethics led him to the unenviable role of whistle-blower. As William Shakespeare observed through the eyes of Queen Cleopatra, people often blame the bearer of bad tidings.[14]

The source of Williams' resolve should be hardly surprising to a pediatrician. Two remarkable and supportive parents who emphasized the importance of individuality, honesty, and forthrightness to their children, William George and Raquel Williams, raised the physician-poet. For example, we can reconstruct evidence of strong parental support in two notes Williams' father, William George Williams, dashed off to his son. The first letter acknowledged the "ordeal" Williams was enduring at the hospital but reminded him "truth and justice will prevail" (W. G. Williams, letter to W. C. Williams, M.D., January 15, 1909, Yale University, Beinicke Rare Book Library). The second note, a 3 × 5-inch slip of paper Mr Williams intended for his son to refer to during his meeting with the hospital trustees, offered the following words of advice: "Don't fire unless you are fired on, etc, etc but if there is to be a fight . . . you know the rest"; "Let them do most of the talking"; "Don't let them get you on the run"; "Don't let them ask all the questions; ask a few yourself"; and "Do not close anything final without advice" (W. G. Williams, letter to W. C. Williams, M.D., January 15, 1909, Yale University, Beinicke Rare Book Library).

Alas, as with many young people with a cause, Dr. Williams only partially followed his father's instructions. When the board of trustees told him to either sign the document or resign his post, Williams boldly chose the latter option. All affiliations with Dr. Kerley's fabulous practice evaporated into thin air. Putting on his best face, Williams wrote to his brother Ed about the relief he felt after his resignation was accepted. He stated he could not work for an institution or for physicians he did not respect: "There was nothing to do but crawl too or get out, so I got out" (W. C. Williams, letter to E. Williams, March 18, 1909).[15](p. 75) As Williams recorded some 40 years later in his autobiography: "My days of internship were over. Not a single doctor of the attending staff had stood by me. To hell with them all, I thought."[6](p. 104)

In our era of contentiousness in the workplace, such a move might be seen today as a minor personality conflict. But it is important for the reader of the early 21st century to place him or herself onto the wards of that now defunct children's hospital of a century ago. It was a place where one either followed the orders of one's superiors to the letter or suffered dire consequences. Of course, physicians continue to adhere to a chain of command, but today there is quite a bit more leeway for areas of disagreement and outright instances of bad behavior. In 1909, Williams' actions, which were interpreted as gross insubordination, assured that he would be forever locked out of the elite world of academic medicine to which he aspired. His resignation from the hospital said goodbye to a prestigious Manhattan medical practice and hello to professional obscurity in the backwaters of New Jersey. Williams essentially drummed himself out of the academic corps. This was no youthful tantrum, it was an act of principle for which he knew at the time he would pay dearly.

After resigning from his pediatrics internship, Williams occupied himself by writing, self-publishing his first book of poems, and embarking on a courtship and an impulsive marriage proposal to a 20-year-old woman he nicknamed Flossie.[6] The young physician left New York in July of 1909 to visit the famed *Kinderkliniken* of Leipzig and Vienna and travel through Europe. Williams returned the following year to practice in a ground-floor room of his parents' house in Rutherford, NJ. It was not until 1912 that he married his fiancée of three years, the same Flossie— Florence Herman—whose family is fictionalized in his trilogy of novels, *White Mule, The Build-Up,* and *In the Money.* Together, they had two sons and he, of course, pursued a career that combined the rigors of solo general practice with the sublime pleasures of writing in his spare time and in between patients, deliveries, and house calls. Over the years, he steadily enlarged his practice and took on additional responsibilities as the physician for the Rutherford public school system and attending pediatrician at the Passaic General Hospital, Passaic, NJ. Williams toiled away for almost half a century in northern New Jersey, often taking care of that region's most needy children.[16]

Williams' arduous schedule as a physician, however, did not prevent his steady progress as a poet and author. Beginning by publishing his poems privately and then moving up to the "little magazines," Williams eventually secured a loyal publisher in James Laughlin, the founder of New Directions. By the end of his life, Williams finally reached the large audience he craved since he was a young man. But it is essential to note that Williams' remarkable poetry and prose were inexorably rooted in his daily role and observations as a practicing physician. The physician from Rutherford, NJ, was awarded the National Book Award for poetry in 1950 and, posthumously, the Pulitzer Prize in 1963.

Pediatricians are constantly reminding parents, when dealing with an obstreperous child or teenager, to pick battles wisely. We often extend this advice to our students and training physicians as well. One conclusion of this episode in Dr. Williams' life might be that confrontation with hospital administrators or senior physicians and resignation were not the wisest career choices. Yet even the most disapproving cannot help but be impressed by the courage of his convictions. Accident, chance, character, independence, and ambition led Williams to Rutherford, NJ, and to produce a body of literature that is sometimes overtly medical but always artfully written with the finely honed senses of a physician. This is not to say that Williams would not have written his marvelous poems and novels had he remained a Manhattan specialist, but such hypothetical musings are impossible to address. The fact remains that he did return to northern New Jersey, relied extensively on the people and environment that constituted his practice both for his livelihood and his art, and became the poet-pediatrician we admire today. With regard to the wealthy children of New York City who did not benefit from Dr. Williams' medical acumen, the historical record argues that fate intervened much to American literature's good fortune. There were (and are) plenty of ambitious young physicians who could write prescriptions and complicated formulas for this elite cohort, but only one who could describe life in northern New Jersey or a "red wheelbarrow" so elegantly.[17](p. 224)

This originally appeared as: Markel, H.: Blowing the Whistle: The Internship of William Carlos Williams, M.D. and his Abrupt Resignation from the New York Nursery and Child's Hospital. Archives of Pediatrics and Adolescent Medicine 2000; 154:952–955.

REFERENCES

1. Bliss, M.: *William Osler: A Life in Medicine.* (New York, NY: Oxford University Press, 1999).
2. *A Century of Service to Mothers and Children* [pamphlet]. (New York, NY: Centennial Committee of the New York Nursery and Child's Hospital, 1923).
3. Markel, H.: Academic pediatrics: the view from New York a century ago. *Acad Med.* 1996; 71: 146–151.
4. Markel, H.: Caring for the foreign born: the health of immigrant children in the United States, 1890–1925. *Arch Pediatr Adolesc Med.* 1998; 152: 1020–1027.
5. Halpern, S.: *American Pediatrics: The Social Dynamics of Professionalism.* (Berkeley: University of California Press, 1988).
6. Williams, W.C.: *The Autobiography of William Carlos Williams.* (New York, NY: Random House, 1951).
7. Leopold, J.S.: Abraham Jacobi, 1820–1919. Veeder, B., ed., *Pediatric Profiles.* (St Louis, Mo: C.V. Mosby Co., 1957), pp.13–21.
8. Holt, L.E.: *The Care and Feeding of Children.* (New York, NY: D. Appleton, 1894).
9. Holt, L.E.: *The Diseases of Childhood and Infancy.* 3rd ed. (New York, NY: D. Appleton, 1907).
10. Markel, H.: Henry Koplik, M.D., the Good Samaritan Dispensary of New York City, and the description of Koplik's spots. *Arch Pediatr Adolesc Med.* 1996; 150: 535–539.
11. Kerley, C.G.: *Short Talks With Young Mothers on the Management of Infants and Young Children.* 7th ed. (New York, NY: G.P. Putnam's Sons, 1922).
12. Kerley, C.G.: *Where Is My Mother?* (New York, NY: Robert Haas, 1935).
13. Obituary of Dr. C.G. Kerley. *New York Times.* September 8 1945.
14. Shakespeare, W.: *Antony and Cleopatra.* Act 2, scene 5, lines 22–90.
15. Mariani, P.: *William Carlos Williams: A New World Naked.* (New York, NY: McGraw-Hill Co Inc., 1981).
16. Coles, R. *William Carlos Williams: The Knack of Survival in America.* (New Brunswick, NJ: Rutgers University Press, 1975).
17. Williams, W.C.: *Collected Poems of William Carlos Williams, Volume I: 1909–1939.* (New York, NY: New Directions, 1986).

CHAPTER 7

∾

Sinclair Lewis' *Arrowsmith*

The Great American Medical Novel of Medicine

A s we trudge the rocky road that is the 21st century, an era in which one is del-
uged daily by a torrent of information on medical discoveries, public health,
and the conquest of disease, it may be surprising to recall that it was only a little less
than a century ago that a medical scientist first entered American literary consciousness in the exalted role of hero. Sinclair Lewis's 1925 novel, *Arrowsmith*, chronicles
a physician's relentless search for truth. Unlike other novels of this period or before
it, the main character, Martin Arrowsmith, is no cleric, writer, or philosopher. He
is not even a particularly great doctor. Lewis, aware of the wide public interest in
medical progress—not unlike our current fascination with all things genomic—
introduced millions of American readers to a young man who dedicated himself to
the singularly hottest scientific field of his day: bacteriology. And in an age in which
the authority of science is as much a part of our world view as an even "higher"
authority once was for our grandparents, a hero inspired to stamp out disease is,
as historian Charles Rosenberg observed, "one appropriate to twentieth-century
America."[1]

The novel's influence extends well beyond its immediate critical and popular
success. I well recall how as a first year medical student I raptly read about the
adventures of Martin Arrowsmith when I should have been committing to memory
the intricacies of the brachial plexus. Somehow it was comforting to recognize the
same traits among Martin, his fellow students, and teachers—from the purely mercenary to the honorable—that I witnessed daily in the lecture halls and hospital
wards. My battered paperback copy of *Arrowsmith* is annotated throughout with the
same pen-scrawled comment: "Still true!" I am hardly alone: from its publication
to the present, countless men and women have been inspired to pursue careers in

Literatim: Essays at the Intersections of Medicine and Culture. Howard Markel, Oxford University Press (2020).
© Oxford University Press.
DOI: 10.1093/oso/9780190087647.001.0001

research because of Martin's intense devotion to science. Indeed, it would be a fascinating (if difficult to properly design) study to survey physicians, medical scientists, and public health workers whose career paths were directed by Martin Arrowsmith over the past eight decades.

The novel records and predicts many of the successes and problems that torment the medical profession to this very day, including the competition of needs, goals, and resources between those who identify themselves as clinicians and those who are scientists; the commercial interests of pharmaceutical companies in the development of new medications and vaccines versus the need to seek out and verify scientific truth; the inherent political and social difficulties in developing programs that protect a community's public health; and the evolving role of the doctor in American society. In addition to being an enduring work of literary art and a scathing satire of the medical profession, *Arrowsmith* is a vibrant document of the history of American public health and medicine during the first two decades of the 20th century. The history behind the creation of this literary and historical document is a fascinating one.

After his stunning critical and popular success in 1920 with *Main Street* and shortly before the publication of *Babbitt* in 1922, Sinclair Lewis cast his literary eye on the American labor movement. That summer he began planning a novel with a protagonist based on Eugene Debs. Two friends and admirers, H.L. Mencken, the famed journalist (a notorious hypochondriac and aficionado of all things medical), and Dr. Morris Fishbein, the editor of the *Journal of the American Medical Association,* convinced him to turn instead to the world of medical research, the medical profession, and the role that science was beginning to play in daily American life.

Mencken and Fishbein then introduced Lewis to an unemployed bacteriologist named Paul DeKruif, who had earned his Ph.D. from the University of Michigan in 1916 and was recently been dismissed from the Rockefeller Institute for Medical Research (now Rockefeller University) when it became clear that his hands itched for a fountain pen instead of test tubes. DeKruif was fired from his post by the Rockefeller's director, Simon Flexner, for writing a four-part series of articles on the medical profession entitled "Our Medicine Men," published in *The Century* magazine.[2] The scientist was still several years away from his string of best-selling books, including *The Microbe Hunters,* that popularized health topics ranging from germs to sex hormones. But as of the summer of 1922, he was officially at liberty to give up the dull drudgery of late nights in the laboratory for what he perceived to be the exciting life of a medical journalist.[3]

Fishbein, Lewis, and DeKruif went to lunch, and they began drinking, first at one bar and soon at another. After a long, alcoholic day that included a narrow escape from a barroom brawl and a fruitless attempt to visit Eugene Debs, then convalescing in a sanitarium outside of Chicago after one of his frequent collapses from physical exhaustion, DeKruif and Lewis agreed to collaborate on a medical novel. Within weeks the two sold the book to Lewis's publishers Harcourt and Brace and booked passage on a steamship to the West Indies where they could work without distractions.

According to DeKruif's memoirs, *The Sweeping Wind*,[3] the original contract he signed with publishers Harcourt and Brace specified that Lewis and DeKruif were to be listed as the novel's co-authors. Soon enough, Lewis had second thoughts about sharing the limelight with an unknown and convinced DeKruif that a "collaboration" might hurt book sales. Aware of his 25 percent stake in what would become a best-selling novel, DeKruif wisely kept silent and allowed Lewis to be listed as sole author. Nevertheless, by January, 1923 Lewis was exclaiming to his publishers that DeKruif was "perfection ... in all there's a question as to whether he won't have contributed more than I shall have."[4] There can be no debate over the fact that DeKruif was essential to the execution of the novel. Nearly all the scientists, physicians, and medical institutions portrayed in *Arrowsmith* were drawn from his experience as a graduate student at the University of Michigan and, later, as a research investigator at the Rockefeller Institute for Medical Research. And while DeKruif did not receive the authorial credit he most likely deserved, Lewis did dedicate the novel to him in a rather splendid manner:

> To Dr. Paul H. DeKruif, I am indebted not only for most of the bacteriological and medical material in this tale but equally for his help in the planning of the fable itself—for his realization of the characters as living people, for his philosophy as a scientist. With this acknowledgement I want to record our months of companionship while working on the book, in the United States, in the West Indies, in Panama, in London and Fountainebleau. I wish I could reproduce our talks along the way, and the laboratory afternoons, the restaurants at night, and the deck at dawn as we steamed into tropic ports.[5]

Given Lewis's genius to mine the rich quarry of the American Middle West, it is not surprising that the favorite son of Sauk Centre, Minnesota (and the actual son of a doctor) sets much of *Arrowsmith* in the heartland. For example, Martin's medical school, the University of Winnemac, is a precise pen-portrait of the University of Michigan during the first decade of the 20th century:

> It is not a snobbish rich-man's college, devoted to leisurely nonsense. It is the property of the people of the state, and what they want—or what they are told they want—is a mill to turn out men and women who will lead moral lives, play bridge, drive good cars, be enterprising in business, and occasionally mention books, though they are not expected to have time to read them. It is a Ford Motor Factory, and if its products rattle a little, they are beautifully standardized, with perfectly interchangeable parts.[5]

Many of Martin Arrowsmith's professors are easily identifiable from the faculty roster of the University of Michigan Medical School during this period, even down to the material they presented in their lectures. It is also at the University of Winnemac where Martin comes under the spell of an immunology professor named

Max Gottleib, who is an amalgam of DeKruif's mentor at Michigan, the professor of bacteriology Frederick Novy, and his idol at the Rockfeller, biologist Jacques Loeb. It is while toiling in Gottleib's laboratory late at night and into the early hours of the morning that Martin first decides to devote his life to the pursuit of scientific knowledge. Before doing so, however, Martin makes a few detours, including completing his internship at the Zenith General Hospital, marrying a student nurse he meets there named Leora Tozer, and a brief sojourn as a general practitioner in Leora's hometown, Wheatsylvania, North Dakota. Lewis's descriptions of the rigors, politics, and boredom of general medical practice during this era are as good as one is going to find. For example, Martin drives back and forth 50 miles late one night to obtain diphtheria anti-toxin for a 7-year-old patient, only to administer the life-saving elixir too late. This compelling scene combines the high drama of a life and death situation with the advent of a new biological agent that could potentially cure an all-too-common killer:

> . . . the healer bulked in the room, crowding out Gottlieb the inhuman perfectionist. Martin leaned nervously over the child on the tousled bed, absent-mindedly trying her pulse again and again. He felt helpless without the equipment of Zenith General [Hospital], its nurses and [his medical colleague] Angus Duer's sure advice. He had a sudden respect for the lone country doctor.[5]

But general practice does not hold Martin's interest and he is soon drawn to a position as a junior public health officer in Nautilus, Iowa, under an enthusiastic physician named Almus Pickerbaugh, who "looked somewhat like President Roosevelt, with the same squareness and the same bristly mustache."[5] Although Pickerbaugh understands the need for scientific research in improving the health of a community, he is a firm subscriber of the "Billy Sunday" approach to spreading the gospel of public health. To this end, he has organized his eight daughters into the Healthette Octette, who sing "health hymns" at county fairs, has made countless, rousing speeches on hygiene at YMCA picnics and other public gatherings; and has written a series of public health poems earning him the sobriquet, "the two-fisted fightin' poet-doc." One excellent example of Pickerbaugh's literary *metier* should suffice:

> Boil the milk bottles or by gum
>
> You better buy your ticket to Kingdom Come.[5]

While Dr. Pickerbaugh leads a health crusade that by the novel's end lands him a post in the President's Cabinet as the "first Secretary of Health and Eugenics," Martin becomes enamoured with the daily drudgery of a working public health officer. The young physician eagerly sets about testing local milk supplies, performing Wasserman syphilis tests, making vaccines and performing diphtheria cultures for the local doctors. Sadly, after Pickerbaugh is elected to the U.S. House of Representatives and leaves the Nautilus health department under the charge of his assistant, Martin becomes a bit overzealous in protecting the town's public health and the town elders dismiss him from his position. Although this section of the novel is a splendid example of Lewisian satire pointed at local health departments and the public's resentment of too much encroachment on their private (if unhygienic) lives, Pickerbaugh's bombastic crusades and carnival-like approach also represent a fairly accurate mirror of these institutions throughout the United States during the early decades of the 20th century.

Eventually, Martin is called to a post at the prestigious McGurk (read Rockefeller) Institute in New York, where his former mentor, Max Gottlieb, is now a prominent research director. Again, DeKruif's experience shines in terms of Lewis's descriptions of the search for scientific knowledge, the philosophy of the research investigator, the sumptuously plush research facilities courtesy of the greatest robber baron of them all, and some rather hilarious caricatures of such medical luminaries as Simon Flexner, Peyton Rous, and others.

Perhaps the novel's greatest strength is its veracity of detail about a life in medicine, from the conflicts that arise between commerce and altruism to the design of scientific experiments. Nowhere is this more clearly drawn than during a bubonic plague epidemic raging on the mythical island of St. Hubert in the West Indies that affords Martin an opportunity to test his newly discovered magic bullet, bacteriophage. Martin's wife, Leora, insists on joining him on this dangerous trip. Soon enough, Martin immerses himself in a meticulous experiment in which half the island's inhabitants receive bacteriophage and the rest a placebo. Bacteriophage was no fictional device. A viral parasite that kills bacteria, it was the talk of the bacteriology world soon after its real-life discovery by Felix d'Herelle of the Pasteur Institute in Paris in 1917.[6,7] One of many marchers in the parade of great medical hopes that continues to the present, bacteriophage was eventually cast aside for something even more miraculous: antibiotics.

Late one night, a lonely Leora finds a cigarette Martin left behind on his makeshift laboratory bench. Unaware that the housekeeper had accidentally spilled some plague culture on the cigarette, she smokes it in an effort to be closer to her absent husband and dies a miserable death before sunrise. Overwhelmed with grief, Martin damns science and gives bacteriophage to all who want it. While the epidemic wanes and he receives international acclaim, Martin knows he botched the experiment. Here we encounter DeKruif's touch in this plot twist. In February 1901, DeKruif's bacteriology professor, Frederick Novy, returned to Ann Arbor with some specimens after investigating a plague epidemic in San Francisco's Chinatown. Some weeks later his laboratory assistant, a second-year medical student named Charles B. Hare, who rolled his own Bull Durhams, unknowingly contaminated a cigarette he was about to smoke. As a result he developed the pneumonic form of plague in early April 1901. Hare was quarantined in the pest house behind the University of Michigan Hospital for several weeks, where he was treated by the eminent internist, and one of William Osler's favorite former pupils, George Dock. Unlike the fictional Leora, however, Hare did recover and graduated from

Michigan with his medical degree in 1905. His bout with plague, however, caused severe heart damage, and Dr. Hare died at the age of 50.[8]

Integral to the novel was Lewis's insistence that Martin be both a physician and a scientist, personifying a conflict that continues to trouble doctors and their patients to the present. Who is more important in the conquest of disease: the compassionate, sympathetic healer caring for a sick individual or the cold, obsessive investigator trying to ascertain the cause of disease and, if successful, render the doctor obsolete?

Interestingly, the other best-selling book about medicine published in 1925 was Dr. Harvey Cushing's painstakingly detailed *Life of Sir William Osler*.[9] It was published only a few years after Osler's death, but Osler had already entered the pantheon of medical heroes. Both books won the Pulitzer Prize in 1926 (though Lewis, famously, turned his down). To the forward-thinking scientists revered by Lewis and DeKruif, the frock-coated, mustachioed Dr. Osler was a quaint relic. As Michael Bliss notes in his biography, *William Osler: A Life in Medicine*, Cushing accepted his prize hoping Osler's benevolent bedside manner would overshadow *Arrowsmith's* glorification of medical research.[10] But Cushing misinterpreted the exquisite tension that Martin negotiates as both a healer and a scientist. Martin understands the imperative to conduct objective experiments that definitively prove a hypothesis. But unlike many of his laboratory-based colleagues, Martin often sides with the healers when confronted by the immediate demands of the sick bed.

While hilariously assailing the Babbittry of the medical profession, Lewis captures the absolute passion for discovery required of a successful scientist. This is no mere job. It's a religion. One of *Arrowsmith's* most moving scenes depicts Martin in his laboratory praying:

> God give me unclouded eyes and freedom from haste. God give me a quiet and relentless anger against all pretense and pretentious work and all work left slack and unfinished. God give me a restlessness whereby I may neither sleep nor accept praise till my observed results equal my calculated results or in pious glee I discover and assault my error. God give me strength not to trust in God![5]

A satire of Judeo-Christian expressions of the ideal life, perhaps, yet one cannot help but be troubled by how much things have changed over the past century. Up until recently, scientists worked decidedly toward the greater good of humankind. The opportunity to contribute to the battle against illness was reward enough for an exciting and honored position in society. Sadly, today, one cannot fathom a research scientist praying for anything so noble when there are patent applications for newly discovered genes to fill out and stock options to consider. As the ties between medical scientists and the biotechnology industry become increasingly intertwined, the doctor in me wishes he could prescribe a page or two of *Arrowsmith* each day to his more profit-driven colleagues. Perhaps "Dr. Lewis" could restore some health to the ailing condition of scientific idealism.

[*This essay originally appeared as: Markel, H.: Reflections on Sinclair Lewis's "Arrowsmith": The Great American Novel of Public Health and Medicine. Public Health Reports 2001; 116:371–375; an earlier and more abbreviated version appeared as "Prescribing Arrowsmith" in The New York Times Book Review, September 24, 2000, Section 7, p. 35.*]

REFERENCES

1. Rosenberg CE. Martin Arrowsmith: the scientist as hero. In: *No Other Gods: On Science and American Social Thought.* (Baltimore: Johns Hopkins University Press, 1976), pp. 123–131.
2. DeKruif P. *Our Medicine Men.* (New York: Century, 1922).
3. DeKruif P. *The Sweeping Wind: A Memoir.* (New York: Harcourt, Brace and World, 1962).
4. Smith H, editor. *From Main Street to Stockholm: The Letters of Sinclair Lewis, 1919–1930.* (New York: Harcourt, Brace and Co., 1952).
5. Lewis S. *Arrowsmith.* (New York: Harcourt, Brace, 1925).
6. D'Herelle, F. Bacteriophage as treatment in acute medical and surgical infections. *Bull NY Acad Med.* 1921; 7: 329–348.
7. Summers, W.C. *Felix d'Herelle and the Origins of Molecular Biology.* (New Haven: Yale University Press, 1999).
8. Entry for April 26, 1901. In: Clinical notebooks of Dr. George Dock, Professor of Medicine at the University of Michigan. Vol. II: 1900–1901. University of Michigan at Ann Arbor, Bentley Historical Library, Michigan Historical Collections. pp. 783–803.
9. Cushing H. *The Life of Sir William Osler.* Volumes I and II. (Oxford, UK: Oxford University Press, 1925).
10. Michael B. *William Osler: A Life in Medicine.* (New York: Oxford University Press, 1999).

ADDITIONAL READING OF INTEREST

ON THE FIRST MEETING OF LEWIS AND DEKRUIF:

Schorer M. *Sinclair Lewis: An American Life.* (New York: McGraw-Hill Co., 1961), pp. 337–341; 361–373.
Mencken HL. *My Life as an Author and Editor.* (New York: Alfred A. Knopf, 1993), pp. 275–282.
Fishbein M. *Morris Fishbein, M.D.: An Autobiography.* (Garden City, NY: Doubleday, 1969), pp. 99–104.
Lewis GH. *With Love from Gracie. Sinclair Lewis, 1912–1925.* (New York: Harcourt, Brace and Co., 1955).

FOR A DESCRIPTION OF EUGENE DEBS'S FREQUENT BOUTS OF DEPRESSION:

Salvatore N. *Eugene Debs: Citizen and Socialist.* (Urbana, IL: University of Illinois Press, 1982).

FOR BIOGRAPHICAL MATERIAL ON NOVY:

Garrett C.G.B. Frederick Novy. In: Garraty J, editor. *Dictionary of American Biography,* Supplement 6, 1956–1960. (New York: Charles Scribner's Sons, 1980), pp. 481–482.

FOR BIOGRAPHICAL MATERIAL ON LOEB:

Pauly P.J. *Controlling life: Jacques Loeb and the engineering ideal in biology.* (New York: Oxford University Press, 1987).

DeKruif PH. Jacques Loeb, the mechanist. *Harpers.* 1923: 146; 182–190.

DeKruif, P.H. Jacques Loeb. *The American Mercury.* 1925: 5; 273–279.

On the Rockefeller Institute:

Corner G.W. *A History of the Rockefeller Institute, 1901–1953: Origins and Growth.* (New York: Rockefeller Institute Press, 1964).

Brown E.R. *Rockefeller Medicine Men: Medicine and Capitalism in America.* (Berkeley, CA: University of California Press, 1979).

On Charles B. Hare's case of bubonic plague:

Bubonic Plague File, Frederick Novy Papers, Bentley Historical Library, The University of Michigan, Ann Arbor, MI.

Benscoter, W.A. Ann Arbor's case of bubonic plague. *Detroit News-Tribune,* April 12, 1901; p. 2.

Davenport, H.W. *Doctor Dock: Teaching and Learning at the Turn of the Century.* (New Brunswick, NJ: Rutgers University Press, 1987), pp. 255–259.

Cummings, J.G. The plague: a laboratory case report. *Military Med.* 1963: 128; 435–439.

Davenport, H.W. *Not Just Any Medical school: The Science, Practice and Teaching of Medicine at the University of Michigan, 1850–1941.* (Ann Arbor: University of Michigan Press, 1999), p. 46.

CHAPTER 8

⌘

Living (and Practicing) in the Shadow of the House of God

Every physician recalls with relative clarity his or her first day of medical school. A quarter of a century after mine, I can still conjure up images of entering the dimly lit, badly ventilated auditorium that became my class' central headquarters and *ad hoc* clubhouse. In particular, I recollect my intense anticipation as I took my assigned position in the anatomy suite that afternoon—a passage representing both physically and symbolically my entry into the medical profession.

My class's initiation began with the dramatic entrance of our anatomy professor, a revered and skilled dissector who reeked of formaldehyde and was armed with a holster containing 57 varieties of colored chalk and pencils that he used to illustrate his pedagogic lectures. The rotund, precise anatomist sternly announced at this first formal gathering and, at each class thereafter, that we were charged with attaining an absolute intellectual mastery of the human body's architecture. Indeed, he empha‐ sized, our patients' lives would depend on it, since anatomy was the foundation for understanding the function and dysfunction of the body and the manipulation of it by therapeutic means and procedures.

But somewhere during the professor's macabre discourse on the myriad means of skinning a cadaver, my laboratory partner—a clownish guy I had known since high school and who later made a fortune selling nutritional supplements to the worried well—nudged me with a broad grin on his face and a dog-eared paperback in hand. "Have you read it?" he asked. "It's called *House of God* and all the third- and fourth-year medical students say it's practically required if you want to understand what it's really like to be a doctor."

House. Of. God. Those three words, and the many thousands more that com‐ prised its raunchy, troubling, and, at times, hilarious text have spoken to millions of medical students and physicians-in-training over the past 30 years. Indeed, it

Literatim: Essays at the Intersections of Medicine and Culture. Howard Markel, Oxford University Press (2020).
© Oxford University Press.
DOI: 10.1093/oso/9780190087647.001.0001

has served as the essential underground travel guide to the once closely guarded lives of interns and residents at prestigious hospitals across the United States.[1] Written by a psychiatrist named Stephen Bergman, under the *nom de plume* of Samuel Shem, the novel was based on his experiences as an intern at one of Harvard Medical School's teaching hospitals, the Beth Israel Hospital (now Beth Israel Deaconess Hospital).

Publisher Richard Marek was so confident of the novel's literary merit that at its 1978 debut he took the unconventional step of distributing 10,000 copies to bookstores and book reviewers, free of charge; when that generous supply ran out, Marek produced and distributed three more printings of 5,000 each.[2] While the reviews of this "brutally frank account" ran the gamut from enthusiastic to uneasy,[3–5] the first 25,000 copies initiated a buzz that continues to hum to the present and has resulted in the sales of millions of copies.

The daily activities of interns, residents, and attending physicians in busy hospitals has been a staple of U.S. popular culture since 1925, when Sinclair Lewis published his glorious Pulitzer Prize–winning medical chronicle, *Arrowsmith*.[6,7] On its heels came a flood of novels, stories, plays, motion pictures, radio and television dramas, documentaries, and docudramas.[8] In recent years, medical fiction has been overwhelmed by medical memoir as an increasingly large number of glib students and interns (many of them, it seems, from Harvard) describe their experiences and the potentially crushing effects that graduate medical education can have on the humanity of those who deliver as well as those who receive health care.[9–15] This veritable library barely scratches the surface of the growing cadre of physician-scribes currently writing books and articles on virtually every aspect of the medical life.[16,17] But none of these volumes has had as universal an impact on U.S. physicians during the late 20th century. Perhaps it is because *The House of God* is a direct descendant of the wildly popular *Catch-22*, Joseph Heller's absurdly satirical exploration of the insanity of war. As with all soldiers who read Heller's literary vision of military life, virtually every medical reader who has spent time on the wards of the largest U.S. hospitals in the last 30 years will recognize profound, albeit disturbing, veracity in the pages of *The House of God*.

Shem describes the emotionally and physically draining experiences of an intern named Roy Basch during the 1973-1974 academic year, an era when attending physicians were ethereal presences in the hospital at night and the intern's mandated 80-hour workweek was merely a gleam in the eye of the most radical of medical reformers. Somehow, thanks to a supportive girlfriend, Berry, who inexplicably puts up with Roy's roller-coaster and sleep-deprived emotions; a disgustingly ribald yet warm senior resident known only as "the Fat Man," who will forever be remembered in medical literature for coining the term GOMER ("Get Out of My Emergency Room") in reference to the elderly, chronically ill patients he did not want to admit to his service; an orgy of sexual affairs with sundry nurses; and some of the bleakest (if not side-splitting) medical hijinks ever recorded on the written page, Roy completes his internal medicine internship. By the book's end, however, Roy (as well as the author) rejects and leaves the internists, once considered to be the elite ruling class of academic medical centers, for a residency in psychiatry.

Often vulgar and crudely sexist, it is difficult to deny the novel's raw accuracy in documenting the realities of the academic medical center as they existed in the early 1970s.[18] The education of Roy Basch coincides with a historical moment that witnessed the twilight of the civil rights movement, the crumbling of the Nixon White House, and the corrosive social effects that Watergate had on the public's perceptions of once-trusted institutions and so-called role models. As Shem later explained this fomenting ethos, his cohort of interns came of age in an era of protest. When confronted with what they considered to be inhumane medical practices, "We stuck together and used classic, nonviolent methods—including humor—to resist."[19]

These years also marked the explosive expansion of academic medical-industrial complexes in every corner of the nation. But at the same time the most august physicians promised great scientific and therapeutic hopes to their colleagues, patients, and patrons, the profession was forced to contend daily with the realities of powerfully stubborn chronic diseases and a growing awareness of the limits of scientific medicine. For many, it seemed that every clinical success was countered by 10 greater skirmishes, marred by diminished access to health care for those who needed it most, exponential growth in health care costs, and the emergence of a plethora of complex ethical, social, and legal dilemmas related to caring for elderly, young, and dying patients.

On several evenings in early September 1982, after definitively shutting my textbooks and capping my highlighters, I turned to a used copy of *The House of God* I had purchased for 75 cents. Always an avid re-reader, I returned to that volume during my third year of medical school and again as an intern. Some might recall this period as Ronald Reagan's "go-go eighties," but those entering the halls of medicine at this point seemed much more preoccupied with how U.S. hospitals and physicians were scrambling to adapt to the newly mandated diagnosis related groups (DRGs) and their severely prescribed hospital length of stays and billing expectations for specific disease processes. I can recall chuckling at how *The House of God* predicted the DRG tidal wave with its outraged descriptions of an attending physician named Dr. Putzel (which, probably not coincidentally, is a bastardization of the Yiddish word for a diminutive male sex organ). Putzel was infamous at the House of God for admitting patients for weeks on end and racking up insanely high bills by ordering useless batteries of diagnostic tests. Little wonder that hospitals of the late 1960s and early 1970s, swimming downstream in that great river of medical revenue occasioned by Medicaid, Medicare, and the rise of health care benefits for the employed, loved the Dr. Putzels of the world.

Born in 1960, I missed the endless protest marches and political causes that characterized Shem and his generation's high school and college years. Yet in my day there still existed a wary, if not adversarial, relationship between medical students and faculty that permeated the classrooms and, later, the wards as students were examined for intellectual fitness with questions we dismissed as trivial "rat-facts" having little to do with "real doctoring" or confronting the looming economic and social storm we now refer to as "the health care crisis." In this miasma of professional insecurity and hostility, *The House of God* proved simultaneously thrilling and disturbing.

Like many first-year medical students, I often awoke feeling as inconsequential as Sisyphus after a grueling day of hauling an enormous rock up some hill only to watch its predictable downward slide each evening. By turning to *The House of God*, instead of memorizing the pages of Lehninger's *Biochemistry* or *Grant's Atlas of Anatomy*, I grew envious and inspired by the adventures of Roy and his fellow "terns." These were the guys who thumped on the chests of arresting GOMERS; "turfed" the patients they did not want to admit; "buffed" and "polished" the charts of patients they desperately wanted to transfer to the care of others; ignored the LOL in NAD ("Little Old Lady in No Apparent Distress") admitted at the whim of mercenary attending physicians; entertained and then dismissed obscure or "zebra" diagnoses; and spoke truth to the pompous, potbellied, long-coated cadre of men who once controlled the internal medicine professoriate. And then there were those hilarious 13 laws of the *The House of God* (p. 420) that seeped into daily conversations in the hospital cafeteria with appropriate changes depending on what specialty one was pursuing.

By the time I became a pediatrics intern in 1986, my internal medicine colleagues had grown weary of the term GOMER and instead concocted the acronym HONDA ("Hypertensive, Obese, Noncompliant, Diabetic, Asthmatic"); patients once considered to be "going sour" were now charted as CTD ("Circling The Drain"). But the internists were hardly alone in creating disrespectful and unbecoming nicknames for patients they were obliged to care for. Late at night when our attending pediatricians were tightly tucked in their beds at home, I must confess to laughing at the coinage of the term "gomette," in reference to the neonatal intensive care survivors, chronically ill, and neurologically impaired minors who resided in virtually every U.S. children's hospital during this era. Astoundingly, we either never admitted to ourselves that there was something remarkably wrong in our behavior, or we blithely dismissed it as sophomoric sarcasm, a mere Freudian defense mechanism.

Years later, I came to understand our dehumanizing *lingua franca* as a convenient shorthand for the ethical, and often bizarre, quandary we found ourselves actively participating in during this discrete period of medical history. We would gladly "play God" in extending a child's life, often without regard to the quality of life they or their parents would experience as a result of our medical heroism; at the same time, we fervently vowed never to play God in the negative sense of simply not doing anything, let alone the traditionally more unmentionable act of withdrawing life support.

At the medical school where I teach, there is a student society devoted to the history and philosophy of medicine. Every month since 1929, a few withered faculty and a dozen or so medical students have met for discussion and refreshment. In ambitious years we tackle a novel or two about medicine and, frequently, we read *The House of God*. While pouring over the same, and increasingly fragile, copy I bought so long ago and listening to medical students comment with revulsion about Roy Basch's picaresque but horrifying experiences, I recall a youthful, positive energy I once commanded. In its place is a disappointment over those long-ago moments when I was a student or intern and did devolve to using such epithets as GOMER or gomette. This was shameful and, like many physicians, I need to say a slew of *mea culpas*. Fortunately, I have that opportunity with every new medical school class and each time we read *The House of God* together.

The best books, after all, are those we read at several points in our lives. Unlike earlier literary attempts to describe the intense and often traumatic rite of passage called internship and residency, *The House of God* neither sugarcoats nor ignores a host of bad medical behaviors that existed long before the novel was even published. Revisiting and reconsidering the anger and derisive verbal cracks we once expressed at patients who refused to bend to our efforts to "cure" them reminds us that such so-called defense mechanisms have the potential to harm the very people we once took an oath to heal.

[This essay originally appeared as: Markel, H.: The House of God: 30 Years Later. Journal of the American Medical Association. 2008; 299 (2):227–229.]

REFERENCES

1. Shem S. *The House of God*. (New York, NY: Richard Marek, 1978).
2. Lask T. Bookends: Giveaway. *New York Times Book Review*. January 28, 1979: 11.
3. Stacey J. *House of God*—It's grim, but it's life. *Chicago Tribune*. September 28, 1978: A4.
4. Vonnegut M. An intern's ordeal. *Washington Post Book World*. October 12, 1978: D8.
5. Fuller E. A sampler of recent, variable fiction. *Wall Street Journal*. September 11, 1978: 24.
6. Lewis S. *Arrowsmith*. (New York, NY: Harcourt Brace, 1925).
7. Markel H. Prescribing *Arrowsmith*. *New York Times Book Review*. September 23, 2000: 35.
8. Dans PE. *Doctors in the Movies: Boil the Water and Just Say Aah*. (New York, NY: Medi-Ed Press, 2000).
9. Doctor X. *Intern*. (New York, NY: Fawcett Crest Books, 1965).
10. Hasteline F. *Woman Doctor: The Internship of a Modern Woman*. (Boston, MA: Houghton Mifflin Co, 1976).
11. LeBaron C. *Gentle Vengeance: An Account of the First Year at Harvard Medical School*. (New York, NY: Penguin Books, 1982).
12. Hoffman S. *Under the Ether Dome: A Physician's Apprenticeship at the Massachusetts General Hospital*. (New York, NY: Scribner's, 1986).
13. Verghese, A. *My Own Country: A Doctor's Story*. (New York, NY: Vintage Books, 1995).
14. Rothman EL. *White Coat: Becoming a Doctor at Harvard Medical School*. (New York, NY: HarperCollins, 1999).

15. Konner M. *Becoming a Doctor: A Journey of Initiation in Medical School.* (New York, NY: Elisabeth Sifton Books, 1987).
16. Markel H. Patients are discovering "my doctor, the author." *New York Times.* August 22, 2000: D7.
17. Mullan F, Ficklen E, Rubin K. *Narrative Matters: The Power of the Personal Essay in Health Policy.* (Baltimore, MD: Johns Hopkins University Press, 2006).
18. Mullan F. *White Coat, Clenched Fist: The Political Education of an American Physician.* (Ann Arbor: University of Michigan Press, 2006).
19. Shem S. Fiction as resistance. *Ann Intern Med.* 2002; 137: 934–937.

PART II

—◦◦◦—

Medical Texts

CHAPTER 9

ᦀ

The Stethoscope and the Art
of Listening

Laënnec, R.T.H., *De l'Auscultation Médiate ou Traité du Diagnostic des Maladies des Poumons et du Coeur.*

(Paris: Brosson and Chaude, 1819).

Laënnec, R. T. H.; Forbes, John, Sir, (trans). *A Treatise on the Diseases of the Chest and on Meditate Auscultation.*

(New York: Samuel Wood & Sons, 1835).

M any physicians cling to Asclepios's staff as the quintessential insignia of our craft, no doubt debating endlessly whether it should have one or two ascending snakes. Some doctors cherish instead the symbolism of the white coats they don daily, which impart a hygienic air. Still others tightly clutch their beaten black-leather doctor's bags, once indispensable accessories for bygone house calls.

But with all due respect to these and a host of other treasured tokens, I contend that the stethoscope best symbolizes the practice of medicine. Whether absent-mindedly worn around the neck like an amulet or coiled gunslinger-style in the pocket, ever ready for the quick draw, the stethoscope is much more than a tool that allows us to eavesdrop on the workings of the body. Indeed, it embodies the essence of doctoring: using science and technology in concert with the human skill of listening to determine what ails a patient.

Many doctors will gladly bore you with the details of their first stethoscope, and I feel compelled to make a disclosure of sorts. Mine was actually a "gift" from one of the pharmaceutical industry representatives who clogged the corridors of my medical school during the 1980s, routinely tempting medical students with coveted

Literatim: Essays at the Intersections of Medicine and Culture. Howard Markel, Oxford University Press (2020).
© Oxford University Press.
DOI: 10.1093/oso/9780190087647.001.0001

freebies that are now strictly and deservedly prohibited. Just before graduating, however, I did the honorable thing and purchased a top-of-the-line, cardiologist's stethoscope, with all the bells and diaphragms, which I still own. Alas, I do not use it much these days, but I still cling to the clinical conceit that I can distinguish between a diastolic murmur and a split second heart sound.

Long before Hippocrates (ca. 460–380 B.C.E.) taught his disciples the importance of listening to breath sounds, references to its usefulness appeared in the Ebers Papyrus (ca. 1500 B.C.E.) and the Hindu Vedas (ca. 1500–1200 B.C.E.). Nevertheless, it was not until the early 19th century that physicians began to explore in a systematic way the precise clinical meanings of both breath and heart sounds by correlating data gathered during patient examinations with what was ultimately discovered on the autopsy table.[1]

This was the period when Paris reigned as the international center for all things medical. Drawing from a system of hospitals affording limitless access to what was then referred to as "clinical material," the Paris Medical School boasted a talented faculty that represented the vanguard of medicine.

One of the brightest stars in this firmament was the man credited with creating the stethoscope, René Théophile Hyacinthe Laënnec (1781–1826). Long before he assumed the position of chief of service at the teeming Necker Hospital in 1816, Laënnec became adept at a technique called percussion, which involves striking the chest with one's fingertips in search of pathologic processes. Leopold Auenbrugger, the physician-in-chief of Vienna's Holy Trinity Hospital, first described the method in his 1761 treatise *Inventum novum*, but it was largely ignored until 1808, when Laënnec's professor and Napoleon's favorite physician, Jean-Nicolas Corvisart, translated Auenbrugger's text into French and began teaching it to his students and colleagues.

Yet neither percussion nor the time-honored technique of listening to breath sounds by placing an ear against a patient's chest satisfied Laënnec's demand for diagnostic precision. He was especially critical of his inability to hear muffled sounds emerging from the chest of an obese person, and he balked at what he described as the "disgusting" hygiene of his patients, many of whom were unwashed and lice-ridden.

We do know that one day in the fall of 1816, Laënnec was scheduled to examine a young woman who had been "laboring under general symptoms of diseased heart."[2] He was running late, according to the most charming version of the tale, and so took a shortcut through the courtyard of the Louvre, where a group of laughing children playing atop a pile of old timber caught his attention. Laënnec became especially entranced by a pair of youngsters toying with a long, narrow wooden beam. While one child held the beam to his ear, the other tapped nails against the opposite end; all had a jolly good time transmitting sound.[3] Whether or not this instructive event ever occurred, Laënnec would later record that his invention was inspired by the science of acoustics and, in particular, the fact that sound is "conveyed through certain solid bodies, as when we hear the scratch of a pin at one end of a piece of wood, on applying our ear to the other."[2]

Fortunately, all can agree that what eventually transpired was one of the great moments in the history of medicine. On entering his patient's room, Laënnec asked for a quire of paper and rolled it into a cylinder. Placing it against the patient's chest, the doctor was amazed to find how well he could "perceive the action of the heart in a manner much more clear and distinct than [he had] ever been able to do by the immediate application of the ear."[3]

Between 1816 and 1819, Laënnec experimented with a series of hollow tubes that he fashioned out of cedar or ebony, arriving at a model approximately 1 foot in length and 1.5 inches in diameter, with a 1/4-inch central channel. He would name his invention the stethoscope, derived from the Greek *stethos,* meaning chest, and *skopein,* meaning to observe.

A superb flautist who often used music to console himself during his own long and ultimately losing battle against tuberculosis, Laënnec pursued his studies with a vigor that belied the frailty of his frame. He became the first physician to distinguish reliably among bronchiectasis, emphysema, pneumothorax, lung abscess, hemorrhagic pleurisy, and pulmonary infarcts. He also opened the door to our modern understanding of cardiac maladies by describing their associated heart sounds and various murmurs.[4]

Initially, his magnum opus, *De l'Auscultation Médiate,* published in 1819, caused hardly a stir in the medical world—even at the price of 13 francs, with a stethoscope thrown in for an extra 3 francs. By the late 1820s, however, the book had been reprinted and translated into other languages and had managed to triumph over poor publicity and distribution. This success, combined with the gradual acceptance of the stethoscope by practicing physicians, allowed Laënnec to revolutionize clinical medicine.[5]

Although historians of medical technology consider the golden age of the stethoscope to have run from the publication of Laënnec's treatise to the death of Sir William Osler in 1919, the tool continues to be of great clinical value to those who take the time to learn how to use it. But as with all technological advances, its days were numbered from the start. To be sure, the stethoscope has not yet achieved quaintness, like the medieval physician's urine flask, but it is safe to assume that it, too, will someday be relegated to a museum shelf.

Yet even the stethoscope's predicted obsolescence is instructive and cautionary. After all, its creation initiated an irreversible trend in medicine by physically separating diagnosing physicians from their patients, albeit only by the length of a hollow tube. Today, with our advanced capabilities for noninvasive imaging and a host of other techniques that afford stunningly accurate glimpses into the human body, that distance has grown exponentially. Perhaps, then, as a reminder of how separation can alter the enduring task of physicians—listening to our patients—we ought to hang on to our stethoscopes a bit longer than practical usefulness dictates.

[This essay originally appeared as: Markel, H.: The Stethoscope and the Art of Listening. New England Journal of Medicine 2006; 354:551–553].

REFERENCES

1. Bishop, P.J. Evolution of the stethoscope. *Journal of the Royal Society of Medicine (London).* 1980; 73: 448–456
2. Laënnec, R.T.H. *A Treatise on Diseases of the Chest.* J. Forbes, trans. (London: Underwood, 1821), pp. 284–285.
3. Sigerist, H.E. *The Great Doctors: A Biographical History of Medicine.* (New York: W.W. Norton, 1933), pp. 283–290.
4. Nuland, S.B. *Doctors: The Biography of Medicine.* (New York: Vintage Books/Random House, 1995), pp. 200–237.
5. Duffin, J. *To See With a Better Eye: A Life of R.T.H. Laënnec.* (Princeton, N.J.: Princeton University Press, 1998).

CHAPTER 10

∿

"Experiments and Observations"

How William Beaumont and Alexis St. Martin
Seized the Moment of Scientific Progress

Beaumont W. *Experiments and Observations of the Gastric Juice and the Physiology of Digestion.*
(Plattsburgh, NY: F.P Allen, 1833).

N estled along the clear blue straits between the great lakes called Michigan and Huron is an oblong and verdant island. Centuries ago, the Chippewa and Ottawa tribes named it Michilimackinac, or "the great turtle." Referred to today as Mackinac but pronounced "Mackinaw," this tiny land mass attracts tourists by the millions seeking its calming waters, grand hotels, attractive vistas, bicycle paths, and tons of a sticky, sweet confection made of butter, milk, sugar, cocoa, and a touch of vanilla, called Mackinac fudge.

In 1670, the French Jesuit missionary Father Jacques Marquette and his intrepid interpreter Louis Joliet fled St. Ignace, Michigan, to settle on the "Great Turtle" in the name of their homeland.[1] Less than a century later, in 1759, the British took control of the island from the French and, in 1783, after signing the Treaty of Paris, Great Britain relinquished it to the fledgling United States, which had to defend and regain it during the War of 1812. The French pursued fur trapping there with vigor and cunning. But it was John Jacob Astor, the first U.S. multimillionaire, who put Mackinac Island on the map in 1817, when he chose the island as the main trading post of his fabled American Fur Company, a pelt empire that spanned from the Great Lakes to the Mississippi River.[2]

Literatim: Essays at the Intersections of Medicine and Culture. Howard Markel, Oxford University Press (2020).
© Oxford University Press.
DOI: 10.1093/oso/9780190087647.001.0001

Every June, the American Fur Company hosted a convention on Mackinac for thousands of trappers eager to sell or barter the bounty they had hunted the previous winter. The rest of the year, the island's population hovered at a mere 500. Situated on the southeast cliff a few hundred feet above the shoreline was a limestone fortress built by the British in 1761 and subsequently occupied by the U.S. Army to protect the island's commerce and trade.[3]

In 1820, one of the military officers stationed there was a young physician named William Beaumont. In 1810, he began a two-year apprenticeship to a well-established Vermont physician named Benjamin Chandler and in 1812 passed that state's qualification examination. The same year, Beaumont enlisted with the U.S. Army in search of adventure and clinical experience and served as a surgeon's mate in the War of 1812. After the end of that conflict in 1815, he resigned his post to set up a private practice in Plattsburgh, New York. Five years later, he turned his practice over to a cousin and re-enlisted in the Army, which assigned him to Fort Michilimackinac.[4]

At this distant frontier outpost, Beaumont began the work that culminated in a remarkable, if not outright revolutionary, book—*Experiments and Observations on the Gastric Juice and the Physiology of Digestion*.[5] But he hardly accomplished this gargantuan task alone. Indeed, Beaumont had the help and the body of a French Canadian fur trapper named Alexis St. Martin.

The story of Beaumont and St. Martin has been recounted so often it has acquired the finely burnished patina of hagiography. Yet even when stripped of its most sensational layers, their collaboration remains an inspiring and cautionary tale about the boundaries between physician and patient and medical investigator and human participant.

On the morning of June 6, 1822, as the annual pelt swapping jamboree was under way, a 20-year-old St. Martin waited in line at the American Fur Company's store to make some trades. What began as a rudimentary exercise in capitalism erupted into a medical emergency when a shotgun accidentally discharged. As one eyewitness described, "the muzzle was not over three feet from [St. Martin]—I think not more than two. The wadding entered, as well as pieces of his clothing; his shirt took fire; he fell, as we supposed, dead."[6]

The gun's contents entered just under St. Martin's left breast, fractured several ribs, lacerated his diaphragm, and left a gaping hole through which portions of the lung and stomach protruded. Beaumont quickly arrived and administered first aid amid the stunning sights and smells of St. Martin's breakfast leaking from the wound. Thanks to Beaumont's quick-witted and precise ministrations, St. Martin did survive the event, albeit with a fistula leading directly into his stomach that remained patent until his last day of life. It was a medical intervention that would soon change medicine.[7]

For much of the next few years, Beaumont provided daily care and attention to his fascinating patient. Although the wound partially healed, St. Martin remained weak and miserable and refused any attempts by Beaumont to somehow suture the hole shut. As a result of his critical injuries and lengthy rehabilitation, St. Martin was also penniless.

Medical historians and ethicists have long argued over Beaumont's motives in caring for St. Martin. Alas, the historical record obscures more than clarifies the physician's thinking and intent, as does the striking passage of time, custom, and class, not to mention vast changes in the social understandings of the rights of patients and the obligations of physicians. Assessing the motives and ethical impulses of those long dead is a difficult task for even the most adept historians. Clearly, Beaumont and St. Martin's was a complex relationship consisting of more than sympathy and science. It also included ambition and careerism on Beaumont's part; dependence and need from the ailing St. Martin; and a huge reserve of negative and positive human actions, emotions, and feelings that occupied both men in the years to come.

On May 30, 1823, for example, Beaumont first recorded his inkling that major scientific observations in this case were possible after introducing a cathartic via a glass funnel into St. Martin's fistula and stomach. "I gave a cathartic, administered, it is presumed, as never medicine was administered to man since the creation of the world." The next day, however, Beaumont described taking a destitute and sickly St. Martin into his own home "from mere motives of charity, and a disposition to save his life or at least to make him more comfortable."[8]

Others, however, have pointed out that a local woman named Mary LaFleur first boarded St. Martin through the spring of 1823, and it was not until after Beaumont discovered the ease with which food and medications could be inserted into St. Martin's stomach for further study that he eagerly welcomed the trapper into his home.[7]

On August 1, 1825, St. Martin finally felt well enough to allow Beaumont to formally begin the studies that served as the basis of his soon-to-be famous book. As Beaumont gleefully recorded, at "12 o'clock [noon], I introduced through the perforation, into the stomach, the following articles of diet, suspended by a silk string, and fastened at proper distances, so as to pass in without pain-viz. A piece of high seasoned *a la mode beef*; a piece of *raw, salted, fat pork*, a piece of *raw, salted, lean beef*; a piece of *boiled, salted beef*; a piece of *stale bread*; and a bunch of *raw, sliced cabbage* [the italics are Beaumont's]."[5(p125)] During this and subsequent experiments, Beaumont also withdrew copious amounts of gastric fluids and chyme for analysis and elaboration.

Beaumont employed St. Martin as an aide and servant in his subsequent military medical posts and continued to care for him at his own expense. By the summer of 1825, however, St. Martin grew tired of being a human guinea pig and abruptly fled to Canada. It was not until 1829 that physician and patient were reunited after St. Martin made a heroic canoe trip extending from northern Canada to Fort Crawford in Prairie du Chien, Wisconsin, where Beaumont was stationed. A second series of experiments briefly transpired until a homesick and tired St. Martin returned to Canada. Many pleas and years later, the two met again in Plattsburgh and Washington between 1832 and 1833 for a final round of studies.

When Beaumont published his treatise in 1833, there was great debate among the medical community about the precise mechanisms of digestion. Similarly, the lay public on both sides of the Atlantic were obsessed with every episode of dyspepsia, flatulence, and heartburn they experienced, resulting in a huge demand for panaceas from their physicians. Many medical experts advocated their own theory of how humans digested their meals, but until Beaumont encountered the ailing St. Martin, no one had firsthand access to a living, secreting stomach.[9]

Although sales were slow initially, *Experiments and Observations* eventually generated great excitement in Europe. By 1850, Beaumont enjoyed the status of being the first American-born medical scientist to achieve international renown. No less an authority than Claude Bernard, the Parisian physiologist whose work led to the concept of homeostasis, credited Beaumont with initiating "a new era in the study of this important organ and those associated with it." Across Europe and beyond, physiologists looked for individuals with similar fistulas or created them, experimentally, in animals as they labored to elucidate the digestive process. Ironically, like so many prophets in their own land, in the United States Beaumont's theories were initially met with indifference by a medical profession less enthralled with scientific method than their peers in Britain, France, and Germany. By the mid-19th century, however, even his countrymen reconsidered and initiated a cult of hero worship that remains intact to the present day.[4,7,10–12]

After the publication of *Experiments and Observations*, Beaumont hoped to conduct another round of experiments, but St. Martin refused all such requests. The constant poking and insertion of food, drinks, medications, tubes, and thermometers into his fistula was hardly enjoyable, let alone comfortable. Moreover, he missed his family and life in Canada and was experiencing the ravages of alcoholism.

St. Martin's refusal to cooperate must have frustrated Beaumont; undoubtedly, Beaumont's relentless coercion and pleading irritated St. Martin. At various points in their collaboration, St. Martin demanded a formal contract. In return for allowing experiments to be conducted exclusively by Beaumont, St. Martin received financial compensation, medical care, and a modicum of respect and attention to his wishes and comfort.[7,13] Yet even after refusing additional experiments with Beaumont in 1833, St. Martin steadfastly rebuffed the requests of other scientists eager to employ him in search of some additional data. In 1856, three years after Beaumont's death, the financially strapped St. Martin finally did consent to participate in a short-lived traveling exhibition show with a quack physician named G. T. Bunting.[14]

After St. Martin died on June 20, 1880, his family kept the body from being buried or embalmed for four days. The corpse decomposed so badly that the odiferous coffin could not even be brought into the church. He was interred on June 24, in a grave 8 feet deep and covered with 2 feet of stones and another 6 feet of dirt to prevent medically inspired grave robbers from exhuming his body for further inquiry.[3]

Apparently, St. Martin meant what he said when he told his faithful and persistent healer William Beaumont that enough was enough. Unlike the soil placed over his grave, however, neither refusal nor death could cover the stunning contributions he had already made to the medical literature and, more broadly, medical history. Both St. Martin's wound and his willingness to work with Beaumont literally opened the path for a field of study that continues to benefit humankind to the present day.

[This essay originally appeared as: Markel, H.: Experiments and Observations: How William Beaumont and Alexis St. Martin Seized the Moment of Scientific Progress. Journal of the American Medical Association. 2009; 302 (7):804–806].

REFERENCES

1. Dunbar W.F. May GS. *Michigan: A History of the Wolverine State.* 3rd ed. (Grand Rapids, MI: William B. Eerdmans Publishing Co, 1995).
2. Madsen A. *John Jacob Astor: America's First Multimillionaire.* (New York, NY: John Wiley, 2001).
3. Leblond S. The life and times of Alexis St. Martin. *Can Med Assoc J.* 1963; 88: 1205–1211.
4. Horsman R. *Frontier Doctor: William Beaumont, America's First Great Medical Scientist.* (Columbia, MO: University of Missouri Press, 1996).
5. Beaumont W. *Experiments and Observations of the Gastric Juice and the Physiology of Digestion.* (Plattsburgh, NY: F.P Allen, 1833).
6. Osler W. William Beaumont: a pioneer American physiologist. *J Am Med Assoc.* 1902; 39: 1223–1231.
7. Numbers R.L. William Beaumont and the ethics of human experimentation. *J Hist Biol.* 1979; 12(1): 113–135.
8. Beaumont W. *Sundry Cases of Practice, 1822–1825; and Notebook.* (Located at: William Beaumont Collection, School of Medicine Library, Washington University, St Louis, MO).
9. Bylebyl J.J. William Beaumont, Robley Dunglison, and the "Philadelphia Physiologists." *J Hist Med Allied Sci.* 1970; 25(1): 3–21.
10. Myer J.S. *Life and Letters of William Beaumont.* (St Louis, MO: C.V. Mosby & Co, 1912), p. 289.
11. Numbers R.L. Orr WJ Jr. William Beaumont's reception at home and abroad. *Isis.* 1981; 72(264): 590–612.
12. Rosen G. *The Reception of William Beaumont's Discovery in Europe.* (New York, NY: Schuman's, 1942).
13. Rutkow I. Beaumont and St. Martin: a blast from the past. *Arch Surg.* 1998; 133(11): 125.
14. Bensley E.H. Alexis St. Martin and Dr. Bunting. *Bull Hist Med.* 1970; 44(2): 101–108.

CHAPTER 11

∽

On John Snow

John Snow. *On the Mode of Communication of Cholera.*
(London: John Churchill, 1849, first edition; 1855, second edition).

March 15, 2013 marked the 200th birthday of John Snow, the singular genius who created the modern science of epidemiology. Without fear of historical hyperbole, the occasion merited a global pause of reflection and honor, even if very few of us noticed.

Born in York, England, John Snow chose a life in medicine at a relatively young age. At 16, he began an apprenticeship under William Hardcastle, a surgeon who practiced in Newcastle-upon-Tyne. A few years later, in 1831, Snow first encountered cholera, which entered Newcastle via the seaport of Sunderland and decimated his town.

By 1836, Snow moved to London, where he furthered his medical studies at Westminster Hospital and earned his membership in the Royal College of Surgeons and as a licentiate of the Society of Apothecaries. In 1843, he took his bachelor's degree in medicine and, the following year, received his doctorate in medicine, both at the University of London. He "hung his shingle" or, as the British like to say, "nailed up his colours" in Soho, a raucous neighborhood where he cared for working-class patients for the rest of his career.[1]

After its demonstration at the Massachusetts General Hospital in 1846, ether anesthesia became the surgical rage on both sides of the Atlantic. In 1847, Snow wrote a superb book on its use, *On Ether*, before focusing his attention on another anesthetic called chloroform. Since at least the days of the Old Testament, medical doctrine assumed that childbirth was destined to be a painful and a laborious event. Yet many physicians like Snow insisted this need not be the case. Snow's opinion

Literatim: Essays at the Intersections of Medicine and Culture. Howard Markel, Oxford University Press (2020).
© Oxford University Press.
DOI: 10.1093/oso/9780190087647.001.0001

became common practice on April 7, 1853, when he was chosen to administer chloroform to Queen Victoria as she delivered Prince Leopold.

It is difficult, if not impossible, for most modern readers to fathom how badly London smelled in the mid 19th century. Every day was a constant negotiation against the odiferous waste left behind by more than 300,000 horses, hundreds of thousands of pigs, sheep, cows, and other livestock waiting to become somebody's meal, and 2.4 million Londoners. With the paucity of modern sewage systems, water closets in wealthier homes expelling streams of stool and urine into the streets and the Thames River, and countless outhouses, privies, and cesspools, the city positively stunk.[2]

When confronted with cholera epidemics in the years before medical scientists elucidated the role microbes play in infectious diseases, many of Britain's finest medical minds took a page from Hippocrates and associated cholera with the foul-smelling gases produced by mounting piles of rotting garbage and raw sewage. *Miasma* (from the Greek, for *pollution*) was thought to contaminate the atmosphere. When inhaled, this noxious air upset the balance of an individual's body humors and led to an abundance of *choler*, or yellow bile, which the body did its best to expel, even if it meant overwhelming dehydration and death.

Snow's genius was his uncanny ability to connect the dots, so to speak, of disease causation. A keen observer of the diffusion of gases, gained from his work on ether and chloroform, Snow began to doubt the miasma theory during the 1848 cholera epidemic that ruthlessly carted off thousands of Londoners to the graveyard. If foul-smelling gases caused cholera, he queried in his landmark 1849 book, *On the Mode of Communication of Cholera*, why were those closest to the emanations, such as garbage removal workers and night-soil men (those who emptied privies), not disproportionately affected? Conversely, given that the concentration of a gas tended to dissipate and decline as it traveled over a distance, how could one miasmic source infect people living far from it, let alone an entire city? The accepted dogma that cholera was inhaled through the air via the respiratory tract—even though the disease clearly struck the gastrointestinal tract with an ugly vengeance—simply made no sense to the inquiring Dr. Snow.[3]

Although there were many miasmatists and anticontagionists who scoffed at Snow's thesis, the good doctor seized his opportunity during London's 1854 cholera epidemic. He began by meticulously surveying every case and their contacts, even to the point of verifying their water source by checking each home's water bills. Snow discovered that Londoners who drew water from the Southwark and Vauxhall Water Company, which came from the fecal-contaminated Thames River, were infected nine times more than those living in areas supplied by the Lambeth Company, whose water originated from an upstream, and less contaminated, source.[4]

Snow's greatest scientific moment, however, resulted from an even more detailed study of the cholera's spread in Soho. After carefully charting some 500 cases in his district, Dr. Snow noted that most of the cholera victims had been consuming water from a well located in Broad Street. Unfortunately for those frequenting the hand pump–operated well, it was contaminated with sewage from a nearby house where cholera had previously visited. Snow convinced the parish councilors to remove the well's pump handle, thus making it inoperable. Soon after disabling the pump, the cholera rate plummeted, allowing Snow a well-deserved *quod erat demonstrandum*. The doctor concluded that a specific water-borne "poison" capable of self-reproduction was in the excreta of cholera patients who, in turn, tainted the water supply. His solution: careful washing of the hands, decontaminating soiled linens, and boiling all drinking water.[5]

John Snow died of a cerebral hemorrhage on June 16, 1858. He was 45. Twenty-five years later, in 1883, Robert Koch, who along with Louis Pasteur is credited with demonstrating the germ theory of disease, proved Snow correct. While battling a cholera epidemic in Egypt, Koch identified *Vibrio cholerae*, teeming in fecal-contaminated water supplies, as the microbial cause of cholera. Yet even before Koch's great discovery, Snow was on an upward trajectory toward permanent, albeit posthumous, acclaim in the history books.[6]

In the summer of 2012, I had the pleasure of taking my then-12-year-old daughter, Bess, on a trip to London. A few hours before a much-anticipated high tea at the Ritz Hotel, Bess asked, "Dad, if you could take me to the most important historical sight in London, where would we go?"

With a spring to my middle-aged step, I escorted her across Piccadilly, past the Royal Academy of Art, and through Soho to Broadwick Street, as Broad Street is presently known. In front of a facsimile of the Broad Street pump, I told Bess how Snow helped usher in the modern world by insisting that we clean up after our own excrement. Yet as great as that contribution was, I added, this basic health requirement has still not been met for, at least, 783 million people living in the developing nations of Africa, Asia, and South America who do not have daily access to clean drinking water; 2.6 billion people do not have access to adequate sanitation. Every year, more than 1.5 million people, mostly children younger than 5 years, die because of water-borne diarrhea, including cholera, which modern medicine has known how to prevent, or at least attenuate, since the mid 19th century.[7]

Bess's eyes opened widely as she exclaimed an impressed "Wow!"

Wow, indeed.

Thank you, Dr. Snow. Two centuries after your birth, you still have the power to change the world. If only everyone had the access and wherewithal to follow your life-saving prescriptions.

[*This essay originally appeared as Markel, H.: Happy 200th Birthday Dr. Snow. Journal of the American Medical Association. 2013; 309 (10): 995–996*].

REFERENCES

1. Thomas K.B. John Snow. In: *Dictionary of Scientific Biography*. Vol 12. (New York, NY: Charles Scribner's Sons, 1973), pp. 502–503.

2. Snow J. *Snow on Cholera: Being a Reprint of Two Papers by John Snow With a Biographical Memoir.* (New York, NY: Hafner, 1965).

3. Wohl A.S. *Endangered Lives: Public Health in Victorian England.* (London, England: JM Dent & Sons, 1983).

4. Markel H. *When Germs Travel: Six Major Epidemics That Invaded America Since 1900 and the Fears They Unleashed.* (New York, NY: Pantheon Books, 2004).

5. Johnson S. *The Ghost Map: The Story of London's Most Terrifying Epidemic and How It Changed Cities, Science and the Modern World.* (New York, NY: Riverhead Books, 2006).

6. Rosenberg C.E. *The Cholera Years: The United States in 1832, 1849, and 1866.* (Chicago, IL: University of Chicago Press, 1962).

7. World Health Organization. *U.N.-Water Global Analysis and Assessment of Sanitation and Drinking-Water (GLAAS)2012Report: The Challenge of Extending and Sustaining Services.* (Geneva, Switzerland: World Health Organization, 2012).

CHAPTER 12

❧

Dr. Osler's Relapsing Fever

Pratt J.H. *A Year With Osler, 1896–1897:*

Notes Taken at his Clinics in the Johns Hopkins Hospital.
(Baltimore, MD: Johns Hopkins University Press, 1949).

Minutes before noon on October 7, 1896, the medical students hurriedly took their seats in a spanking-new, cherrywood-paneled amphitheater charged with the energy of youthful excitement and professional ambition.[1] The topic to be discussed was fever, a vital sign that had vexed and fascinated physicians since the dawn of recorded medical history.

These physicians-to-be represented America's, indeed the world's, best and brightest hopes for a healthy future. Their medical school, Johns Hopkins (named for the dyspeptic, cranky, but decidedly wealthy Quaker merchant who endowed it), had only opened its doors three years earlier in provincial Baltimore, Maryland. But it had immediately assumed the vanguard of *fin de siècle* Western medicine as the profession leaped from blind allegiance to centuries-old, not infrequently toxic, medications and heroic surgical measures to the laboratory-based enterprise that characterizes modern medical practice.[2]

The room instantly hushed as the professor entered the room. About to speak was none other than William Osler—the perfect escort for nascent physicians hoping to learn every aspect of fever, from its history and theory to its clinical permutations and precise connections to specific maladies.

There was a lot to discuss. Baltimore led the nation in typhoid fever deaths and was annually visited by a plethora of other contagious crises. Consequently, a standard feature of Osler's classroom was an elaborate series of interlocking blackboards that meticulously summarized every case of typhoid fever, and its

Literatim: Essays at the Intersections of Medicine and Culture. Howard Markel, Oxford University Press (2020).
© Oxford University Press.
DOI: 10.1093/oso/9780190087647.001.0001

myriad complications, in patients admitted to the Johns Hopkins Hospital that year. As an academic bonus, Professor Osler was internationally regarded as a vociferous advocate for public health reforms essential to the containment of contagion.

Surely, as the students opened their notebooks and unscrewed their fountain pens, some must have been mentally reviewing "the Chief's" recent address on fever to the American Medical Association, which on publication in the *Journal of the American Medical Association* in the fall of 1896, soon became one of the most widely quoted papers of its time. It was during this speech to a multitude of physicians convening in Atlanta, Georgia, that Osler famously declared, "Humanity has but three great enemies: fever, famine, and war; of these by far the greatest, by far the most terrible, is fever."[3]

Osler's was an era, of course, when clinicians spent significant time and energy diagnosing and battling infectious diseases. In the days before the microbiological etiology of a particular infectious entity was identifiable, the exact nature of a patient's fever curve often served as a key to accurate diagnosis. No wonder, then, of all the topics with which to begin the academic year, Osler chose fever.

Medical textbooks, lectures, and clinical pedagogy from well before Osler's era until after the close of World War II emphasized knowing the difference between a tertiary and quotidian fever, relapsing from intermittent, and the importance of charting the fever's ascent, highest point—the *fastigum* (Latin, for ridge)—and decline. Even in the years immediately after the advent of antibiotics, the spiky fever curve remained a standard feature of the patient's chart, often prominently displayed at the foot of the bed and popularized in movies, books, and magazine cartoons.[4]

To be sure, physicians have recognized the importance of fever since antiquity. But before the rise and fall of body temperature could be used as a window into pathological processes, a reliable means to measure it was needed. Many historians credit Galileo Galilei with inventing a crude water thermometer around 1593–1595. Duke Ferdinand II of Tuscany experimented with an alcohol-based thermometer during the 1640s. Sir Isaac Newton developed a linseed oil thermometer around 1700; and Daniel Gabriel Fahrenheit unveiled his mercury-based thermometer in 1714. These are but a few of the prominent scientific minds who worked on this critical device, not to mention several distinguished physicians of these eras, including Santorio, Boerhaave, de Haen, Willis, and Allbutt, who each applied their own variations of the thermometer in their clinics.[5]

But the undisputed patriarch of the scientific study of fever was Carl Wunderlich, the venerable professor of medicine in Leipzig, Germany. In 1868, he published his magisterial book, *Das Verhalten der Eigenwarme in Krankheiten (On the Course of Temperature in Diseases)*.[6] Having collected millions of temperature readings in approximately 25,000 patients with different diseases, Wunderlich had the quantitative evidence he needed to lay one of the medical world's great conundrums to rest—was fever, as many older physicians insisted, a disease in and of itself, or was fever simply a sign of disease?[6] After Wunderlich demonstrated that fever varied in characteristic patterns for different diseases, it was only a short time before physicians routinely measured their patients' temperatures.

Approximately three hours before the medical students eagerly assembled for their lecture, a horse-drawn cab carrying Osler made its way past the gates and up the cobblestone circular driveway of the Johns Hopkins Hospital. The great physician, impeccably dressed in a charcoal gray morning coat, accessorized by a silk cravat, a freshly cut flower in his lapel, and an imperious gold chain hanging from his expansive waistcoat, exited the coach and bounded up the steps of the hospital's main entrance.[7]

Handing his gloves, top hat, and umbrella to a waiting nurse, Osler warmly greeted the weary resident physician on duty who was eager to report about the patients he had admitted during the night. From there, Osler strolled around an enormous marble rendering of *Christus Consolator* (the Divine Healer) and up the enormous quartersawn oak staircase centered in a domed octagonal atrium that, quite possibly, constitutes the grandest hospital lobby in the history of medicine.[8]

After poking his head into the hospital's library and offering salutations to an admiring gaggle of employees, Osler descended the stairs and made his way to the wards to visit his patients and enlighten the training physicians and student clerks (always pronounced with Anglophilic devotion as "clarks") assigned to their care.

Most days, Osler finished clinical rounds at approximately 1 p.m. before settling down to a cold luncheon. The meal was followed by 20 minutes of rest and then several more hours of remunerative consultations with private patients and reflective time writing the lengthy list of medical articles and best-selling textbooks that comprised his bulging *curriculum vitae*. But on this Wednesday, as the clock struck noon, Osler gracefully excused himself from the task at hand and negotiated a path into the amphitheater to meet with his medical students of the second class to enter Johns Hopkins.[9]

One of them, Joseph H. Pratt, dutifully recorded Osler's presentation of four patients with different infectious diseases and hence markedly different fever patterns.[10] From other accounts of Osler's teaching, it is clear that the professor "hammered incessantly into his students" every conceivable detail about the three great plagues of the day: typhoid, tuberculosis, and pneumonia (the latter, incidentally, provided the clinical coda of Osler's life in 1919).[11] Reading Osler's copious oeuvre on fever, it is entirely reasonable to assume he "hammered" into his students' heads that the control of fever and the prevention of contagious diseases were their generation's holy grails to seek.

In the decades that followed, these lofty goals seemed eminently obtainable. Therapeutics were developed to eradicate infection and a cornucopia of antipyretics emerged to subvert the inflammatory processes underlying fever, attenuating its rise. Vaccines were created to wholly prevent many of the maladies that routinely caused deaths or harm to millions annually. In addition to building hospitals, clinics, and research laboratories, U.S. and European communities constructed modern sewage and water systems. Thanks to these and a host of other sanitary measures, many old-time scourges were, perhaps prematurely, assigned the status of relics.[12,13]

Ironically, these successes—the very ones Osler exhorted his students to pursue—led to a mentality that can only be described as a profound amnesia of contagious scourges past. Thus, by the late 20th century, many physicians and patients blithely assumed that infectious diseases, and the fevers that often accompanied them, had been completely conquered.

Today, few physicians would be so bold to articulate this assumption.[14] In a world where 1,500 individuals die every hour of an infectious disease, where many impoverished nations cannot provide their citizens clean water and food on a daily basis, and, more troubling, where newly emerging and reemerging infectious diseases are again stalking the planet, Osler's advice to pay close attention to all aspects of fever—from the bedside to its global ramifications and from its causes to its effects—is as vital today as it was a century ago.

[This essay originally appeared as: Markel, H.: Dr. Osler's Relapsing Fever. Journal of the American Medical Association 2006; 295:2886–2887].

REFERENCES

1. Billings J.S. Description of the Johns Hopkins Hospital. (Baltimore, MD: Johns Hopkins University Press, 1890).
2. Chesney A.M. The Johns Hopkins Hospital and the Johns Hopkins University School of Medicine: A Chronicle: Volume I, Early Years, 1867–1892. (Baltimore, MD: Johns Hopkins University Press, 1943).
3. Osler W. The study of the fevers in the south. JAMA. 1896; 26: 999–1004.
4. Sigerist H. Carl August Wunderlich, 1815–1877. In: The Great Doctors. (New York, NY: Dover Publications, 1971), pp. 329–334.
5. Estes J.W. Quantitative observations on fever and its treatment before the advent of short clinical thermometers. Med Hist. 1991; 35: 189–216.
6. Wunderlich C.A. Das Verhalten der Eigenwarme in Krankheiten. (Leipzig, Germany: O. Wigand, 1870).
7. Bliss M. William Osler: A Life in Medicine. (New York, NY: Oxford University Press, 1999), pp. 208–258.
8. Harvey A.M., et alia. A Model of its Kind: A Centennial History of Medicine at Johns Hopkins. (Baltimore, MD: Johns Hopkins University Press, 1989).
9. Bulletin No. IX of the International Association of Medical Museums and Journal of Technical Methods: Sir William Osler Memorial Number: Appreciations and Reminiscences. (Montreal, Canada: Murray Printing Co., 1926), pp. 250–321.
10. Pratt J.H. A Year With Osler, 1896–1897: Notes Taken at his Clinics in the Johns Hopkins Hospital. (Baltimore, MD: Johns Hopkins University Press; 1949), pp. v–xx, 4–7, 199–201
11. Cushing H. The Life of Sir William Osler. Vol 1. (Oxford, UK: Oxford University Press; 1925), pp. 378–381, 431–433.
12. Winslow C.E.-A. The Conquest of Epidemic Disease: A Chapter in the History of Ideas. (Princeton, NJ: Princeton University Press, 1943).
13. Zinsser H. Rats, Lice and History. (Boston, MA: Little Brown & Co Inc, 1935).
14. Markel H. When Germs Travel: Six Major Epidemics That Have Invaded America Since 1900 and the Fears They Have Unleashed. (New York, NY: Pantheon Books, 2004).

CHAPTER 13

∽

The Extraordinary Dr. Biggs

Biggs H. Public Health is Purchasable. Monthly Bulletin of the Department of Health of the City of New York. October 11, 1911:225–226.

Although not quite a household name, during the late 19th and early 20th centuries Hermann M. Biggs (1859–1923) commanded enormous power and influence. Throughout his career at the helm of the Health Department of the City of New York and later as Commissioner of the New York State Department of Health, Biggs was world-renowned for developing innovative and effective policies that both protected the public's health and respected the needs of the ill.

While still a young man in the early 1880s, Biggs' intellectual life was indelibly shaped by the exciting discoveries being made about bacteria and the then-novel germ theory of disease.[1] A signal event that occurred during Biggs' medical student days at New York City's Bellevue Hospital Medical College superbly illustrates the cultural and intellectual wedge then being driven between antiquated medical practices and the scientific revolution in healing that continues to the present.

One of Biggs' favorite medical school professors at Bellevue was William Henry Welch, a brilliant young pathologist and bacteriologist just beginning his meteoric rise to becoming one of the founders of the Johns Hopkins Hospital and Medical School and the leading medical statesman of his generation. One spring afternoon in 1882, Welch lectured to his pathology class, of which Biggs was a promising member, about Robert Koch's monumental discovery of the tubercle bacillus as the cause of the white plague of tuberculosis. So inspired was Biggs by this pedagogic moment that he ran to Bellevue's senior professor of medicine, the redoubtable and bespectacled Alfred L. Loomis, to tell him about the remarkable information.

A few days later, the aging Loomis, author of scores of textbooks that made him famous among medical students and practitioners alike, ascended the lecture

Literatim: Essays at the Intersections of Medicine and Culture. Howard Markel, Oxford University Press (2020).
© Oxford University Press.
DOI: 10.1093/oso/9780190087647.001.0001

platform of the Bellevue Hospital amphitheater, looked merrily about the vast room, and boldly declared: "People say there are bacteria in the air, but I cannot see them." Many of the medical students laughed uproariously at Loomis' witty denunciation, as they are wont to do whenever their professor makes the slightest attempt at humor. Yet when Biggs later told Welch about the episode, the pathologist shook his head with an equal mixture of sadness and whimsy. "That's too bad," Welch quipped, "Loomis is such a nice man"; in other words, time had passed Loomis by, and his old notions about disease causation and prevention had been, or were about to be, superseded by new ones. And by refusing to accept the evidence supporting the germ theory, Loomis had virtually guaranteed his transition into a medical relic. It was a cautionary tale of change over time that impressed Biggs to the end of his life.[2]

Biggs was one of many young physicians in the late 19th century who embraced the effects that the new science of bacteriology would have on public health and preventive medicine. Unlike many of his peers, however, Biggs put those concepts into action. For example, during the late 1880s Biggs consulted with the New York Quarantine Station on the application of cholera culture methods among incoming immigrants. He continued to act as a consultant to the New York Quarantine Station, the largest and busiest facility of its kind in the United States, throughout his career. In September 1892, when there was fear of a major cholera pandemic reaching American shores, Biggs was asked to organize and direct the Department of Pathology and Bacteriology of the New York City Health Department. Medical historians have long argued over which U.S. city was the first to develop a bacteriological laboratory (Lawrence, Massachusetts, Ann Arbor, Michigan, and Providence, Rhode Island, all had such laboratories established in the late 1880s); nevertheless, New York City's municipal bacteriology laboratory was the first of its kind to not only test the purity of food and water but also to apply bacteriological methods to the diagnosis of disease.[3–5]

For 22 years, Biggs maintained leadership roles with the New York City Health Department, one of the most advanced and innovative municipal health departments in the history of public health. The match was a perfect fit. In 1894, for example, with the assistance of William H. Park, he introduced the use of diphtheria antitoxin to the United States. Under Biggs, the Health Department Bacteriology Laboratory was extraordinarily entrepreneurial, raising a stable of horses that were routinely injected with diphtheria toxin, and licensing and selling the antitoxin product to health departments, physicians, and hospitals across the United States.[6,7]

Biggs also was active in the prevention and amelioration of tuberculosis. During the early part of the 20th century, tuberculosis was among the major killers of Americans between the ages of 20 and 40 years. Biggs and his associates at the city health department, and later on a statewide level, worked arduously to set up prevention programs based on analysis of the sputum of patients suspected of having tuberculosis, notification and reporting processes, care facilities—including nursing home care—for those stricken with tuberculosis, and the mandatory isolation of recalcitrant patients.[8]

One of Biggs' greatest skills was his political adeptness in steering so many public health reforms within a milieu of partisan infighting, burgeoning social problems among the impoverished and immigrant populations, and "good old-fashioned" urban graft and patronage. For Biggs, the operative word of every public health venture was "public." He understood that without generating a strong consensus among the multitudes constituting a community, little could be accomplished in any attempt to rein in disease.

Decades after their time together at Bellevue, William H. Welch was assigned the emotionally draining task of delivering the eulogy for his former pupil in 1923. Speaking with admiration and pride, Welch observed that Biggs was "tenacious of principles in which he believed, patiently perseverant and fearless, without aggressiveness, constructive and clear in vision, with a sure sense of the immediately attainable."[9]

Twelve years earlier, at the occasion of the 1911 opening of a new, modern tuberculosis treatment facility, Biggs declared his credo even better in what may well be the most important speech in the history of American public health:

> Disease is largely a removable evil. It continues to afflict humanity, not only because of incomplete knowledge of its causes and lack of adequate individual and public hygiene, but also because it is extensively fostered by harsh economic conditions and by wretched housing in congested communities. . . . No duty of society, acting through its governmental agencies, is paramount to this obligation to attack the removable causes of disease. . . . Public health is purchasable.[10]

Our current era, unfortunately, is characterized by huge financial inequities between the richest and poorest citizens, the drastic dismantling of governmental agencies devoted to the public good, and far too great a reliance on the free market to perform the jobs all rely on to keep society healthy and secure. When reflecting on the life of Hermann M. Biggs, then, we are all well advised to recall the visionary concepts he declared a century ago.

[This essay originally appeared as: Markel, H. The Extraordinary Dr. Biggs. Journal of the American Medical Association. 2011; 305 (23):2473–2474].

REFERENCES

1. Markel H. When Germs Travel: Six Major Epidemics That Have Invaded America and the Fears They Have Unleashed. (New York, NY: Pantheon, 2004), pp. 205–214.
2. Flexner S., Flexner J.T. William Henry Welch and the Heroic Age of American Medicine. (New York, NY: Viking Press, 1941), p. 119.
3. Markel H. Quarantine! East European Jewish Immigrants and the New York City Epidemics of 1892. (Baltimore, MD: Johns Hopkins University Press, 1997), pp. 119, 125–126.

4. Biggs H.M. The diagnostic value of the cholera spirillum, as illustrated by the investigation of a case at the New York quarantine station. *N Y Med J*. 1887; 46: 548–549.

5. Biggs H.M. History of the recent outbreak of epidemic cholera in New York. *Am J Med Sci (New Series)*. 1893; 105: 63–72.

6. Oliver W. *The Man Who Lived for Tomorrow: A Biography of William Hallock Park, M.D.* (New York, NY: E.P. Dutton, 1941).

7. Markel H. Long ago against diphtheria, the heroes were horses. *New York Times*. July 10, 2007: D6.

8. Fox D.M. Social policy and city politics: tuberculosis reporting in New York, 1889-1900. *Bull Hist Med*. 1975; 49(2): 169–175.

9. Winslow C.E.-A. *The Life of Hermann Biggs, M.D., D.Sc., LL.D.: Physician and Statesman of the Public Health*. (Philadelphia, PA: Lea & Febiger, 1929), p. xii.

10. Biggs H. Public Health is Purchasable. *Monthly Bulletin of the Department of Health of the City of New York*. October 11, 1911: 225–226.

CHAPTER 14

∽

Sigmund Freud's Long Line of Cocaine

Part I. Carl Koller

Sigmund Freud. 'Über Coca' *Centralblatt für die ges. Therapie.* 1884; 2: 289–314.

I n the spring of 1884, a 28-year-old Viennese neurologist named Sigmund Freud
published *Über Coca*, a superb medical analysis of cocaine hydrochloride.[1,2]
Although the monograph was an early career milestone for the ambitious physician, it also represented a missed opportunity. Using himself as his experimental
subject over several months, Freud consumed a great deal of cocaine as he recorded the drug's physiological effects and potential therapeutic uses. However,
he skimmed over cocaine's most important clinical use as a local anesthetic. In a
hurried last paragraph, a postscript really, Freud noted that "cocaine and its salts
have a marked anesthetizing effect when brought into contact with the skin and
mucous membrane in concentrated solution." Without offering any additional data
or experiments, Freud merely concluded that these properties "should make it suitable for a good many applications."[2]

The person who did capitalize on describing cocaine's anesthetic properties
was Freud's colleague Carl Koller, an *aspirant* (intern) in ophthalmology at the
Vienna Allgemeines Krankenhaus (General Hospital).[3] That Koller became so
interested in local anesthesia was a direct result of the operation he frequently
performed: cataract removal. Although practiced since antiquity, it remained a
dreaded procedure in 1884. After all, without pharmaceutical assistance, cataract
removal was not only excruciating, it required a patient to watch as the surgeon,
literally, poked him or her in the eye. Few have re-created the operation's awful
immediacy as well as the British novelist Thomas Hardy: "It was a like a red-hot

Literatim: Essays at the Intersections of Medicine and Culture. Howard Markel, Oxford University Press (2020).
© Oxford University Press.
DOI: 10.1093/oso/9780190087647.001.0001

needle in yer eye while he was doing it. But he wasn't long about it. Oh No. If he had been long I couldn't ha' beared it. He wasn't a minute more than three quarters of an hour at the outside."[4]

With the advent of ether and chloroform in the mid-19th century came great hopes among ophthalmologists for making cataract removal less traumatic. But these anesthetic agents often induced vomiting in patients—which in turn created alarmingly high pressures in the abdomen, chest, and head that are not conducive to performing delicate eye surgery.

During the summer of 1884, Koller slaved over a formal address on cocaine for the International Ophthalmological Congress to be held that September at Heidelberg. Too poor to afford the travel expenses to Germany, he asked Josef Brettauer, a 49-year-old ophthalmologist, to read his paper at the meeting—a common practice in an era when travel was both costly and arduous. The presentation was nothing short of spectacular.

As the world's most distinguished eye surgeons took their seats in the auditorium, Brettauer approached the podium. After explaining what Koller had been working on for the past few months, Koller's surrogate snapped his fingers and called for a diener to wheel in a gurney bearing a large dog. With a theatrical flair, the physician showed the audience that the animal was alert, comfortably seated on a cushion, and loosely tied down on the gurney.

He then took a calibrated dropper full of cocaine solution, delicately held the canine's left eye open with his thumb and forefinger, and introduced 3 or 4 drops of the elixir. Brettauer let 1, then 2, minutes pass in silence—a period that seems like a lifetime when giving a lecture before a crowded room. Satisfied that the cocaine had taken effect, he thrust a forceps toward the dog's eye. While the animal's right eye blinked in response to this threat, the left eye remained still. Brettauer deftly touched the canine's left eye with the surgical instrument and the results were astonishing: nothing happened! No whimpering, no barking, not even a flinch—that is, until the crowd sighed in relief that no harm had come to the dog and burst into uproarious applause.[5]

The development of a topical agent that could safely render a patient insensate to the surgeon's pointedly sharp manipulations while completely awake was earthshaking. It was front-page news that captured the attention of just about every physician (and dentist) in the world. It also enabled pharmaceutical companies to make a fortune marketing cocaine and, later, safer local anesthetics like procaine hydrochloride (Novocain) and lidocaine hydrochloride (Xylocaine).

Freud, understandably, was less than thrilled about Koller's achievement. Working in the same hospital, where gossip of successes and failures traveled quickly, could not have been an easy cross for the young, sensitive physician to bear. Whenever the topic of cocaine came up, it was Koller's name and not Freud's that generated adulation.

Initially, the jealous Freud claimed that he and Leopold Königstein, a Viennese ophthalmologist, were already working on cocaine anesthesia and that it was Freud who introduced the idea to Koller; few bought such claims. Months later, in January 1885, he dismissively declared that his cocaine work was merely a scientific trifle he executed in the "chase after money, position and reputation."[6] Another barometer of Freud's feelings about his scientific rival can be summarized by his later contention that a joke is never really a joke.[7] In 1885, Freud inscribed a copy of his *Über Coca* for Carl Koller: "To my dear friend, Coca Koller, from Sigmund Freud"—a mildly demeaning sobriquet that, much to the ophthalmologist's chagrin, followed Koller well after his death in 1944.[8]

Nor did it end there. In 1895, Freud experienced a dream in which he received due credit for the "discovery" of cocaine. It occurred around the time when Freud had arranged for his father to undergo surgery for glaucoma with the benefit of cocaine anesthesia. In 1900, he reported in *The Interpretation of Dreams* that during this particular dream, Koller congratulated both him and Königstein for being members of the medical triumvirate who introduced local anesthesia to the world.[9] The dream may have been based on a real experience or, more likely, was merely a wish.

Even 40 years after the event, while musing over this period of his life in his 1925 autobiography, Freud went as far as to blame Martha, his then-fiancée and later wife, for distracting him from his cocaine experiments.[10]

It hardly required the genius of a Freud to inquire why touching his tongue and lips with cocaine created such powerfully numbing sensations; this is, after all, a key characteristic of ingesting it. With his frequent cocaine use, it is difficult to explain why he did not value this particular action of the drug as much as he did its ability to alter one's mood, blood pressure, breathing rate, and many other physiological and sensational parameters. Perhaps Freud was so preoccupied with completing his paper and rushing it into print that he simply neglected this particular drug action. Maybe his lack of interest in pain-inducing, surgical procedures blocked his view to such a critical finding. An even more possible explanation might be that the exhilarating effects of cocaine—the high rather than the physical numbness—dominated his thoughts and actions. Whatever the reason, he made a colossal blunder by overlooking what proved to be a historic scientific discovery.

The annals of medical history, of course, are littered with tales of investigators bested by others in the aggressive quest for discovery. The striking difference in this case was that Freud had the talent and determination to transcend his early defeat. Only a few years later he would unveil his own signature discoveries of psychoanalysis and "the talking cure."

[This essay originally appeared as: Markel, H.: Über Coca: Sigmund Freud, Carl Koller, and Cocaine. Journal of the American Medical Association. 2011; 305 (13): 1360–1361].

REFERENCES

1. Markel, H. *An Anatomy of Addiction: Sigmund Freud, William Halsted, and the Miracle Drug Cocaine.* (New York, NY: Pantheon Books, 2011).
2. Freud, S. Über Coca. *Centralblatt für die ges. Therapie.* 1885; 2: 289–314.
3. Becker, H.K. Carl Koller and cocaine. *Psychoanal Q.* 1963; 32: 309–373.
4. Hardy, F.E. *Early Life of Thomas Hardy, 1840–1891.* (New York, NY: Macmillan, 1928), p. 200.
5. Beckhard, A.J., Crane, W.D. *Cancer, Cocaine and Courage: The Story of Dr. William Halsted.* (New York, NY: Julian Messner Inc, 1960), pp. 119–121.
6. Letter from Sigmund Freud to Martha Bernays. January 7, 1885. In: Freud S, ed. *Letters of Sigmund Freud.* Stern T, Stern J, trans. (New York, NY: Basic Books, 1960), pp. 132–133.
7. Freud, S. *The Joke and Its Relation to the Unconscious.* Crick J, trans. (New York, NY: Penguin Classics, 2002).
8. Byck, R, ed. *Cocaine Papers.* (New York, NY: Stonehill, 1974), pp. 95–109.
9. Freud, S. *The Interpretation of Dreams.* Strachey J, trans. (New York, NY: Penguin Books, 1991), pp. 255–256, 259, 262, 309, 387.
10. Freud, S. *An Autobiographical Study.* Strachey J, trans. (New York, NY: W.W. Norton & Co, 1989), p. 13.

CHAPTER 15

꙰

Sigmund Freud's Long Line of Cocaine

Part II. The Accidental Addict

Sigmund Freud, Über Coca.*Centralblatt für die ges. Therapie.* 1884; 2: 289–314.

ﬞll stories of addiction are tragic. Some addictions are so well concealed that, when discovered, they initially appear to be inconceivable. One of the most remarkable tales of a concealed drug addiction began more than a century ago and involves a brilliant young doctor. Talented, well educated, and socially prominent, he was a swift and decisive operator when speed was of paramount importance to surgical prowess. But by the age of 33, the physician faced both professional and literal extinction because of a losing battle against a relentless addiction to cocaine.

Yet less than a decade after reaching what recovery experts today might call his "bottom," he was appointed professor of surgery at an illustrious medical school and enjoyed international renown as one of the greatest surgeons ever to wield a scalpel. Today, his name is recognizable by even the most casual observer of American medical history: William Stewart Halsted of the Johns Hopkins Hospital. But one question has haunted many historians: Did Dr. Halsted ever vanquish his addiction, as he claimed? Sadly, as is true of so many people caught in the vortex of a disease that attacks the mind, body, and soul, he did not.

In 1884, cocaine, the alkaloid derivative of the coca plant treasured by the Incas, became all the rage among the medical cognoscenti. In July of that year, Sigmund Freud published a detailed monograph on cocaine. Although Freud's series of experiments on himself and others demonstrated many of cocaine's effects, in the monograph he glossed over a critical one that had immediate applications, the drug's properties as a local anesthetic. But one of Freud's contemporaries, an

Literatim: Essays at the Intersections of Medicine and Culture. Howard Markel, Oxford University Press (2020).
DOI: 10.1093/oso/9780190087647.001.0001

ophthalmologist named Karl Koller, did recognize this potential and that autumn announced his findings to an international congress of eye surgeons gathered in Heidelberg, Germany. Because so many surgeons around the world were engaged in the search for an anesthetic agent that was safer and simpler to use than ether, there was great excitement about the ramifications of Koller's discovery.[1]

In late October of 1884, Halsted, who was practicing in New York City, began his own experiments with this "wonder drug." Most important, he demonstrated how infiltrating sensory nerves and blocking major nerve trunks safely facilitated both mildly invasive and general surgical operations. Yet his description of these findings in the September 12, 1885, issue of the *New York Medical Journal* was so disjointed and overwrought that it could only have been written under the influence of cocaine.[2] Within months after beginning his exploration of the drug and heroically enlisting himself as a human subject, Dr. Halsted had accidentally transformed himself into an addict.

By early 1886, one of his closest colleagues, an exuberant pathologist named William Henry Welch, took it upon himself to institute an *ad hoc* treatment plan for Halsted's deteriorating condition. First on the agenda was a sea voyage, which was then considered highly therapeutic for men of means who were suffering from a broad range of maladies. During February and March of 1886, Halsted sailed on a schooner bound for the Windward Islands. Ever the crafty addict, he had secreted a large supply of cocaine in the sincere hope of gradually cutting down his dose. Despite his calculations, Halsted could not satisfy his addictive hunger and ran out of cocaine long before the ship pointed its bow north for the voyage home. Late one night, thousands of miles out at sea, the cocaine-obsessed Halsted lay awake in his rocking hammock until his bunkmates' telltale snoring indicated slumber. Audibly assured that they would not witness his actions, Halsted sneaked out of the cabin and prowled about until he located the captain's medicine chest. It was only minutes before this scion of privilege was reduced to breaking into the locked container for a much-needed fix.

After his return to New York, Halsted remained unable to quit a habit that was clearly destroying him; he therefore admitted himself to the highly regarded Butler Hospital for the Insane in Providence, Rhode Island. Ashamed of his addiction and afraid that public knowledge of it might adversely affect his career, he signed the hospital's register as "William Stewart."

From May to November of 1886, Halsted surrendered to the dictates of his "alienists" (i.e., psychiatrists)—seclusion, fresh air, exercise, a healthful diet, and a gradual withdrawal from cocaine. Agitation and insomnia were managed with hot wet packs and doses of alcohol, chloral hydrate, and bromides. At that time, the approach of choice for weaning an addict from cocaine was the liberal use of morphine as a substitute agent. Sadly, this drug, too, would cause addictive problems for Halsted in the years to come.

Around this time, Halsted's friend William Welch became a professor of pathology at the newly established Johns Hopkins Hospital in Baltimore. Armed with a hefty endowment, Welch was charged with gathering the talent to launch one of the greatest experiments in modern medicine. Shortly after Halsted's discharge from Butler, Welch urged the troubled surgeon to quit New York and his cocaine-abusing cronies and move to Baltimore to live in Welch's home and work in his laboratory. Welch kept a watchful eye on Halsted, remaining far more attentive than mere friendship or an employer's supervision demanded. One of Welch's principal tasks involved monitoring the surgeon's cash flow to ensure that Halsted did not have enough money to satisfy his cocaine cravings.[3]

During the next few years, Halsted labored in the laboratory, patiently creating new surgical procedures and testing them on dogs. However, in late 1887 he readmitted himself to Butler Hospital for an extended period. By early 1889, he had convinced his colleagues that he was no longer a slave to either cocaine or morphine and could be trusted to care for patients—a claim he firmly maintained for the rest of his life. In February 1889, he was named surgeon-in-chief at the Johns Hopkins dispensary and acting surgeon at the hospital. In 1892, he was appointed the first professor of surgery at Hopkins.

His New York days and his old reputation behind him, Halsted was now revered as a careful, deliberate, and painstakingly slow surgeon. Indeed, many surgeons referred to Halsted's newly adopted technique as the "School of Safety." Others have speculated, however, that this level of patience may have been augmented by the powers of concentration then associated with using cocaine. Nevertheless, it was in Baltimore that Halsted developed several highly regarded surgical procedures, including the use of rubber gloves to advance sterile technique, and launched a rigorous training program for junior surgeons that continues in some fashion to the present.

According to most firsthand accounts of his days at Johns Hopkins, Halsted was moody, elusive, sarcastic, and prone to dropping out in the middle of an operation and leaving his talented resident assistants to complete the procedure that was under way. The excuses he gave were anginal pain or, more troubling, hands that were simply too shaky to operate—a symptom that Halsted blamed on his legendary overconsumption of cigarettes but that could also have been caused by the recent ingestion of cocaine or withdrawal from morphine.

In fact, many of Halsted's colleagues thought something was amiss and worried that his addiction remained active. Most famously, Dr. William Osler recalled in 1890 that he had seen the surgeon having severe chills. Suspecting that Halsted was still addicted to morphine and was going through withdrawal, Osler gained the surgeon's trust and confidence. In a secret diary that Osler kept sometime between 1902 and 1905, which was not unsealed until 1969, the great physician wrote, "[Halsted] has never been able to reduce the amount to less than three grains [of morphine] daily, on this he could do his work comfortably and maintain his excellent physical vigor.... I do not think that anyone suspected him—not even Welch."[4]

Although Halsted's nieces and his longtime secretary said that they never saw any evidence of drug addiction, another close observer, his former chief resident

George Heuer, suggested that "the real truth of the matter is that he never conquered" his cocaine addiction.[5] Definitive answers to questions such as "how much,"
"what," and "when" will probably never be found. But in addition to Halsted's erratic behavior in the operating room, circumstantial evidence—ranging from his
frequent absences from the hospital when his whereabouts were unknown to his
avoidance of close colleagues when he walked the wards (perhaps because he was
under the influence and did not wish to be scrutinized by those who might recognize this), his going home daily at 4:30 p.m. and locking himself in his study for 90
minutes before dinner, his curious habit of sending his soiled linen to an exclusive
laundry in Paris (which may or may not have sent back more than clean shirts), and,
most troubling, his easy access to morphine and to the cocaine that was used in his
operating room throughout this period—suggests that he continued to abuse morphine and, I suspect, cocaine to the end of his life.[5]

Halsted's affliction was no less real than others' addictions simply because it
occurred "accidentally" in the name of advancing science. No one becomes an
addict on purpose. Unfortunately, society's view of drug addiction has remained
largely unchanged since Halsted's time; the disease, which today has reached epidemic proportions, is still too often met with secrecy, denial, and shame.

*[This essay originally appeared as: Markel, H.: The Accidental Addict. New England
Journal of Medicine 2005; 352:966-968.]*

REFERENCES

1. Freud S. *Uber Coca.* In: Byck R, ed. *Cocaine Papers.* (New York: Stonehill, 1974), pp. 48–73,
   107–109, 263–319.
2. Halsted, W.S. Practical comments on the use and abuse of cocaine. *New York Medical Journal.*
   1885; 42: 294–295.
3. Olch, P.D. William S. Halsted and local anesthesia: contributions and complications.
   Anesthesiology 1975; 42: 479–486.
4. Osler, W., Bates D.G., Bensley E.H. The Inner History of the Johns Hopkins Hospital. *Johns
   Hopkins Med J* 1969; 125: 184–194.
5. Heuer, G.W. Dr. Halsted. *Bulletin of the Johns Hopkins Hospital.* 1952; 90: Suppl 2: 1–105.

CHAPTER 16

c√o

Exploring the Dangerous Trades With Dr. Alice Hamilton

Hamilton, A. *Exploring the Dangerous Trades: The Autobiography of Alice Hamilton, M.D.* By Alice Hamilton.

(Boston, MA, Atlantic Monthly Press/Little Brown, 1943).

A few months after the Armistice was signed and World War I came to a screeching halt, a 50-year-old physician named Alice Hamilton received an assignment from the U.S. Department of Labor. She was to investigate the working conditions of copper miners in Arizona, many of whom had sustained various hand and finger injuries from the overuse of air jackhammers, a problem she had already studied in stonecutters.[1] She was also to assess the miners' exposure to poisonous arseniureted hydrogen gases. Predictably, in an era when profit was paramount and the health of those who toiled in the industrial beehive a distant second, she was not warmly welcomed by the men who controlled the mining camps.

As Hamilton recalled in her autobiography:

"There were no neutrals anywhere ... I asked the hotel clerk ... about physicians in the camp, or lawyers, or clergymen, whom I could interview, only to be told: 'All the doctors here are copper ... the lawyers are copper too ... most of the ministers are copper'" (pp. 210–211). Undaunted, Hamilton put on overalls and a miner's cap, crawled and stooped through the labyrinthine spaces, bumped her head repeatedly on the low "ceiling" of the mines, and crossed precipitously deep pits on rails "which were so far apart I felt sure I could fall between them" (p. 217).

This is just one of hundreds of episodes worth reading and relishing in Alice Hamilton's memoir, *Exploring the Dangerous Trades*. The book first appeared to critical acclaim and popular sales in 1943 but is currently out of print (although

Literatim: Essays at the Intersections of Medicine and Culture. Howard Markel, Oxford University Press (2020).
© Oxford University Press.
DOI: 10.1093/oso/9780190087647.001.0001

reprint editions and library copies are available).[2] It is her scrupulous attention to detail about the specific conditions, people, causes, events, and social injustices she encountered both personally and professionally that make this volume such an illuminating historical document.

Take, for example, her recollections of that 1919 copper mining investigation in Arizona. One night, in the Mexican border town Ajo, Hamilton had no choice but to sleep in a shed consisting of two rows of "rooms" separated by a passageway. "The rooms were really much more like horse stalls," she writes, "the walls were only about eight feet high, having a free space above, and there was no door, only a heavy canvas curtain. However, the very casualness was reassuring, and after all the room was as much shut in as a Pullman berth. Anyway our night was very much undisturbed and we woke to see sunrise over the desert" (p. 212).

This dutifully recorded recollection may well have been a personal reminder that she was not always so lucky. During her career, she snuck into factories against the wishes of their owners, treated workers to beers in saloons after their shifts to learn about their work, and exposed herself to multiple hardships and risks. On at least one occasion, while sleeping in an unlocked mining shack, she was mistaken for a prostitute. A modest Hamilton shrugged her shoulders as she told an oral historian about these incidents in 1963, "I used to have to do those things."[3,4]

In fact, she did. Probably no individual was more instrumental in warning Americans about the health risks of the workplace than Alice Hamilton. During the first decades of the 20th century, few physicians were willing to engage in the intense political, scientific, and economic battles necessary to keep workers safe and healthy. Elite academic physicians had bigger intellectual fish to fry; and, for those in private practice, such pursuits simply did not pay enough. But for a woman trying to carve out a niche in medicine, it was a unique opportunity.

During her distinguished career, Hamilton wrote dozens of seminal monographs that remain classics of scientific concision and investigative elegance. The list of topics she tackled reads like a murderer's row of dangerous working conditions once the norm for laborers in this country.[5] She inspected pottery plants,[6] smelters,[7] printing plants,[8] steel mills, mines, and munitions factories and scientifically demonstrated the health risks of lead, carbon monoxide,[9] phosphorus, benzene, picric acid, and various other toxic substances that permeated many workplaces. In so doing, she helped prevent countless cases of lead poisoning, benzene-induced malignancies,[10] black lung disease, anemia, munitions factory mishaps, and other toxic exposures.[11,12]

Hamilton's *Curriculum Vitae* provides a sterling illustration of the modern medical scientist at the *fin de siècle*. It is all the more remarkable considering she was entering her profession in an era when few women practiced medicine and fewer still taught at universities.[13] She earned her medical degree from the University of Michigan in 1893, where she garnered the attention of world-class scientists such as bacteriologist Frederick Novy, internist George Dock, and biochemist Victor Vaughan.[14] From Ann Arbor, she moved on to internships at Minneapolis' Northwestern Hospital for Women and Children and Boston's New England

Hospital for Women and Children, followed by two years of study in pathology and bacteriology in Leipzig, Munich, and, finally, Baltimore, where she frequently lunched and debated with such Johns Hopkins giants as William H. Welch, William Osler, and Simon Flexner (pp. 38–56).

In 1897, Hamilton was called to teach pathology at Northwestern University's Women's Medical School in Chicago. Forty-six years later, she recalled her joy over landing a job in the Windy City: "At last I could realize the dream I had had for years, of going to live in Hull-House" (p. 53). She was referring, of course, to the world-famous settlement house in Chicago founded by Jane Addams in 1889.[15] Charismatic, indefatigable, and articulate, Addams was internationally known as a powerfully effective defender of the powerless.

Cities of this era were roiled by the problems generated by industrialization, immigration, labor unrest, abject poverty, and overcrowding. In response, an ambitious and superbly educated generation of young, white professionals, particularly in British and U.S. cities, created dozens of settlement houses, wherein university students and graduates lived and worked alongside the poor. Those who populated these institutions were fortified by deeply held religious and political convictions and a 19th-century noblesse oblige sensibility of improving the lives of the impoverished and working classes.[16,17] The settlement houses also served as social policy incubators, spawning new ideas, methods, and approaches to counteract the corrosive changes brought on by the industrial age.

Nine years before moving to Chicago, in 1888, Hamilton graduated from Miss Porter's School in Farmington, Connecticut. While living on her family's estate in Fort Wayne, Indiana, she discovered the works of Richard Ely, a brilliant labor economist who preached the gospel of Christian socialism. Ely espoused a progressive political philosophy that interpreted the teachings of Christ as the natural precursors to the aims of socialism. Hamilton's empathy for the oppressed, defeated, and disenfranchised inspired her to pursue a career in medicine because "I could go anywhere I pleased—to far-off lands or to city slums—and be quite sure that I could be of use anywhere" (p. 38).

All of these hopes, aspirations, and convictions took on greater clarity at a lecture Hamilton attended with her sister Agnes at their Methodist church in the spring of 1895. The speaker was Jane Addams. For Hamilton, it was one of the most important afternoons of her life: "I only know that it was then that Agnes and I definitely chose settlement life. . . . This was not so easy as it sounds" (pp. 39, 54).

Working at a settlement house exemplified the adage of doing well by doing good and often led to much greater career opportunities for young urban professionals of this era. Consequently, positions at Hull-House were extremely competitive, even if the applicant typically had to pay his or her own room and board.

When Hamilton arrived in Chicago in spring of 1897, there were no vacancies at Hull-House. During her summer vacation on Michigan's Mackinac Island, however, she received a letter from Addams informing her of an opening that autumn. The brief missive began a 22-year residence at Hull-House, initiating important working relationships with Addams, Julia Lathrop (an expert on infant mortality and, in 1912, the first chief of the U.S. Children's Bureau), and Florence Kelley (a leading child labor law and minimum wage advocate), as well as many others representing the vanguard of Progressive Era social reforms.

One of Hamilton's first duties was to conduct a well-baby clinic. Blessed with a profound sense of humility and awareness, Hamilton recorded the clash of cultures that transpired daily as she examined the children of immigrants:

> Miss Addams let me use the shower-bath room in the basement of the gymnasium and provided a dozen little bathtubs, with soap and bathing towels, for most of the work of the "clinic" was bathing the children. Some of them came all sewed into their clothes for the winter, but I found I could get past the Italian mothers' dread of water if I followed the bath with an alcohol rub and anointing with olive oil. Then I gave what I had been taught was the best advice about feeding babies—nothing but milk till their teeth came. When I see the varied diet modern mothers give their babies, anything apparently from bacon to bananas, I realize that those Italian women knew what a baby needed far better than my Ann Arbor professor did. I cannot feel I did any harm, however, for my teachings had no effect. (p. 69)

Although committed to settlement house life, Hamilton quickly grasped that neither medical practice nor a cloistered laboratory life would fulfill her passion and aspirations. Hence, she investigated typhoid fever and tuberculosis outbreaks in Chicago and cocaine abuse in the years before federal law made it an illegal substance. Beginning in 1908 with her appointment to the Illinois Commission of Occupational Diseases and, in 1911, to the U.S. Department of Labor, she began a tireless pursuit she called "exploring the dangerous trades."

In 1919, Hamilton became the first woman faculty member at Harvard Medical School, albeit on a part-time appointment. Ironically, at this time women were still not allowed to matriculate into that medical school—nor would they be until 1945. Harvard's hiring a woman professor inspired much comment in several newspapers across the nation. To such critiques, Hamilton sharply rejoined: "Yes, I am the first woman on the Harvard faculty—but not the first one who should have been appointed."[18] Her career hardly ended with these stellar accomplishments; until her death in 1970, Hamilton continued to crusade for the health of all Americans, leaving an indelible mark on medical history.

At the heart of her remarkable life, however, were her experiences at Hull-House; it was there, after all, where she discovered her gift for ameliorating industrial diseases and improving the lives of millions. "Living in a working-class quarter, coming in contact with laborers and their wives," she writes, "I could not fail to hear tales of the dangers that workingmen faced, of cases of carbon-monoxide gassing in the great steel mills, of painters disabled by lead palsy, of pneumonia and rheumatism among the men in the stockyards" (p. 114).

When reading Hamilton's autobiography, a compelling blend of tenacious detective work, courage, and compassion, one cannot help but be struck by the author's indignant, yet elegantly phrased, outrage over the abuse or neglect of human beings in pursuit of profits. Today, in an era when so many lives around the globe are endangered or harmed daily by environmental toxins, dangerous workplaces, and hazardous living conditions; an era where too many consumers silently but aggressively purchase cheaper and cheaper products that have the potential to escalate such practices; it would be wise to recall that Alice Hamilton's genius was entirely dependent on the fact that she listened so attentively to those who barely thought they had a voice and acted so bravely in the world she inhabited.

[This essay originally appeared as: Markel, H.: Exploring the Dangerous Trades with Dr. Alice Hamilton. Journal of the American Medical Association. 2007; 298 (23):2802–2804.]

REFERENCES

1. Hamilton A. *Effect of the Air Hammer on the Hands of Stonecutters*. (Washington, D.C.: U.S. Dept of Labor, 1918).
2. Rukeyser M. Inside some testing places of American democracy [Review of Hamilton A. *Exploring the Dangerous Trades: The Autobiography of Alice Hamilton, M.D.*]. *New York Times Book Review*. April 11, 1943:3.
3. Curran JA. Alice Hamilton, Oral History Interview, November 29, 1963. Located at: Francis A. Countway Library, Rare Book Room, Harvard Medical School, Boston, MA.
4. Sicherman B. *Alice Hamilton: A Life in Letters*. (Champaign-Urbana, IL: University of Illinois Press, 2003), p. 3.
5. Hamilton A. *Industrial Toxicology*. (New York, NY: Harper, 1934).
6. Hamilton A. *Lead Poisoning in Potteries, Tile Works and Porcelain Enameled Sanitary Ware Factories*. (Washington, D.C.: U.S. Dept. of Labor, 1912).
7. Hamilton A. *Lead Poisoning in the Smelting and Refining of Lead*. (Washington, D.C.: U.S. Dept. of Labor, 1914).
8. Hamilton A, Verrill CH. *Hygiene of the Printing Trade*. (Washington, D.C.: U.S. Dept. of Labor, 1917).
9. Hamilton A. *Carbon Monoxide Poisoning*. (Washington, D.C.: U.S. Dept. of Labor, 1922).
10. Hamilton A. *Industrial Poisons in Making Coal-Tar Dyes and Dye Intermediates*. (Washington, D.C.: U.S. Dept. of Labor, 1921).
11. Hamilton A. *Industrial Poisons Used or Produced in the Manufacture of Explosives*. (Washington, D.C.: U.S. Dept. of Labor, 1917).
12. Hamilton A. *Industrial Poisons in the United States*. (New York, NY: Macmillan, 1925).
13. Morantz-Sanchez R. *Sympathy and Science: Women Physicians in American Medicine*. (New York, NY: Oxford University Press, 1985).
14. Davenport H.W. *Not Just Any Medical School: The Science, Practice, and Teaching of Medicine at the University of Michigan, 1850–1941*. (Ann Arbor: University of Michigan Press, 1999).
15. Addams J. *Twenty Years at Hull-House, With Autobiographical Notes*. (New York, NY: Macmillan, 1912).
16. Knight L.W. *Citizen: Jane Addams and the Struggle for Democracy*. (Chicago, IL: University of Chicago Press, 2006).
17. Davis A. *Spearheads for Reform: The Social Settlements & the Progressive Movement, 1890 to 1914*. (New Brunswick, NJ: Rutgers University Press, 1985).
18. Corn J.K. Alice Hamilton. In: Garraty JA, Carnes MC, eds. *American National Biography*. Vol 9. (New York, NY: Oxford University Press, 1999), p. 912.

CHAPTER 17

∾

The Principles and Practice of Medicine

How a Textbook, a Former Baptist Minister, and an Oil Tycoon Shaped the Modern American Medical and Public Health Industrial–Research Complex

William Osler. *The Principles and Practice of Medicine.*

(New York, NY, D. Appleton, 1892).

What constitutes a medical classic? Can the impact of a text be measured solely in terms of sales figures or citation numbers? What about its allegiance to what is believed to be scientific truth? Although Hippocrates and Galen wrote shelves of books that dominated medical thought for centuries, few of their ideas are considered pertinent to medical science today. Yet who would deny either of them their due as authors of medical classics? More critically, one might inquire, what was each particular work's historical trajectory and how did it inspire readers to act on the knowledge it imparted in the generations that followed?

With regard to this last query, perhaps the clearest example of the text's meteoric ascent to the pantheon of classics began in July of 1897. A frequent sight for those swimming that summer in the crystal-blue Lake Liberty nestled in New York's Catskill Mountains was a man on the shore reading and relaxing in a hammock. What might have surprised the casual observer of the gentleman's bucolic pose, however, was the book he was reading: the second edition of William Osler's *The Principles and Practice of Medicine.*

Literatim: Essays at the Intersections of Medicine and Culture. Howard Markel, Oxford University Press (2020).
© Oxford University Press.
DOI: 10.1093/oso/9780190087647.001.0001

Osler, of course, was the distinguished professor of medicine at Johns Hopkins and the most inspiring medical educator of his era. But the reader was neither a physician nor a medical student; he was a former Baptist minister who became the trusted advisor to John D. Rockefeller, founder of the American petroleum monopoly called Standard. The recumbent man's name, entirely coincidental to the surname of one of today's biggest medical benefactors, was Frederick T. Gates.

At the time Gates read Osler's *magnum opus*, his employer was the richest man in the world. A devout Baptist, Rockefeller was actively revising his personal history before he met his maker by giving away large portion of his enormous fortune. The announcement of such beneficent intentions inspired frenzy among the needy and the greedy alike. It also may have caused numerous inguinal hernias among the postal workers who delivered countless heavy mailbags loaded with pleas for cash to his office every week. Charged with sorting though—and making sense of—this morass of misery was Rockefeller's carefully groomed proxy, the exceptionally efficient Gates.[1]

First among Rockefeller's many charitable interests during this period was the promotion of medical research. Such pursuits represented the most productive means of distributing his money in a manner guaranteed to garner praise or, at least, mitigate further diatribes about his ill-gotten riches. But, according to one biographer, a potentially intriguing stimulus might have been related to Rockefeller's upbringing. The son of a ne'er-do-well, hard-drinking, patent medicine salesman named William "Doc" Rockefeller, the oil magnate may have been motivated to atone for the sins of his father by investing in medical science.[2]

Regardless of his boss' inspiration, however, Gates needed to learn a lot about medicine quickly. So that July of 1897, he turned to Osler for comfort and advice. As his hammock swayed to the lake's dulcet breezes, the walrus-mustachioed Gates pored over every paragraph of Osler's elegant prose. Years later, in 1928, Gates warmly recalled the spell Osler's book cast on him: "There was a fascination about the style itself that led me on and, having once started, I found a hook in my nose that pulled me from page to page, and from chapter to chapter, until the whole of about a thousand closely printed pages brought me to the end."[3]p. 180

Gates was hardly the only enthusiastic reader of this influential and beloved textbook. Initially published in 1892, *The Principles and Practice of Medicine*, or "Osler" as it was universally referred to, quickly became a best-seller. More than 500,000 copies were sold over the course of half a century, in 16 editions and reprinted in dozens of languages.[4] At least three generations of physicians, nurses, and other health professionals read, memorized, and clutched this tome to their chests during long, anguished nights before critical examinations. Written in an era when textbook authors were required to master the entire field of medical knowledge they covered and, as a result, write every chapter themselves, to this day the book remains a marvel of diamond-sharp expositions on hundreds of diseases that merits the consideration of anyone interested in the human condition.

But there was a proverbial fly—or, given the location of his summer retreat, mosquito—in the soothing ointment of Frederick Gates' reading pleasure: "To a layman like me, demanding cures, he [Osler] had no word of comfort whatever. I saw clearly from the work of this able and honest man, perhaps the ablest physician of his time, that medicine had in fact . . . with . . . four or five exceptions no cures for disease."[3]

This deleterious situation so disturbed Gates that he abruptly ended his summer sojourn and on July 24, 1897, returned to his Manhattan office. Gates wrote a passionate memorandum to Rockefeller wherein he described the optimistic subtext of Osler's textbook. While the medical arsenal circa 1897 was rather paltry, Gates explained that scientific inquiry had the power to discover and create lifesaving treatments for scourges that had long afflicted humankind.

The essential problem, as Gates correctly understood it, was unleashing that power in an age when most scientists and physicians had little or no funds to support their research. Indeed, few U.S. medical schools expected their faculty to do anything more than practice the dictates of their predecessors and keep the diploma mills grinding away by selling lecture tickets to medical aspirants.[5] Finding a benefactor to underwrite the avalanche of costly scientific discovery that would mark the 20th century was, as Gates later explained to Osler in 1904, a novel request: "This line of philanthropy, now almost wholly neglected in this country, is the most needed and the most promising of any field of philanthropic endeavor."[6]

In the onslaught of his gargantuan responsibilities, however, Gates temporarily handed off this project to a lawyer named Starr Murphy who concocted what Gates later concluded was an "utterly futile" plan calling for Rockefeller to endow grants of $20,000 per annum, for 10 years, to selected individual laboratory workers in various parts of the United States.

Undaunted by this setback, Gates, along with John D. Rockefeller, Jr, continued to lobby Mr. Rockefeller about fulfilling the promise of Osler's medical compendium by endowing an independent medical research institute along the lines of Louis Pasteur's famed laboratory in Paris (founded in 1888) and Robert Koch's equally distinguished workshop in Berlin (founded in 1891). Such action, they predicted, would have a far greater impact beyond the four walls of the proposed structure; it would inspire other philanthropies to donate huge sums in support of lifesaving medical research. Yet, ever careful about where he put his hard-won millions, the senior Rockefeller still wanted to let Gates' big idea develop further before fully committing to it.

After fruitless attempts to partner with, successively, the University of Chicago, Columbia, and Harvard, Rockefeller finally tucked into Gates' tall order in early 1901, albeit it was a decision that had its roots in a family tragedy. Fifty years later, John D., Jr. recalled that his father's decision coincided with the death of a beloved grandson, John Rockefeller McCormick, who died at age three years from scarlet fever. Ironically, that death inspired two research institutions, the McCormick Institution for Infectious Diseases in Chicago, founded by the boy's parents, Harold

F. and Edith Rockefeller McCormick, and the more wide-ranging Rockefeller Institute for Medical Research in New York City.[7]

The following year, 1902, William Welch, who had emerged as the chief advisor of the Rockefeller Institute for Medical Research, approached his favorite pupil, Simon Flexner, a professor of pathology at the University of Pennsylvania (and brother of educator Abraham Flexner, who in 1910 wrote his seminal report on medical education in the United States) to be its founding director.

Institutes of substance require substantial real estate, and accordingly, in 1903, John D. Rockefeller purchased 13 acres on a bluff overlooking Manhattan's East River between 64th and 68th streets for the sum of $660,000. There, the institute assumed its permanent home in May of 1906 and, four years later, opened an adjacent 60-bed hospital that treated, free of charge, anyone afflicted with 1 of the 5 priority diseases under study: poliomyelitis, heart disease, syphilis, lobar pneumonia, and "intestinal infantilism" (celiac disease).

Rockefeller prided himself on awarding his scientists all the resources they required to pursue their intellectual curiosity, predicting that such generosity would produce the discovery of many new and great things. "John," the tycoon told his son, "we have money but it will have value for mankind only if we can find able men with ideas, imagination, and courage to put it into productive use."[8]

He was right. Despite being the son of a quack and a lifelong devotee of homeopathy, John D. Rockefeller remains the pivotal patron of modern medical research. Not surprisingly, the master businessman understood this distinction during his lifetime. As he told *Forbes Magazine* in 1917: "If in all of our giving, we had never done more than has been achieved by the fine, able, honest men of the Medical Institute, it would have justified all the money and all the effort we have spent."[9]

In all, Rockefeller donated more than $61 million to what became a model of the modern biomedical research center. His largesse enabled a number of remarkable discoveries and treatments and—as with any research endeavor—not a few outright flops. By 1955, the institute had become a specialized university offering Ph.D. training and research fellowships. In addition, the Rockefeller Foundation (founded in 1913) gave away hundreds of millions of dollars more to ameliorate hookworm in the United States and abroad, support the creation of the Rockefeller International Health Board, fund full-time academic appointments at several medical and public health schools, and fund a large number of other critical health projects that continue to benefit humankind to this day. Yet even as the Rockefeller Foundation promoted health programs that helped millions around the globe, these programs sometimes did so in a dismissive if not condescending manner toward local cultures and communities. In the most extreme, these endeavors are instructive of some of the pitfalls of international medical efforts that over the past decades have been marred by ethical lapses in human experimentation and colonialist impulses.[10–12]

Nevertheless, all of these consequences, intended and unintended, contain germs of ideas incubated by Mr. Gates and paid for by Mr. Rockefeller. But those in an etiologic frame of mind must also acknowledge (as Gates did to Osler in 1902) that Rockefeller's philanthropic vision—one that revolutionized medical science—all began because of one man reading one book, a bona fide classic, entitled *The Principles and Practice of Medicine*.[13]

[*This essay originally appeared as: Markel, H.: The Principles and Practice of Medicine: How a Textbook, a Former Baptist Minister, and an Oil Tycoon Shaped the Modern American Medical and Public Health Industrial-Research Complex. Journal of the American Medical Association. 2008; 299 (10): 1199–1201*].

REFERENCES

1. Nevins, A. *John D. Rockefeller: The Heroic Age of American Enterprise*. Vols. 1 & 2. (New York, NY: Charles Scribner's Sons, 1940).
2. Chernow, R. *Titan: The Life of John D. Rockefeller*. (New York, NY: Random House, 1998), pp. 470–479.
3. Gates, F.T. *Chapters from My Life*. (New York, NY: Free Press/MacMillan, 1977), pp. 180–181.
4. Golden, R. *A History of William Osler's The Principles and Practice of Medicine*. (Montreal, QC: Osler Library/McGill University and American Osler Society, 2004).
5. Flexner, A. *Medical Education in the United States and Canada*. (New York, NY: Carnegie Foundation for the Advancement of Teaching, 1910).
6. Gates, F.T. Letter to William Osler, April 13, 1904. Allan Nevins Papers. Located at: Butler Library, Columbia University, New York, NY.
7. Corner, G. *A History of the Rockefeller Institute, 1901–1953: Origins and Growth*. (New York, NY: Rockefeller Institute Press, 1964), p. 31.
8. Forsdick, R.B. *John D. Rockefeller, Jr.: A Portrait*. (New York, NY: Harper & Bros, 1956), p. 421.
9. Forbes, B.C. John D. Rockefeller tells how to succeed. *Forbes Magazine*. September 29, 1017.
10. Fosdick, R.B. *The Story of the Rockefeller Foundation*. (New Brunswick, NJ: Transactions Publishers, 1989).
11. Ettling, J. *The Germ of Laziness: Rockefeller Philanthropy and Public Health in the New South*. (Cambridge, MA: Harvard University Press, 1981).
12. Farley, J. *To Cast Out Disease: A History of the International Health Division of the Rockefeller Foundation (1913–1951)*. (New York, NY: Oxford University Press, 2004).
13. Gates, F.T. Letter to William Osler, March 4, 1902. Cushing Papers, Acc. 417, Box 3, Ch. 21: 13. Located at: Osler Library Collection, McGill University, Montreal, QC.

CHAPTER 18

ↅↄↆ

Onward Howard Kelly, Marching as to War

Howard A. Kelly. *A Scientific Man and the Bible.*
(Philadelphia, PA: Sunday School Times Co., 1925).

In 1905, the prominent artist John Singer Sargent was commissioned to paint a portrait of the four founding physicians of the Johns Hopkins Hospital: William Welch, William Osler, William Halsted, and Howard Kelly. That June, Welch, Halsted, and Kelly sailed for Southampton and traveled by rail to London. There they reunited with Osler, who had left Hopkins in 1904 to become the Regius Professor of Medicine at Oxford, and all four made their way to Sargent's studio near the Chelsea Embankment.[1]

Welch, Osler, Halsted, and Kelly posed in their academic robes and hoods. For days, they sat under a skylight in a stifling hot, poorly ventilated room redolent with the noxious fumes of oil paint, turpentine, and sweat. On some afternoons, all four were in the studio; on others, each came alone.

By the time his subjects quit London and returned to their demanding careers, Sargent had succeeded in creating a divine gem of portraiture.[2] On a canvas measuring 327.7 × 271.8 cm (10.75 × 9.08 feet), the four physicians are arranged around a book-strewn reading table and an antique Venetian globe. Osler, the great physician, appears as if about to leap to his feet to aid a patient in distress; Welch, the pathologist and medical statesman, sits supremely satisfied, his fingers resting on the leaves of an open tome; standing in Welch's shadow with a dark, brooding pall cast over his face is the dour, cocaine- and morphine-addicted surgeon, William Halsted. And if you look closely at Kelly, the gynecologist, he seems almost beatific or, at least, the saintliest of men.

Literatim: Essays at the Intersections of Medicine and Culture. Howard Markel, Oxford University Press (2020).
© Oxford University Press.
DOI: 10.1093/oso/9780190087647.001.0001

That is because the central devotion of Kelly's life was his savior Jesus Christ. So tightly intertwined was the connection between Kelly's daily endeavors and his Protestant Episcopalian beliefs that he often knelt in prayer before examining a patient or beginning an operation. Until, that is, many of his uncomfortable colleagues asked him to stop.[3(p216)]

Today, Howard Kelly is best recalled for inventing several operating tools and devices, including the clamp that bears his name and that is still requested in operating rooms all over the world. In his day, however, he was widely regarded as a master of pelvic and genitourinary surgery. Many have credited Dr. Kelly with establishing gynecology as a bona fide specialty, and his superb descriptions of diseases of the urinary tract, appendix, abdomen, and female reproductive organs continue to inform physicians who take the time to go to the library stacks to pull down his richly illustrated textbooks. Kelly also found the time to author or edit several authoritative tomes on history, biography, botany, natural history, mushrooms, snakes, and even canoeing.[4(p143)]

On Osler's recommendation, Welch called Kelly to help establish the Johns Hopkins Hospital and Medical School in 1889. On relocating to Baltimore from the University of Pennsylvania, Kelly also maintained a large private practice and a small hospital attached to his house. One of his major contributions to medicine was the use of radium to treat cervical cancer. Ironically for a man once described as "effulgent as an x-ray tube" and "distinctly phosphorescent" legend has it that long after Kelly's house was abandoned and razed in the 1960s, the radioactive waste left behind was so great that a team of hazardous materials experts had to come in to abate it.[3(p215)]

What is lost from such a recitation of credentials was Kelly's remarkable life as a self-described "Christian soldier" who waged active battle against disease, sin, crime, vice, and dangerous living conditions. For example, Kelly had an odd nocturnal habit of visiting Baltimore's most notorious street corners. Once there, he approached many an unsuspecting prostitute—not in search of a business transaction but instead seeking to facilitate her direct path to the Lord. Other times, when taking a taxi from home to hospital or social events, he tried to entice the cabdriver to attend his Sunday school classes.

Kelly also fought for women's suffrage on the premise that the Lord created all to be equal; for the establishment of Prohibition to combat the sin of drunkenness; and on behalf of Baltimore's most impoverished citizens by advocating housing improvements, clean-milk inspections, tuberculosis control, and the creation of sewage and sanitation systems to prevent the spread of typhoid fever. To ensure that elections and elected officials were held accountable to the constituents who needed them most, he played an active role in the Democratic Party of Maryland because, as he once explained to a colleague, "it is the most active and prominent of the political parties and . . . it is the most corrupt."[5]

A true follower of the Golden Rule, Kelly never met a man or woman he could not love as a treasured neighbor. Indeed, one of Kelly's oddest friendships was with the iconoclastic Baltimore journalist H. L. Mencken, a well-known non-believer. One evening in 1916, Kelly invited Mencken to join him in attending a sermon conducted by the famed evangelist Billy Sunday. Throughout the event, Mencken wisecracked and criticized the preacher as a buffoon and charlatan. Kelly maintained his calm, but at one point during the sermon, he took out a small black notebook and scribbled something in it. Later that evening, Mencken learned that Kelly was amending a list of sinners he would pray for in the coming week; not surprisingly, Mencken's name was at the top of this list.[6]

In 1926, Kelly wrote a popular book, A Scientific Man and the Bible, explaining the compatibility of Christianity with the tenets of modern science. In it, Kelly offered a cogent interpretation of the Bible and explained how he applied its teachings to his life and work. When discussing scientific inquiry, he insisted on the importance of an open mind but also declared that "where the Bible is dishonored, life becomes cheap and science an early victim, or if it survives, in a destructive form . . . our 'Science' is but folly when God is left out and if he is not in all our thoughts."[7]

Mencken reviewed Kelly's book the following year in his influential book column for The American Mercury. Applauding Kelly as a physician and scientist of the first rank, Mencken expressed his amazement at how Kelly placed himself "on exhibition as a Fundamentalist of the most extreme wing, compared to whom Judge Raulston, of Dayton, Tennessee [the judge presiding over the famed Scopes "Monkey Trial" of 1925] seems almost an atheist." Yet despite disagreeing with every sentence of Kelly's book, Mencken begrudgingly offered his respect: "He believes the Bible from cover to cover, fly-specks and all, and he says so (considering his station in life) with great courage."[8] Less impressed was the Pulitzer Prize–winning author and medical aficionado Sinclair Lewis, who snidely wrote the neurosurgeon (and also a Pulitzer Prize–winning author) Harvey Cushing, "my dear Harvey, what does an obstetrician know about the Virgin Birth?"[9]

Although Kelly retired from Johns Hopkins in 1919, he remained socially active, intellectually occupied, and spiritually devout to the end of his life. When he died in 1943 at the age of 85, his last utterance was "My Bible, Nurse, give me my Bible."[4(p3)] One can only hope that his prayers were answered.

[This essay originally appeared as: Onward Howard Kelly, Marching as to War. Journal of the American Medical Association. 2011 14;306(22):2514–2515].

REFERENCES

1. Harvey A.M., et alia. A Model of Its Kind: A Pictorial History of Medicine at Johns Hopkins. Vol 2. (Baltimore, MD: Johns Hopkins University Press, 1989), pp.68–69.
2. McCall N., ed. The Portrait Collection of Johns Hopkins Medicine: A Catalog of Paintings and Photographs at the Johns Hopkins University School of Medicine and the Johns Hopkins Hospital. (Baltimore, MD: Johns Hopkins University School of Medicine, 1993).
3. Bliss M. William Osler: A Life in Medicine. (New York, NY: Oxford University Press, 1999).

4. Davis A.W. *Dr. Kelly of Hopkins: Surgeon, Scientist, Christian.* (Baltimore, MD: Johns Hopkins University Press, 1959).
5. Testimonial dinner to Howard Atwood Kelly on his 75th birthday. *Bull Johns Hopkins Hosp.* 1933; 53(2): 65–109.
6. Rodgers M.E. *Mencken: The American Iconoclast.* (New York, NY: Oxford University Press, 2005), pp.15–151.
7. Kelly H.A. *A Scientific Man and the Bible.* (Philadelphia, PA: Sunday School Times Co; 1925), p. 55.
8. Mencken H.L. Fides ante intellectum. *American Mercury.* 1926; 7(26): 251–252.
9. Fulton J.F. *Harvey Cushing: A Biography.* (Springfield, IL: C.C. Thomas Co., 1946), p. 681.

CHAPTER 19

✣

April 12, 1955

Tommy Francis and the Salk Vaccine

Francis T. Jr., *Evaluation of the 1954 Field Trial of Poliomyelitis Vaccine*.
(Ann Arbor, Mich.: Edwards Brothers and the National Foundation for Infantile Paralysis, 1957).

April 12, 1955, was supposed to be Tommy Francis's day. At 10:20 a.m., the distinguished epidemiologist was scheduled to conduct an international press conference in Rackham Auditorium at the University of Michigan. The topic was the field trial he had just completed—the largest of its kind ever—evaluating the efficacy of the poliovirus vaccine developed by Jonas Salk at the University of Pittsburgh.

It is hardly hyperbole to note that the speech by Dr. Thomas Francis, Jr., was eagerly awaited by most of the world.[1] Few diseases were capable of arousing more fear than poliomyelitis. Almost every summer, polio epidemics left behind a wake of paralysis and death; horrific images of children struggling to walk or trapped inside iron lungs were etched into every parent's brain.

The fight against polio was significantly advanced by President Franklin Delano Roosevelt, the world's most famous polio patient. In 1937, convinced that nothing short of the conquest of the disease was required, Roosevelt announced the formation of a National Foundation for Infantile Paralysis (NFIP) that would "lead, direct, and unify the fight of every phase of this sickness." Soon, millions of Americans were responding to the pleas of the radio star Eddie Cantor to "send their dimes directly to the President at the White House . . . and we could call it the March of Dimes."[2]

Literatim: Essays at the Intersections of Medicine and Culture. Howard Markel, Oxford University Press (2020).
© Oxford University Press.
DOI: 10.1093/oso/9780190087647.001.0001

Although we can justifiably recall the battle against polio as a huge success, it was not without its share of well-publicized and almost disastrous failures. Among the most notorious were two highly touted but flawed vaccines that appeared in the mid-1930s—one, a formalin-killed vaccine, developed by Maurice Brodie and William H. Park of the New York City Health Department, and another, a live attenuated vaccine later derided as "a veritable witch's brew," concocted by John Kolmer of Temple University in Philadelphia.[3] The Kolmer vaccine in particular, and perhaps the Brodie–Park vaccine as well, caused several cases of poliomyelitis but conferred no immunity. More than a decade later, the memory of the fiascoes still inspired widespread concern about the safety of polio vaccines.

These qualms had become tempered by the early 1950s, as scientists made considerable progress toward the creation of a safe vaccine. By the late 1940s, several groups of researchers had independently identified the three distinct types of poliovirus, a microbial distinction that was essential to the development of an effective vaccine.

At Harvard, John Enders, Frederick Robbins, and Thomas Weller developed a method of growing poliovirus in nonneural tissue using a tissue culture of monkey kidneys—a seminal achievement that won them the Nobel Prize in 1954. At the University of Cincinnati, Albert Sabin began work on a live attenuated oral vaccine that he insisted would provide better immunity than a killed-virus vaccine but that would not be ready for widespread use until 1961. Jonas Salk, who relied on older vaccine-production methods involving formalin-killed viral strains, was able to proceed more rapidly. By early 1953, Salk had begun campaigning relentlessly for a national field trial of his vaccine.

For this critical but unglamorous task, the NFIP turned to Salk's former teacher, Thomas Francis, who had introduced Salk to the design of killed-virus vaccines, and his staff of epidemiologists at the University of Michigan School of Public Health. Francis had a sterling reputation as an investigator and was internationally known for his deft direction of complex field trials of influenza virus vaccines during World War II. He agreed to conduct the polio-vaccine field trials if three inviolable rules were followed: there would have to be two study groups, one given vaccine and another, at least as large as the vaccine group, given placebo; the trial would have to be conducted in a double-blind manner; and the NFIP was not to interfere. The study formally began on April 26, 1954, when Randy Kerr, a six-year-old boy from McLean, Virginia, received the first inoculation.

No detail of the field trial escaped Francis's watchful gaze—from complex issues of experimental design to such mundane matters as the packaging of vaccine, the composition of safety instructions for parents, and the selection of the "Polio Pioneers," the 650,000 children who received the vaccine and the 1.18 million who received a placebo. The trial relied for its implementation on some 150,000 volunteers, 15,000 schools, and 44 state departments of health. Francis admirably withstood the strain of conducting an extremely complex, high-stakes experiment in public. Thanks to the relentless campaign of the March of Dimes and the fear that polio and polio vaccines inspired, it was critical that Francis's design be free of bias and confounding variables and that there be no ethical lapses in the conduct of the trial. Everything worked out beautifully.

Coincidentally, Francis's announcement was to be made on the 10th anniversary of Franklin Roosevelt's death, the earliest date by which the University of Michigan's carpenters could complete construction of the long platform that would accommodate the battery of television cameras and radio microphones and the hundreds of photographers and journalists who would cover the event. Before a jam-packed audience of scientists and dignitaries, Francis approached the lectern. He began his speech with two simple declarative sentences: "The vaccine works. It is safe, effective, and potent." He then explained that the Salk vaccine was 60 to 70 percent effective in preventing infection with type 1 poliovirus, the most prevalent strain, and at least 90 percent effective against types 2 and 3.

Thrilling as this news was, there was one person in the auditorium who was visibly unhappy with Francis's report: Jonas Salk. As the diminutive virologist took the podium after Francis's speech, an avalanche of applause greeted him. Yet this public show of appreciation on the part of his scientific peers—a group that had never been accused of being overly effusive—was not enough for Salk, who felt compelled to insist that he had created nothing less than the perfect vaccine. Too flustered even to mention the names of the colleagues who had worked with him at Pittsburgh, Salk assailed the accuracy of Francis's findings. The failures encountered in the trial, he declared, were caused by Merthiolate, a mercury-based antiseptic that had been added to the batches of vaccine, against Salk's wishes, at the express orders of the U.S. Laboratory of Biologics Control. With a dramatic flourish, Salk proclaimed that his new and improved (Merthiolate-free) vaccine might well be 100 percent effective.

Salk's comments created a controversy that his critics used to disparage him for the rest of his career. Backstage, a furious Francis was heard scolding his former postdoctoral fellow. "What the hell did you have to say that for?" Francis railed. "You're in no position to claim 100 percent effectiveness. What's the matter with you?"[4]

Salk's failure to recognize the achievements of his coworkers and his injudicious (albeit ultimately correct) claims aside, the rest of the world was eager to lionize him as a bona fide medical hero. As the journalists scrambled out of the auditorium to call their editors, the spotlight of fame permanently shifted from the epidemiologist to the young creator of the polio vaccine. For many days, there wasn't a front page of a newspaper, a television or radio show, or a newsreel that did not shower Jonas Salk with praise and gratitude. For millions of parents and their children around the world, Salk became the avatar of medical progress. Even so, a decade later, Salk admitted, "I was not unscathed by Ann Arbor."[2]

I recently went to my medical school's library to peruse Francis's published, but rarely checked out, account of the 1954 field trial. The book is written in clear, elegant prose, and even a casual reader will recognize its author as a model of scientific integrity, ethical treatment of human subjects, and thorough attention to epidemiologic detail.[5] Still, even in the face of this impressive historical document, it takes little imagination to understand why April 12, 1955, turned out to be Jonas Salk's day. After all, he developed the first effective vaccine against polio; his teacher merely undertook the chore of testing its efficacy on a mass scale and then confirmed to the world that Salk had succeeded. The annals of medical history are replete with such distinctions.

Yet one of the great benefits of reflecting on the past is the opportunity to adjust one's understanding of events and human interactions. The morning after the announcement, the *New York Times* heralded Francis's vaccine report as a "medical classic." No one has ever refuted this conclusion. History would be well served if Tommy Francis's contributions were restored to view.

[*This essay originally appeared as: Markel, H.: April 12, 1955: Tommy Francis and the Salk Vaccine. New England Journal of Medicine 2005; 352(14):1408–1410*].

REFERENCES

1. Gould T. *A Summer Plague: Polio and its Survivors*. (New Haven, Conn.: Yale University Press, 1995), pp. 150–151.
2. Carter R. *Breakthrough; The Saga of Jonas Salk*. (New York: Trident Press, 1966), pp. 15–16, 269.
3. Paul J.R. *A History of Poliomyelitis*. (New Haven, Conn.: Yale University Press, 1971), pp. 252–262.
4. Smith J.S. *Patenting the Sun: Polio and the Salk Vaccine*. (New York: William Morrow, 1990), pp. 320–325.
5. Francis T. Jr. *Evaluation of the 1954 Field Trial of Poliomyelitis Vaccine*. (Ann Arbor, Mich.: Edwards Brothers and the National Foundation for Infantile Paralysis, 1957).

CHAPTER 20

∽

John Harvey Kellogg and
the Pursuit of Wellness

T.C. Boyle. *The Road to Wellville.*
(New York: The Viking Press, 1993).

In 1888, the powerful Michigan Central Railway erected a Romanesque train station in a remote hamlet in southwestern Michigan called Battle Creek. It was built to accommodate the multitude of health-seeking pilgrims flocking from all over the United States and Europe to "take the cure" at the town's luxurious sanitarium.[1]

Passing under the station's arches of rough-hewn gray granite and Lake Superior brick between 1870 and well into the Great Depression were such luminaries as John D. Rockefeller, Jr, fleeing from the disastrous events in his family's coal mines at Ludlow, Colorado; Thomas Edison and Henry Ford, whenever they were in need of a tune-up or recharge from the stresses of industrial gigantism; Amelia Earhart, before her important flights; Warren G. Harding, before embarking on his presidential run; and Booker T. Washington and Sojourner Truth, nursing wounds fresh from fighting the war against racism.

Unlike the warm mineral baths at Wiesbaden or the saintly waters at Lourdes, the Battle Creek Sanitarium (affectionately known as "the San") possessed no natural physical charms for restoring health. Instead, it became a world-renowned destination of health and healing thanks to the charismatic ministering of its director, Dr. John Harvey Kellogg. A medical celebrity, best-selling author, magazine editor, skilled surgeon, public health expert, popular speaker, and Seventh-day Adventist Christian missionary, Dr. Kellogg was a most impressive man. At 5 feet 4 inches tall, rotund yet athletic, and dressed entirely in white, the bespectacled, pointy-bearded

Literatim: Essays at the Intersections of Medicine and Culture. Howard Markel, Oxford University Press (2020).
© Oxford University Press.
DOI: 10.1093/oso/9780190087647.001.0001

physician proclaimed that God had chosen him to make the world a healthier place.[2,3]

During his storied career, hundreds of thousands of persons with serious illnesses ranging from cancer and cardiac disease to gastric ulcers and debilitating digestive disorders demanded Dr. Kellogg's treatments, which combined modern medicine, surgery, and bacteriology with an eclectic blend of hydropathy, vegetarianism, exercise, and spiritual uplift. Every day, hundreds of sickly passengers stepped off the train platforms for a long line of coaches operated by liveried horsemen. Welcoming them at the stately portico of the San was a veritable army of more than a thousand health soldiers. Included in this number were dozens of attentive physicians and many hundreds of nurses, masseuses, bakers, waiters, cooks, bellhops, orderlies, and attendants—all under the command of the good Doctor Kellogg, who examined every patient and prescribed to each an individualized treatment plan guaranteed to save the body, mind, and soul.

Many hundreds of thousands more, who today might be called the "wealthy and worried well," came to Battle Creek as day visitors. Once there, they sat and learned at the master's feet about the myriad ways they could improve their diets, bodily functions, and mental well-being. Cynical journalists mocked John Harvey Kellogg's followers as "Battle Freaks." Such jibes hardly mattered. Whether he was lecturing in his tinny, flat Midwestern accent to standing room–only audiences, treating patients in his clinic and operating room, or communicating in exuberant prose to millions of readers, Kellogg was without question one of the most famous physicians in the United States.[4-6]

The San's luxurious lobby, richly adorned with thick Persian rugs, brightly lit crystal-and-brass chandeliers, and the finest walnut and oak furniture, was the size of a football field. Attached to this welcoming hall was a lush indoor palm garden with 20-foot banana trees providing fresh fruit daily for its visitors. Throughout the facility were 5 acres of indestructible marble flooring in which, bragged the colorful advertising brochures, "germs and vermin can never find a lodging."[7]

Looming above the main entrance was a 15-story tower housing more than 1,200 well-appointed bedrooms, dozens of hygienically perfect operating suites, and a modern clinic for medical examinations. Alongside this building was a massive power plant that provided the raw energy required for the Sanitarium's insatiable central heating and cooling, refrigeration, cooking, maintenance, laundry, bathing, electric, and lighting needs.

In a separate but connected structure were 8 white-tiled indoor pools and hundreds of baths that would have made the ancient Romans jealous. Down the hall from the bathrooms was Dr. Kellogg's *sanctum sanctorum*, the enema room, stuffed with gleaming "enema machines" that could pointedly deliver 15 quarts of water per minute into a human colon. Dr. Kellogg ordered his patients to produce 4 or more bowel movements a day, just like the healthy apes he observed in zoos all around the globe. The son of a broom manufacturer, John Harvey Kellogg was obsessed with bodily cleanliness, both external and internal. If the water enemas were not enough, he ordered his patients to consume a pint of yogurt each day, followed by a yogurt enema.[8]

High colonics aside, Dr. Kellogg understood the importance of rest and relaxation for his patients and treated them to the finest entertainments and diversions. He constructed a theater and lecture hall to present morality plays, lantern slide shows, and health dialogues; he staffed his ballrooms with a full-time orchestra and choir for nightly dances and musicales; elsewhere on the vast campus were stables housing teams of horses, carriages, and sleighs; an army of bicycles at the ready for rides through the San's labyrinth of wooded trails; a deer park; and manicured fields for all kinds of sporting games.

Throughout his career, Dr. Kellogg warned that consuming meat was the gastronomic equivalent of a death wish. A vegetarian long before that term was commonly used, Dr. Kellogg developed his dietetic theories in protest against that era's standard fare of fatty, salted meats and fried foods.

Every meal served in Kellogg's fabled dining room consisted of his own culinary creations: a version of peanut butter, nut-based meat substitutes, vegetable-. and whole grain–based dishes, artificial coffee made with toasted bran and molasses, and—his most famous contribution to the dining table—corn flakes. He commanded that every bite of these meals be chewed at least 40 times so that a person's saliva would thoroughly mix with the food, thus initiating a healthy process of digestion and preventing overtaxing the stomach and bowels. He also required his patients to drink 8 or more glasses of water each day. Many of his well-heeled, well-intentioned patients simply could not commit to such a dietary regimen. Hence, the flourishing business at a little joint down the road called the Red Onion Tavern, where the incurables inhaled Cuban cigars, chewed sirloin steaks drowned in gravy and onions, and drank tumblers of malt whisky before running back to the San to make the 11 pm curfew.

In keeping with his philosophy of wellness and disease prevention—or, as he called it, "biological living"—Dr. Kellogg insisted on daily, vigorous exercise; plenty of fresh air; and complete abstinence from sex except for procreation, alcohol, caffeine, and tobacco. One of J.H. Kellogg's most popular books, *Tobaccoism*, was published in 1922 and is considered by many medical historians to be the first popular text alerting Americans to the dangers of tobacco smoking.[9]

In recent years journalists, novelists, and screenwriters have lampooned his life and somewhat unconventional theories. None have done so more famously or outlandishly than T.C. Boyle in his imaginative novel *The Road to Wellville*, which in 1994 was transformed into a popular film, starring Anthony Hopkins as a remarkably weird Dr. Kellogg, Matthew Broderick as a dyspeptic neurotic suffering from constipation and autointoxication, and a malevolent George Kellogg, one of Dr. Kellogg's adopted sons, who sets fire to the Sanitarium and burns it to the ground (the fire was real, in 1902; the culprit was never found and George was far too young to be a suspect for what was most likely an electrical fire).

Quack ideas, sexual prudishness taken to the extreme and even his pseudoscientific, racist views on race and heredity aside, John Harvey Kellogg helped give the nation a thorough cleansing from the grime and sickness that characterized the Gilded Age and the Progressive Era.[10,11] Eccentric, perhaps; but just as his Michigan peers Henry Ford and Thomas Edison ruled over their vast empires of automobiles and electricity, in his day John Harvey Kellogg was the industrial king of wellness.

[*This essay originally appeared as: Markel, H., John Harvey Kellogg and the Pursuit of Wellness. Journal of the American Medical Association. 2011; 305 (17): 1814-1815.*]

REFERENCES

1. Whorton, J.C. *Crusaders for Fitness: The History of American Health Reformers.* (Princeton, NJ: Princeton University Press, 1982).
2. Schwarz, R.W. *John Harvey Kellogg: Pioneering Health Reformer.* (Hagerstown, MD: Review & Herald Publishing, 2006).
3. Numbers, R.L. *Prophetess of Health: A Study of Ellen G. White.* 3rd ed. (Grand Rapids, MI: William B. Eerdmans Pub. Co, 2008).
4. Kellogg, J.H. *Plain Facts for Old and Young: Embracing the Natural History and Hygiene of Organic Life.* (Burlington, Iowa: I.F. Segner, 1886).
5. Kellogg, J.H. *The Itinerary of a Breakfast.* (Battle Creek, MI: Good Health Publishing Co., 1918).
6. Kellogg, J.H. *Man, the Masterpiece.* (Battle Creek, MI: Good Health Publishing Co., 1891).
7. Kellogg, J.H. *The Battle Creek Sanitarium: Origin, Purpose, Methods.* (Battle Creek, MI: Good Health Publishing Co., 1924).
8. Green, H. *Fit for America: Health, Fitness, Sport.* (New York, NY: Pantheon Books, 1986).
9. Kellogg, J.H. *Tobaccoism.* (Battle Creek, MI: Good Health Publishing Co, 1922).
10. Carson, G. *Cornflake Crusade: From the Pulpit to the Breakfast Table.* (New York, NY: Rinehart & Co, 1957).
11. I describe Dr. Kellogg's repugnant views on eugenics and "race betterment" in my book, *The Kelloggs: The Battling Brothers of Battle Creek.* (New York: Pantheon Books, 2017).

PART III

Medical Performances

CHAPTER 21

∽

Grasping at Straws

Eugene O'Neill, Tuberculosis, and Transformation

Long before he sat down to compose the dramas that have enlightened and haunted audiences by the millions, Eugene O'Neill contracted tuberculosis. Like most serious illnesses, it forever changed him. In O'Neill's case, the infection was a transformation that enabled him to divine his genius and artistic soul.

Sometime in the fall of 1912, the 24-year-old O'Neill developed a "bad cold" accompanied by tonsillitis that refused to resolve. In the following weeks, he experienced bouts of hemoptysis and pleurisy. By Thanksgiving his physician diagnosed tuberculosis, which in the decades leading up to World War II was the leading cause of death for Americans aged 20 to 45 years.[1] Unlike the lyric and romantic plights portrayed in Verdi's *La Traviata* or Puccini's *La Boheme*, not to mention a slew of Victorian novels, O'Neill understood all too clearly that the bacilli brewing in his lungs posed a serious threat to his longevity.[2]

O'Neill's initial diagnosis with tuberculosis was most famously recounted in his masterpiece *Long Day's Journey Into Night*.[3] Less well known is that one of his earliest plays, *The Straw*, was drawn from his experiences as a patient in a tuberculosis sanatorium.[4] Aptly, O'Neill used the metaphor of the children's game of drawing straws for his title: when it came to tuberculosis, like so many other aspects of life, he insisted, some seemed to randomly draw more short than long straws. Written in 1918-1919 and set in 1910, *The Straw* is a compelling drama depicting a poignant love affair between two patients with tuberculosis and markedly different fates, a young reporter named Stephen Murray and a woman, Eileen Carmody. Aside from its literary merit, the play faithfully documents the daily routines of an early 20th-century tuberculosis sanatorium.

Literatim: Essays at the Intersections of Medicine and Culture. Howard Markel, Oxford University Press (2020).
© Oxford University Press.
DOI: 10.1093/oso/9780190087647.001.0001

The ancient Greeks had a wonderful word to describe the ravages of tuberculosis: *phthisis,* from the root *phote*, which describes a living body that shrivels with intense heat as if placed on a flame. A few centuries later, the Romans used the Latin word *consumare* (to consume or devour) to describe how unchecked tuberculosis consumes with a passionate and incisive energy, slowly and inexorably devouring the structure of the lungs and other critical organs with the single goal of conquering its host—but not until the progeny of the bacillus have had the opportunity to travel to and settle in the lungs of another human being to start the horrific process all over again.[1] Consequently, even as late as the opening decades of the 20th century, physicians and patients still referred to the disease as "consumption."

Eugene's father, James O'Neill, initially elected to send his son to the Fairfield County State Tuberculosis Sanatorium, in Shelton, Connecticut, a few miles from New Haven. Those who could afford it were charged $4 a week; those who could not were admitted free of charge and supported by the state. In 1854, at the age of 9, James immigrated from famine-struck Ireland to the slums of Buffalo, New York. He eventually metamorphosed himself into a successful actor who played on Broadway and across the nation in roles ranging from Shakespearian heroes and villains to, most famously, the Count of Monte Cristo. Long after becoming relatively wealthy, however, James O'Neill could never shake off his difficult years of abject poverty and was notoriously tight-fisted.

Penury aside, the choice of Fairfield suggested that James was not exactly sanguine about Eugene's chances of recovery. When father and son arrived at the seedy institution on December 9, 1912, they found that the physical plant consisted of little more than a ramshackle clinic building and a smattering of cottages housing exceedingly ill patients. Dressed in a brand-new, dark-gray, single-breasted suit that James had hand-tailored for his son, Eugene was admitted but stayed only two days. Eugene's low state of mind combined with an appeal made by his physician inspired James O'Neill to cough up the cash and send the young man to a far posher facility, the Gaylord Farm Sanatorium in Wallingford, Connecticut. There, Eugene's physician advised, "he'd meet a better class of people."[2(p.375)]

Fittingly, the word *sanatorium* comes from the Latin root for a house to which an individual went to be cured. The best of the early 20th-century tuberculosis sanatoria in the United States were bucolic, woodsy encampments of cottages surrounded by fresh air and mountain views, such as the famed Saranac Lake Sanatorium in the Adirondacks, a hospital that catered to wealthy patients including author Robert Louis Stevenson and New York Giants pitching ace Christy Mathewson. In Europe, private tuberculosis hospitals were even more elaborate, such as the Alps-based facility described by Thomas Mann in his novel *The Magic Mountain*.[5] Incidentally, the location of many, but certainly not all, tuberculosis sanatoria at high altitudes was a serendipitous, therapeutic discovery. During the late 19th century, physicians noted that their patients recuperated faster at altitudes where the oxygen content of the air was thin, although it took many decades more for microbiologists to appreciate that *Mycobacterium tuberculosis* thrives best at altitudes with rich oxygen concentrations. The concomitant cold temperatures of these mountain retreats were also thought to be healing, and patients with tuberculosis typically slept in open-air sleeping porches, exposed to the elements.

The exclusive and expensive private sanatoria could never serve the tens of thousands of Americans afflicted with tuberculosis who needed care each year. As a result, there existed a wide range of state- or municipal-run isolation hospitals. Regardless of the medical, economic, or social circumstances of the patients each facility admitted, all tuberculosis sanatoria were framed by strict rules on how patients should act, sleep, dress, and exercise; what and when they should eat; and even with whom they should and should not associate. Relationships between men and women patients were strictly forbidden. Patients endured weekly weigh-ins to make sure their disease was being held in check rather than "consuming" their bodies. Those who failed to improve with the help of the prescribed dietary and fresh-air regimens were often transferred to an "incurables" facility so as not to diminish the "cure rate" of a particular sanatorium, essential to recruiting new and paying customers.[1,6-11]

Epidemiologists and medical historians have suggested that there was a definite public health benefit to these institutions beyond the care offered on an individual basis. Decades before the advent of antibiotics, physicians observed a striking decrease in the incidence of tuberculosis in Europe and the United States. In 1923, the eminent British public health official Sir Arthur Newsholme theorized that the decline of tuberculosis in his country resulted from reduced exposure to infection brought about by the segregation of impoverished and immigrant persons with tuberculosis in Poor Law Infirmaries. This same trend was noted in the United States during the 1930s, when tuberculosis isolation hospitals facilitated the separation of the ill and infectious from the healthy population. This arrangement may have contributed to the steady decline in cases during this period, which only accelerated with the advent of the powerful anti-tuberculosis drugs developed in the late 1940s.[12]

Much of the plot of *The Straw* is based on Eugene's relationship with another Gaylord Farm Sanatorium patient named Catherine "Kitty" Mackay, who hailed from a working class Irish family in nearby Waterbury. Kitty had been treated at Gaylord for 5 months a year earlier, but because her mother was dead and she was the principal caregiver for her 9 younger sisters and brothers, she was prematurely discharged. When Eugene met her in March of 1913, Kitty was 23 and seriously ill. O'Neill was attracted by Kitty's beauty and thirst for knowledge. Of note, there were two major infractions at Gaylord that could lead to immediate discharge. The first was drinking alcohol; the second was love affairs between patients. Between his relationship with Kitty and his legendary consumption of alcohol, Eugene broke both these rules but, apparently, with no repercussions.

By May 1913, 5 months after his admission to Gaylord, Eugene's weight had increased from 148 to 164 pounds, and his physicians declared him cured. After convincing James that he was not a contagious threat to his family and bidding farewell to the physicians, nurses, and Kitty, Eugene returned to his family's cottage in New London, Connecticut, on Long Island Sound, the very home that served as the setting for both *Ah Wilderness!* and *Long Day's Journey Into Night.* He never saw Kitty again. She was discharged 6 months after Eugene but, according to the Gaylord Farm records, died on May 17, 1915.[2 (pp.392,393)]

While no document exists to describe the details of Kitty and Eugene's parting, O'Neill concluded his dramatic version of it in *The Straw* with a cured Stephen returning to the sanatorium to find the desperately ill Eileen. Stephen pledges to return even as Eileen acknowledges the meeting will likely be their last. "I love you—love you—remember," Eileen declares as she runs back into the hospital. Stephen starts after her but stops short, cursing and clenching his hands in "impotent rage at himself and at fate" as the final curtain is rung down.[4 (p.101)]

Seven months after his discharge from Gaylord Farm, O'Neill wrote a note of appreciation to his physician David R. Lyman and expressed the wish to visit the sanatorium: "If, as they say, it is sweet to visit the place one was born in, then it will be doubly sweet for me to visit the place I was reborn in—for my second birth was the only one which had my full approval."

Throughout his life, Eugene O'Neill credited his hospitalization with inspiring him to plumb the depths of his psyche, a tool necessary for a life of composing his profound dramas. In essence, tuberculosis provided O'Neill with a second chance at life, when, as he noted to his physician, "[I] should have been cast down by my fate—and wasn't."[2 (pp.388,389)]

[This essay originally appeared as: Markel, H. Grasping at Straws: Eugene O'Neill, Tuberculosis, and Transformation. Journal of the American Medical Association. 2010; 303 (13): 1316–1317].

REFERENCES

1. Markel H. *When Germs Travel: Six Major Epidemics That Have Invaded America Since 1900 and the Fears They Have Unleashed.* (New York, NY: Pantheon Books, 2004), pp. 14–46.
2. Gelb A, Gelb B. *O'Neill: Life With Monte Cristo.* (New York, NY: Applause Books, 2000), pp. 369–393.
3. O'Neill E. *Long Day's Journey Into Night.* (New Haven, CT: Yale University Press, 1955).
4. O'Neill E. *The Straw.* In: *The Emperor Jones, Diff'rent, and The Straw.* (New York, NY: Boni & Liveright, 1921).
5. Mann T. *The Magic Mountain.* Wood JE, trans. (New York, NY: Vintage Books/Random House, 1996).
6. Trudeau E.L. *An Autobiography.* (Garden City, CA: Doubleday Page & Co., 1916).
7. Ellison D. *Healing Tuberculosis in the Woods: Medicine and Science at the End of the Nineteenth Century.* (Westport, CT: Greenwood Press, 1994).
8. Rothman S. *Living in the Shadow of Death: Tuberculosis and the Social Experience of Illness in American History.* (New York, NY: Basic Books, 1994), pp. 211–241.
9. Feldberg G. *Disease and Class: Tuberculosis and the Shaping of Modern North American Society.* (New Brunswick, NJ: Rutgers University Press, 1995).

10. Ott K. *Fevered Lives: Tuberculosis in American Culture Since 1870.* (Cambridge, MA: Harvard University Press, 1996), pp. 69–86.
11. Dormandy T. *The White Death: A History of Tuberculosis.* (New York, NY: New York University Press, 2000), pp. 147–186.
12. Wilson L.G. The historical decline of tuberculosis in Europe and America: its causes and significance. *J Hist Med Allied Sci.* 1990; 45(3): 366–396.

CHAPTER 22

ᴄᴌᴏ

Men in White

The Operating Room's Debut Into Popular American Culture

Today's television viewers are relentlessly exposed to endless dramas, documentaries, and "reality" shows centered on the operating room. But the dramatization of the surgeon's workshop, replete with urgent calls for scalpels and sponges, represents a rather recent wrinkle in the long history of American popular culture. To be more precise, on September 26, 1933, the operating room made its Broadway debut in Sidney Kingsley's medical melodrama, *Men in White*.[1] Its opening curtain essentially lifted a sluice gate, releasing a torrent of medical shows for public consumption.

The now famous but then barely surviving Group Theatre produced what turned out to be a smashing success. Gushing over the production's realistic portrayal of life in an urban general hospital, critic Brooks Atkinson described the play in the *New York Times* as forceful and "warm with life and high in aspiration . . . it has a contagious respect for the theme it discusses."[2,3] Equally effusive, the crusty Joseph Wood Krutch of *The Nation* categorized *Men in White* as a "genuine work of art."[4] Several months later, the play was awarded the Pulitzer Prize for the best play of 1933.

Lee Strasberg, Harold Clurman, and Cheryl Crawford founded the Group Theatre in 1931. By all accounts it was a hotbed of novel theories on acting and the social role of the theater, petty jealousies, love triangles, and political foment. Inspired by the Stanislavsky system of acting (named for Constantin Stanislavsky, the director of the Moscow Art Players), Strasberg and his colleagues developed a rigorous curriculum that guided generations of successful stage and screen actors.

Literatim: Essays at the Intersections of Medicine and Culture. Howard Markel, Oxford University Press (2020).
© Oxford University Press.
DOI: 10.1093/oso/9780190087647.001.0001

Perhaps Strasberg's most significant albeit controversial contribution to what came to be called "Method Acting" was an emphasis on improvisation and affective or emotional memory.[5-9]

In rehearsals, Strasberg extracted painful psychological moments, or affective memories, from the actor's real life to help animate the raw emotions called for by the script at hand. The process was brutal in its exposure and reduced many actors to tears.[5] He also ordered his actors to trail real physicians in the hospital to gather a realistic sense of the profession. Stage and film director Elia Kazan played the minor role of a young physician named Vitale in the original production of *Men in White*. Fifty-five years later, he chillingly recalled Strasberg's directorial modus operandi:

> [H]e carried with him the aura of a prophet, a magician, a witch doctor, a psychoanalyst, and a feared father of a Jewish home … unswerving, uncompromising, and unadjustable. Lee knew this. He studied other revolutions, political and artistic. He knew what was needed, and he was fired up by his mission and its importance.[10]

Apparently, there was method to this madness; even Kazan begrudgingly admitted that "Lee's production [of *Men in White*], at moments, seemed like a modern ballet; it relied not on words, but on movement, activity, and behavior. In the theatre of the time, this was new."[10]

Historians of the McCarthy era often recall the Group Theatre for its Communist sympathies during the 1930s. These associations became especially controversial in 1952, when Kazan named 8 of his former Group Theatre comrades, and several others, as members of the Communist Party during his testimony to the U.S. House of Representatives Un-American Activities Committee (HUAC).[11]

That said, it is difficult to identify a "party line" from reading the play's text. Instead, the paramount theme of *Men in White* is the beck-and-call relationship between physician and patient. Everything else—loved ones, leisure activities, even sleep—is secondary to the care and treatment of the ill. Exemplifying this professional ideal are a stellar and compassionate intern named George Ferguson and his mentor, the eminent and wise Dr. Hochberg. A masterful surgeon, Hochberg has selected George to become his successor, with the stipulation that he complete many years more of grueling training at the hospital and intensive postgraduate work and research in Vienna. If he accepts, George stands an excellent chance of becoming as great a servant to humanity as Hochberg. The price is the sacrifice of his youth and absolute commitment of his industry.

Early in the first act, the audience is introduced to George's impatient fiancée, Laura Hudson, a beautiful and spoiled socialite whose wealthy father is one of Hochberg's patients and a potential benefactor to the hospital. Unfortunately, Laura shows little tolerance when George's patient responsibilities demand that he break dinner dates with her. Scheming to tempt George into a softer career path free of Hochberg's demands, she asks her father to arrange for George to be prematurely promoted to attending physician rank at the hospital and handed the keys to a profitable private practice for the worried well.

After still another cancelled date, however, Laura truculently calls off the engagement. This romantic rupture sends George into the arms of an attractive and willing student nurse named Mary. Given the theatrical conventions of the day, of course, the real action occurs offstage. The penalty for acting on such lustful impulses is revealed in a subsequent scene, when Mary is urgently admitted to the hospital. Stricken by the sequelae of a frankly described, septic, and presumably illegally performed abortion, George rushes her into the operating room.

One of the most memorable aspects of the original production was a precisely choreographed and brilliantly lit pantomime of surgeons scrubbing, gowning, gloving, and operating. Hochberg invites Laura, and by extension the audience, into the operating room to watch. After accidentally contaminating George by hugging him, she is ushered to the back of the chamber before hurriedly exiting the room. Not even acknowledging her departure, Hochberg dramatically holds out his hand and demands, "Scalpel." Today, the scene would elicit yawns from seasoned couch potatoes and medical drama buffs who have been entertained by such surgical derring-do for decades. But in 1933, this stunning scene made theatrical history as it introduced large audiences to a *sanctum sanctorum* once accessible only to surgeons and nurses. Producer Cheryl Crawford recalled years later that it was "as painful as the scalpel making the incision."[12]

Understandably upset over discovering George's sexual indiscretion with Mary, Laura is shocked to further learn that George's surgical efforts to save Mary's life have failed: a few hours after the operation, Mary died of embolism. Remarkably, Laura—glowing with pride over George's intention to answer his professional calling—rises to the occasion, and a vague but promising rapprochement occurs. Predictably, the loudspeaker trumpets still another urgent page for George and interrupts their final goodbye. Laura sends George on his way and coyly suggests that he call her while in Vienna. A repentant George nods and returns to his medical tasks, followed by the closing curtain, boisterous applause, and multiple bows.

Attracted by the play's rave reviews and, more pragmatically, the long lines of theatergoers at the Broadhurst Theatre on West 43rd Street, agents for William Randolph Hearst came knocking on the stage door. In late 1933, his Cosmopolitan Pictures, a unit of Hollywood's famed Metro-Goldwyn-Mayer Studios (MGM), purchased the motion picture rights. On April 6, 1934, while the play was still running on Broadway, MGM released their version of *Men in White*. It starred a strikingly young Clark Gable, *sans* moustache, as George; the frosty yet fetching Myrna Loy as Laura; and the avuncular and Teutonic Jean Hersholt as Hochberg.[13,14] The director assigned to the film was a Russian émigré named Richard Boleslavsky, a prized pupil of Stanislavsky's who taught Lee Strasberg and Harold Clurman at the American Laboratory Theatre School in New York in the early 1920s. Although an entertaining and superbly produced motion picture, little in the footage suggests that Gable or Loy submitted to the deep psychological introspection required by Method Acting.

Method aside, one of the most exciting scenes in both the play and the film depicts a 10-year-old girl with diabetes mellitus who suddenly becomes pale, clammy, cold, and unresponsive after complaining of hunger. Her physician, a pompous fop named Cunningham, misdiagnoses her condition as a diabetic coma and orders a hefty dose of insulin to counteract what he perceives to be the effects of hyperglycemia and ketoacidosis. George instantly recognizes that the little girl is actually experiencing the reverse condition, the diabetic shock of severe hypoglycemia, and countermands the call for insulin, knowing it will only worsen the situation. A fierce argument ensues, with Cunningham severely reprimanding George as the little girl's clinical condition continues to deteriorate. Ignoring the commands of his superior, George assumes control and barks for syringes filled with glucose and adrenaline. The girl is dramatically brought back from the brink of death thanks to George's ministrations, as Cunningham slithers off the stage, stethoscope in hand.

Admirers of both the play and the film will discover some elements lost in translation. For example, Mary's septic abortion is never explicitly mentioned in the movie, and Mary and George's illicit relationship is handled with allegiance to the prevailing motion picture code of morality, even though the attentive viewer will understand what occurred between them. Strasberg's stage pantomime–ballet of the operating room is transformed in the MGM production into a visually pleasing kaleidoscopic montage shot of autoclaves in action and surgeons at work.

Today, *Men in White* is rarely read, viewed, or performed. Adding insult to obscurity, a crude parody is far better recalled than the original. In 1934, Columbia Pictures released a Three Stooges short called *Men in Black*.[15] Legions of Stooges fans over the past 8 decades have squealed with delight when hearing the episode's most memorable line: "Calling Doctor Howard, Doctor Fine, Doctor Howard." Even though this line uses the surnames of Moe and Curly (Howard) and Larry (Fine), it was a direct steal from the play and film, in which the hospital's public address system constantly called physicians to duty. In their inimitable fashion, the Stooges soon become frustrated by the nonstop barrage of pages and attempt to disable the dispatch transmitter. Despite their worst, slapstick efforts, the machine assumes a life of its own and continues to belt out pages. In desperation, Larry, Moe, and Curly each pulls out a pistol and shoots it dead, "for duty and for humanity."

History has the power to play cruel tricks on many a creative endeavor, distorting the perceptions and opinions of subsequent generations. Although the spoof did garner the comedy trio's only Academy Award nomination (in 1934, for best short comedy subject), surely the literary legacy of *Men in White* deserves better than manipulation and ridicule by The Three Stooges. Indeed, as modern medicine negotiates its own tenuous slice of history, an era twisted and threatened by a battery of political, technological, ethical, economic, and social woes, the work of Sidney Kingsley, Lee Strasberg, and the Group Theatre as well as of Clark Gable, Myrna Loy, and MGM warrants thoughtful consideration by practitioners and consumers of medicine alike. Even from the distance of more than three-quarters of a century, their quest to idealize those noble instances when a physician sacrifices all for the good of patients remains both inspiring and powerful.

[*This essay originally appeared as: Markel, H.: Men in White: The Operating Room's Debut Into Popular American Culture. Journal of the American Medical Association. 2009; 302 (21):2376–2378.*]

REFERENCES

1. Kingsley S. *Men in White*. (New York, NY: Crown Publishers, 1933).
2. Atkinson B., The Play: men of medicine in a Group Theatre drama. *New York Times*. September 27, 1933:24.
3. Atkinson B. Medicine men. *New York Times*. October 1, 1933, Section 9, page 1.
4. Krutch J.W. Review of *Men in White*. *The Nation*. 1933; 137(3562): 419–420.
5. Clurman H. *The Fervent Years: The Group Theatre and the 30's*. (New York, NY: Harcourt Brace & Jovanovich, 1975), p. 62.
6. Strasberg L. *A Dream of Passion: The Development of the Method*. (Boston, MA: Little Brown, 1987), p. 7.
7. Adams C.H. *Lee Strasberg, the Imperfect Genius of the Actors Studio*. (New York, NY: Doubleday, 1980).
8. Schickel R. *Elia Kazan: A Biography*. (New York, NY: Harper Collins, 2005).
9. Smith W. *Real Life: The Group Theatre and America, 1931-1940*. (New York, NY: Alfred A Knopf, 1990).
10. Kazan E. *Elia Kazan: A Life*. (New York, NY: Alfred A Knopf, 1988), pp. 61–62, 103.
11. Testimony of Elia Kazan. April 11, 1952. In: Bentley E, ed. *Thirty Years of Treason: Excerpts From Hearings Before the House Committee on Un-American Activities, 1938–1968*. (New York, NY: Viking Press, 1971), pp. 482–495.
12. Crawford C. *One Naked Individual: My Fifty Years in the Theatre*. (Indianapolis, IN: Bobbs-Merrill, 1977), p. 65.
13. *Men in White* [DVD]. Hollywood, CA: Metro-Goldwyn-Mayer Studios; 1934.
14. Hall M. Clark Gable, Myrna Loy and Jean Hersholt in a film of "Men in White." *New York Times*. June 9, 1934:18.
15. *Men in Black* [DVD]. (Hollywood, CA: Columbia Pictures; 1934).

CHAPTER 23

∾

Not So Great Moments

The "Discovery" of Ether Anesthesia and
Its "Re-Discovery" by Hollywood

One of the truly great moments in medical history occurred on a tense fall morning in the surgical amphitheater of Boston's Massachusetts General Hospital. It was there, on October 16, 1846, that a dentist named William T. G. Morton administered an effective anesthetic to a surgical patient. Consenting to what became a most magnificent scientific revolution were John Warren, an apprehensive surgeon, and Glenn Abbott, an even more nervous young man about to undergo removal of a vascular tumor on the left side of his neck. Both Warren and Abbott sailed through the procedure painlessly, although some have noted that Abbott moved a bit near the end. Turning away from the operating table toward the gallery packed with legitimately dumbstruck medical students, Warren gleefully exclaimed, "Gentlemen, this is no humbug!"[1]

Morton named his "creation" Letheon, after the Lethe river of Greek mythology. drinking its waters, the ancients contended, erased painful memories. Hardly such an exotic elixir, Morton's stuff was actually sulphuric ether. Regardless of composition, Letheon inspired a legion of enterprising surgeons to devise and execute an armamentarium of lifesaving, invasive procedures.[2]

Yet while the discovery of anesthesia was a bona fide blessing for humankind, it hardly turned out to be that great for either its "discoverer," William Morton, or the Hollywood director Preston Sturges, who, a century later, decided to make a film about it.

Morton began his dental studies in Baltimore in 1840. Two years later he set up practice in Hartford, ultimately working with a dentist named Horace Wells.

Literatim: Essays at the Intersections of Medicine and Culture. Howard Markel, Oxford University Press (2020).
© Oxford University Press.
DOI: 10.1093/oso/9780190087647.001.0001

At this time, surgeons could offer patients little beyond opium and alcohol to endure the agonizing pain engendered by scalpels. From the late 18th century well into the 1840s, physicians and chemists experimented with agents such as nitrous oxide, ether, carbon dioxide, and other mind-altering chemicals without success. In an era before the adoption of daily dental hygiene and fluoride treatments, excruciating tooth extractions were also a common part of the human experience. Consequently, dentists joined the holy grail–like search for substances to conquer operative pain.[3]

Around this time, Morton and Wells conducted experiments using nitrous oxide, including a demonstration at Harvard Medical School in 1845 that failed to completely squelch the pain of a student submitting to a tooth-pulling, thus publicly humiliating the dentists. Although Morton and Wells amicably dissolved their partnership, Morton continued his search for anesthetic agents.

A year earlier, in 1844, during studies at Harvard Medical School (which were cut short by financial difficulties), Morton attended the lectures of chemistry professor Charles Jackson. One lecture was on how the common organic solvent sulphuric ether could render a person unconscious and even insensate. Recalling these lessons during the summer of 1846, Morton purchased bottles of the stuff from his local chemist and began exposing himself and a menagerie of pets to ether fumes. Satisfied with its safety and reliability, he began using ether on his dental patients. Soon, mobs of tooth-aching, dollar-waving Bostonians made their way to his office. Morton relished his financial success but quickly perceived that Letheon was good for far more than pulling teeth.[4]

Morton's remarkable demonstration at the Massachusetts General Hospital transmogrified his status from profitable dentist to internationally acclaimed healer. But the half-life of his celebrity turned out to be *molto presto*, followed by an interminable period of infamy. In particular, he was lambasted for insisting on applying for an exclusive patent on Letheon. In the United States of the mid-19th century it was considered unseemly, if not greedy, for members of the medical profession to profit from discoveries that universally benefited humankind, particularly from a patent for what turned out to be the easily acquired sulphuric ether. As long as he stuck to dentistry, many physicians argued, Morton could do as he liked; but if he desired acceptance of Letheon by physicians and surgeons, he needed to comply with what they considered their higher-minded ideals and ethics. Morton aggressively rejected all such suggestions, much to his detriment. There was also the issue of credit. Horace Wells demanded his share. So did Crawford W. Long, a Georgia practitioner who claimed to have used nitrous oxide and ether as early as 1842 but who was too busy to publish his findings. Morton's former professor, Charles Jackson, argued that he, too, deserved a piece of the action.[1–5]

While many toyed with anesthetic agents, it was Morton who first developed a novel delivery instrument to enable ether inhalation during an operation. The device consisted of a glass flask with a wooden mouthpiece that could be opened and closed depending on the patient's state of consciousness. This was critical because other experimenters, including Wells and Long, could not ensure rapid reversibility of the anesthetic state and often overdosed their patients. Morton's genius resided not only in his observations of the power of ether but also in his development of a crude but scientific method of regulating its inhalation, thus creating the field of anesthesiology.

Not everyone saw it that way. Vigorously combating the whispered and shouted campaigns against him, the dentist spent his remaining days trying to restore his sullied reputation. Morton died broke and embittered in 1868. This controversial episode continues to fascinate historians, but it was most famously, and melodramatically, recounted in a best-selling 1938 book called *Triumph Over Pain* by René Fülöp-Miller.[1]

The publication of Fülöp-Miller's book coincided precisely with a period when Hollywood was hungry for motion pictures about medical research, such as Samuel Goldwyn's *Arrowsmith* (1931), Warner Brothers' *The Life of Louis Pasteur* (1936), and MGM's *Yellow Jack* (1938). Consequently, Paramount Pictures purchased an option on Fülöp-Miller's book and the property soon caught the eye of the studio's white-hot screenwriter-director, Preston Sturges.[6]

Between 1939 and 1944, Sturges created an acclaimed series of precisely timed, one liner–laden, screwball comedies. His Academy Award–winning *The Great McGinty* (1940), *The Lady Eve* (1941), *Sullivan's Travels* (1942), *Hail the Conquering Hero* (1944), and *The Miracle of Morgan's Creek* (1944) are among the most hilarious motion pictures ever committed to celluloid.[7,8] At first glance, wedding the story of anesthesia to a slapstick artiste seems mismatched. Yet as Sturges' biographer James Curtis observed, it was the "kind of dark, everything-right-gone-all-wrong story" that had long appealed to the director's sensibility and that, as it turned out, characterized his personal biography.[9]

Because Sturges simultaneously maintained a full production schedule while running a posh Hollywood restaurant-haunt, he did not get around to filming the anesthesia story until spring of 1942. Despite Sturges' sterling track record, Buddy DeSylva, Paramount Pictures' production chief, waged an abusive verbal war against the project. For DeSylva, the subject, the script, even the original title (eventually changed to *The Great Moment*), was "repulsive." On the one hand, Sturges feared DeSylva because of his boss' well-deserved reputation for capriciously wielding power in the hierarchical Hollywood studio system of the 1940s. But Sturges also considered DeSylva to be a know-nothing hack who was "full of beans."[9] Consequently, Sturges assumed that he could both win an artistic debate and convince the mogul of the film's social importance and enormous financial potential.[10,11]

Although Sturges took great literary license with Fülöp-Miller's popular historical potboiler, the contours of the story remain somewhat accurate. But instead of presenting Morton's life in chronological order, from birth to death, Sturges ended the film with Morton's "great moment" of October 16, 1846. In the dramatic closing scene, Warren demands that Morton tell him the ingredients of Letheon before administering it to his patient, as protection against quackery or worse. Morton understands that such a declaration would jeopardize his exclusive financial claim to ether but provides it anyway. The camera dissolves to a tableau of Morton's impoverished widow seated with a former dental patient, accompanied by the classic Hollywood prompt, "The End."

Defending his screenplay, Sturges wrote that "Unfortunately, I was not around in 1846 to direct Dr. Morton's life. I had to take it as I found it or construct an entirely fictitious story far removed from fact, as Pasteur was presented with a piece of Semmelweis's work in the Warner Brothers picture.... Dr. Morton's life, as lived, was a very bad piece of dramatic construction. He had a few months of excitement ending in triumph and twenty years of disillusionment, boredom and increasing bitterness."[9] Because the audience had already witnessed scenes from Morton's later life earlier in the film, the director argued, they would leave the theater inspired by his selfless gift of anesthesia to the world.

Predictably, DeSylva and the various pooh-bahs on the Paramount lot disagreed, complaining that the jumbled chronology culminating with a scene depicting the "middle" of Morton's life would confuse, if not alienate, moviegoers. Knowing that he had control over the final cut, DeSylva patiently waited until Sturges completed the film and then ruthlessly slashed footage from each reel. This was not the first time he had hacked away at one of Sturges' masterpieces, and his interventions were already a source of great resentment for the director. Nevertheless, the released 1944 version does end with a slightly trimmed scene depicting Morton's "great moment" pretty much as Sturges intended.[12]

The reviews ran the gamut from dismayed to disgusted and, true to DeSylva's prognosis, the film flopped. Soon after, Sturges entered negotiations to renew his contract with Paramount. Banking on the successes of his other 1944 films, *Hail the Conquering Hero* and *The Miracle of Morgan's Creek*, Sturges demanded unprecedented free reign to make his motion pictures without the studio's interference. DeSylva, focusing on the failure of *The Great Moment*, declined and Sturges left for the proverbial greener pastures. Never quite finding them, the director eventually realized that while healthy disagreement was essential to his craft, he sorely lacked the ability to handle the "dangerous aftermath" with his bosses. "The only amazing thing about my career in Hollywood," he admitted in 1959, "is that I ever had one at all."[9,13]

Sturges made several more films, first for an ill-fated company he ran briefly with Howard Hughes and, later, for other studios. But never again was he accorded the accolades that had accompanied his brief shining moment as Hollywood's King of Comedy. Over the next two decades, Sturges oscillated from false start, to flop, to near miss. Working on his memoirs, *The Events Leading Up to My Death*, he died alone in a hotel room in New York City in 1959.[13]

Morton and Sturges were men of different eras, sensibilities, and backgrounds. Yet, in an ironic twist of life imitating art, their biographies depict how one man's search to conquer pain and another's desire to record that struggle turned out to be so painful for both. Although Morton and Sturges were men of great accomplishment, they were also all too human. And like many human beings, Morton and Sturges aggressively hunted for fame, glory, professional success, and ego gratification at the expense of judiciously contemplating the consequences of their actions.

[This essay originally appeared as: Markel, H.: Not So Great Moments: The "Discovery" of Ether Anesthesia and its "Re-Discovery" by Hollywood. Journal of the American Medical Association. 2008; 300 (18):2188–2190].

REFERENCES

1. Fülöp-Miller R. *Triumph Over Pain*. Paul E, Paul C, trans. (New York, NY: Literary Guild of America, 1938).
2. Fenster J.M. *Ether Day: The Strange Tale of America's Greatest Medical Discovery and the Haunted Men Who Made It*. (New York, NY: Harper Perennial, 2002).
3. Nuland S. *Origins of Anesthesia*. (Birmingham, AL: Classics of Medicine Library, 1983).
4. Fulton J.F. William T. G. Morton. In: Malone D, ed. *Dictionary of American Biography*. Vol 13. (New York, NY: Charles Scribners Sons, 1934), pp. 268–271.
5. Morton W.T.G. *The Invention of Anesthetic Inhalation: or Discovery of Anaesthesia*. (New York, NY: D. Appleton & Co, 1880).
6. Dans PE. *Doctors in the Movies: Boil the Water and Just Say Aah*. (Bloomington, IL: Medi-Ed Press, 2000).
7. Sturges P. *Preston Sturges: The Filmmaker Collection: Sullivan's Travels, The Lady Eve, The Palm Beach Story, Hail the Conquering Hero, The Great McGinty, Christmas in July, and The Great Moment* [7-disk DVD]. (Los Angeles, CA: Universal Studios, 2006).
8. Sturges P. *The Miracle of Morgan's Creek* [DVD]. (Los Angeles, CA: Paramount Studios, 2005).
9. Curtis J. *Between Flops: A Biography of Preston Sturges*. (New York, NY: Harcourt Brace Jovanovich, 1982), pp. 168–193.
10. Jacobs D. *Christmas in July: The Life and Art of Preston Sturges*. (Berkeley: University of California Press, 1994).
11. Spoto D. *Madcap: The Life of Preston Sturges*. (Boston, MA: Little Brown & Co, 1990).
12. Henderson B. Introduction: *Triumph Over Pain/The Great Moment*. In: Sturges P. *Four More Screenplays by Preston Sturges*. Berkeley: University of California Press, 1995), pp. 241–364.
13. Sturges, P. *Preston Sturges by Preston Sturges: His Life in His Words*. (New York: Touchstone Books, 1991).

CHAPTER 24

⟨⟩

"Calling Dr. Kildare"

The Literary Lives of Frederick Schiller Faust, a.k.a. Max Brand

My earliest dreams of becoming a physician began while sitting far too close to a big, boxy Admiral television set and watching the 1961-1966 NBC series *Dr. Kildare*. As a boy, I was astounded at how the bright intern James Kildare, played by Richard Chamberlain, and his irascible but wise mentor, Dr. Leonard Gillespie, portrayed by Raymond Massey, always managed to cure their patients and send them on their merry way in a span of 60 minutes, including commercials.

Years later I learned that this television show hardly represented the first time Dr. Kildare had commanded a national audience. During my college days, a local cinema society presented the 9 Dr. Kildare films produced by Metro-Goldwyn-Mayer (MGM) between 1938 and 1942 and starring Lew Ayres as Kildare and Lionel Barrymore as Gillespie. Also showing were the 6 Dr. Gillespie films MGM made from 1942 to 1947. These subsequent movies did not include Dr. Kildare— or rather Lew Ayres—because the actor declared himself to be a conscientious objector during World War II. Even though Ayres subsequently distinguished himself as a noncombatant medical corpsman, the studio dropped his contract.

Over the course of a Michigan winter, I saw all 15 films. At the conclusion of each, I exited the auditorium into the frigid night, warmed by the prospect of someday walking the wards of a hospital, like Kildare and Gillespie, for the benefit of humankind.

I was reminded of these idealistic impressions by the DVD release of the first Dr. Kildare film, *Internes Can't Take Money*, produced by Paramount in 1937. Featuring Joel McCrea as Kildare and Barbara Stanwyck as an ex-convict and single

Literatim: Essays at the Intersections of Medicine and Culture. Howard Markel, Oxford University Press (2020).
© Oxford University Press.
DOI: 10.1093/oso/9780190087647.001.0001

mother in search of her stolen child, this fast-paced melodrama exemplifies how much medicine has changed over the past eighty years.[1]

Its most memorable scene involves a gangster who staggers into a bar after being gunned down. Bleeding profusely and in need of urgent medical attention, he cannot risk going to a hospital for fear of being incarcerated. Dr. Kildare, who happens to be enjoying a glass of beer between cases, instantly assesses the situation, plucks the strings off of a patron's violin for sutures, shouts for boiling water, cutlery, and rum, and commences to operate in the bar's back room. As the bartender admiringly exclaims during the procedure, "The kid's got eyes in his fingers." The next day, Kildare nobly refuses the mobster's offer of $1,000, saying, "I'm not allowed to take money. Internes can't do that while they're serving time at a hospital. If we took money, then the patient who couldn't pay wouldn't get the same care."

Despite excellent reviews, Paramount relinquished the literary rights to the Kildare stories, leaving them for its rival, MGM, to snap up. The MGM films that followed were equally inspirational in emphasizing that caring for patients trumped all other considerations, incorporating realistic details of clinical medicine, solving every diagnostic dilemma, and always ending happily without serious complications. For nearly a decade, millions of moviegoers clamored to see each installment.[2,3]

Sadly, few recall that Dr. Kildare was the creation of Frederick Schiller Faust. This improbable moniker undoubtedly led to his adopting 18 pseudonyms during his literary career, the most famous being Max Brand. Although he remains best known for his tales about the American West, many of which are still in print, Faust also wrote popular mysteries, historical fiction, romances, sea stories, science fiction, and medical novels featuring Dr. Kildare.[4]

Born in 1892, Faust grew up on a wheat ranch near Stockton, California, after his mother died in 1900 and his father left him in the care of an uncle. As a boy, he voraciously read Greek poetry and drama, mythology, medieval legends, and the works of Homer, Dante, and Shakespeare, all of which influenced his literary oeuvre.

Faust entered the University of California at Berkeley to study literature in 1911 but was dismissed during his junior year for drunkenness, poor attendance, and fighting with the university's president. In 1915, he joined the Canadian Army, hoping to be among the first Yanks to fight in the European trenches. After being denied this assignment, he deserted the ranks in 1916 and moved to New York City. There he took up writing and, in 1917, married his Berkeley sweetheart, Dorothy Schilig. The thrill of battle called again in 1918 as the nation geared up for World War I, but his U.S. Army hitch was restricted to Virginia.

In 1919, Faust published his first novel, a western called *The Untamed*. The book's popularity inspired him to embark on a decades-long production of fiction, during which he typed out more than 2000 words an hour, 10 hours a day. Faust also managed to entangle himself in numerous extramarital affairs, nonstop travel across Europe, and too many all-night parties, stimulants, sedatives, and bottles of liquor. The dizzying pace caught up with him in 1921, when he had a severe heart attack—an experience that both stimulated his interest in medicine and left him with debilitating cardiac disease.[5]

Despite his infirmities, Faust regularly earned more than $100,000 a year, writing stories for some of the best magazines of the day as well as novels and even a few volumes of poetry. Nevertheless, for much of the 1920s and 1930s, his profligate spending habits, penchant for servants, and upkeep of his villa in the hills of Florence reliably drained his bank account. Having long sworn against Tinsel Town, Faust moved his wife and 3 children from Italy to Hollywood in 1937. There he toiled on screenplays and movie ideas for MGM, from 1938 to 1941; between 1941 and 1944, he put in stints at Columbia, Warner Brothers, and RKO.

Faust left Hollywood in spring 1944 to become a war correspondent for *Harper's Magazine*. Doctoring his congestive heart failure with whiskey and digitalis, Faust covered the U.S. Army's 351st Infantry Regiment, 88th division on the Italian front during the bloody "Battle for Rome." On May 12, 1944, he was killed by German artillery near Santa Maria Infante.[6]

With hundreds of novels and stories to his credit, Faust's readers have long debated which one was his best. But for those who carry a stethoscope, the Kildare films—as well as the novels, radio shows, comic books, and television series that followed—signal his claim to posterity. To be sure, they helped spawn an industry of popular entertainment centering on the hospital and its inhabitants that continues to this day. More difficult to appreciate and quantify is the multitude of youngsters who were inspired by Kildare and his fictional cohort to pursue careers in medicine.

The astute reader of history knows that there were no "good old days" in American medicine. Waxing nostalgically about the past is a fool's errand. The Kildare films gloss over the health care inequities of their era in the cause of entertainment, but of course these inequities did exist and harmed many. Moreover, unlike Kildare in his fictional practice, real-life physicians rarely have the pleasure of solving their patients' problems so quickly and to everyone's satisfaction. Yet in these troubled times, when many physicians feel beleaguered or dissatisfied by their profession and when many more patients worry about paying their medical bills, it is comforting, if not advisable, to watch these optimistic films boldly declare that the soul of medicine is about healing rather than the expenditure of dollars. I suspect this is precisely what Dr. Kildare—and Frederick Schiller Faust—would have ordered.

[*This essay originally appeared as: Markel, H. "Calling Dr. Kildare": The Literary Lives of Frederick Schiller Faust, a.k.a Max Brand. Journal of the American Medical Association. 2010: 304 (13): 1501–1502*].

REFERENCES

1. *Internes Can't Take Money.* Hollywood, CA: Paramount Pictures, 1937. DVD Rereleased in *The Barbara Stanwyck Collection* (*Universal Backlot Series*). (Universal City, CA: Universal Studios, 2010).
2. Kalisch P.A., Kalisch B.J. When Americans called for Dr. Kildare: images of physicians and nurses in the Dr. Kildare and Dr. Gillespie movies, 1937–1947. *Med Herit.* 1985; 1(5): 348–363.
3. Dans P.E. *Doctors in the Movies: Boil the Water and Just Say Ahh.* (Bloomington, IL: Medi-Ed Press, 2000), pp. 64–74.
4. Gale R.L. Faust, Frederick Schiller. IN: Garrity JA, Carnes M.C., eds. *American National Biography.* Vol 7. (New York, NY: Oxford University Press, 1999), pp. 767–768.
5. Easton R. *Max Brand: The Big "Westerner."* (Norman, OK: University of Oklahoma Press, 1970).
6. Nolan W.F., ed. *Max Brand: Western Giant: The Life and Times of Frederick Schiller Faust.* (New York, NY: Popular Press, 1985).

CHAPTER 25

∽

"Gotta' Sing! Gotta' Diagnose!"
A Postmortem Examination of Rodgers and Hammerstein's Medical Musical *Allegro*

I magine going to the theater to see a musical pageant about a young physician's professional trials and tribulations, a play that explores the decisions he makes about how he practices medicine and where; the meanings and obligations of the physician's social contract; and even the risks of medical error. Let us extend this fantasy by hiring a trendsetting team of producers, an equally accomplished choreographer and set designer, and an army of professionals to mount the production. And while we are at it, we should invite Richard Rodgers and Oscar Hammerstein II, perhaps the greatest writing duo in the history of musical theater, to write the words and music.

As it happened, if you were a theater devotee more than 70 years ago, all you had to do was walk over to the Majestic Theatre on Manhattan's West 44th Street to see such a production. Opening night seats for *Allegro*, a now obscure medical musical, were the hottest tickets of the 1947 Broadway theatrical season. Heralded on the covers of *Time* and *Life*, Rodgers and Hammerstein's creative success or failure was heatedly debated for weeks by a teeming ant farm of gossip columnists, critics, and show biz beat reporters across the nation.[1-3] Featuring a cast of 78 and an orchestra of 35, *Allegro* was entirely *moderne* in concept, boasting a set consisting of multiple curtains, rotating flats, and lantern slides, a singing "Greek chorus," and 4 integrated ballet scenes depicting and commenting on the life of Dr. Joseph Taylor, Jr., from his birth until age 35 years.[1]

Literatim: Essays at the Intersections of Medicine and Culture. Howard Markel, Oxford University Press (2020).
© Oxford University Press.
DOI: 10.1093/oso/9780190087647.001.0001

The historian's task of re-creating this version of "Everydoctor" is somewhat vexing. The first flop to flow from the golden pens of Rodgers and Hammerstein, *Allegro* ran on the Great White Way for only nine months (314 performances), and its huge cast and staggering weekly budget precluded any profit. There is no film version of the play or even a complete original cast recording (the extant version contains only ten of *Allegro*'s songs and none of the choral narratives). Rarely performed today, the libretto and score are nevertheless easily acquired at any decent library, and the more scholarly will find a fairly evocative collection of photographs of the original production safely reposing at the New York Public Library for the Performing Arts.[4-7] These documentary remnants, plus a modicum of dramatic imagination and, if you are fortunate, the talents of a friendly pianist, immediately demonstrate an insightful navigation of the Scylla and Charybdis between demanding professional careers and personal choices.

The play opens on the day of Joe's birth and, soon enough, the audience is introduced to his father, a rural general practitioner struggling to build a modern hospital for his impoverished and underserved patients. As the father picks up his newborn son, he mellifluously declares the infant to be his clinical successor. In subsequent scenes, the audience is treated to lilting descriptions of Joe's developmental milestones, from his first steps to matriculation into college. There are, however, foreboding hints of a series of increasingly wrong choices to come. These discordant tones begin to peal loudest during his courtship and marriage to a beautiful young woman, Jenny Baker, who derides Joe's aspirations to become a country practitioner and pressures him into finding more lucrative ways to make a living. Indeed, Jenny exhibits a dedicated selfishness that literally induces a fatal myocardial infarction in Joe's morally superior mother; all the while, Jenny seduces Joe into abandoning the family business of doing the most good where most needed.[4]

After several sexually charged ultimatums from Jenny, Joe leaves his father's practice for the glittering lights of the big city. There, amidst the distracting whirl of parties, soliciting donors to fund new patient pavilions, ceremonial ribbon cuttings, and making a mint giving vitamin injections to the worried (and wealthy) well, Joe discovers that his bored and neglected wife is having an affair with the chairman of the hospital trustees. Disillusioned but undefeated, Joe, in true Broadway musical fashion, manages to resolve his ambivalences and stresses just before the fall of the closing curtain. Turning down a promotion to become the youngest ever physician-in-chief of his prestigious city hospital, Joe instead opts for what Rodgers and Hammerstein believed to be the purer life as lone practitioner in the small town where he was born.[4]

In the show's final moment, Joe's shocked employer plaintively asks what he should inform the newspapers regarding Joe's inexplicable declension of the coveted position of physician-in-chief. One powerful hospital trustee suggests telling the press that Joe is "sick." Joe tunefully counters them both, "Tell them I'm just getting well," as the libretto's stage directions prescribe that he "walk away, out into the sunlight," joined by his adoring nurse.[4]

Although they each had enormous popular success with different collaborators, the team of composer Richard Rodgers and lyricist-librettist Oscar Hammerstein II first came to international acclaim in 1943 with *Oklahoma!*, a musical play that astonished and transformed audiences around the world with its seamless integration of story, acting, dance, and dozens of songs that demanded to be whistled upon exiting the theater and for weeks thereafter. In 1945, the duo wrote the songs for the treacly motion picture *State Fair* and created the bittersweet but brilliant musical *Carousel*, both to remarkable critical and popular acclaim. Around the same time, they produced a string of hit Broadway shows, including Irving Berlin's *Annie Get Your Gun*.[8-12] That, of course, was only the start of their impressive partnership; to quote the editors of *Variety*, the Bible of show business, the Rodgers and Hammerstein imprimatur invariably translated into "boffola box office."[13]

Consequently, Rodgers and Hammerstein's announcement in summer 1947 of their next masterpiece-to-be, *Allegro*, inspired a whopping $750,000 in advance ticket sales before rehearsals even began. This was an era, by the way, when the most successful shows had, at best, a $100,000 advance and the top orchestra seat sold for about $6.[1,14] But that anticipation was also heavily compounded with an unhealthy dose of schadenfreude. As *Time* reported on *Allegro*'s world premier at the fabled Shubert Theatre in New Haven, "the faintly malicious question in almost everyone's mind was 'would the wonder boys do it again?' "[2]

Without fear of contradiction, *Allegro* endured the most hazardous if not the worst opening night in the history of the American theater. At the root of these risks was the musical's innovative set, which relied on an intricate set of tracks and grooves embedded in the stage. Early in the first act, a dancer caught his foot in one of the grooves and essentially destroyed his knee. Eyewitness accounts vary from his collapsing offstage into the arms of a fellow thespian to being carried off the stage in front of the audience.[1,8-12]

During the song "A Fellow Needs a Girl," a flat began to fall on the head of the actor playing Joe's father who, fortunately, had the presence of mind to croon and hold up the set simultaneously. Almost as soon as that disaster was averted, smoke began to seep into the auditorium, understandably alarming the audience. Some 60 playgoers hurriedly took to the aisles before famed director Joshua Logan, who was attending the performance that night as a potential play-doctor and would ultimately direct and coauthor Rodgers and Hammerstein's 1949 smash hit *South Pacific*, commandingly bellowed, "It's just an alley fire! Everybody sit down!" Logan later admitted he was only guessing as to the smoke's origins; fortunately for the immediate health of the audience, he was correct.[1,10]

After intermission, crisis struck again at the close of a scene depicting Joe's fascination with the schmoozing requisites of high society at the expense of his medical practice. After his nurse saves Joe from missing the diagnosis of a bleeding gastric ulcer in a patient, she begins a melodic lament of unrequited love entitled "The Gentleman Is a Dope." But before the song reached its refrain, the actress playing the nurse caught her foot in one of the embedded stage grooves and lurched into the string section of the orchestra. Falling at the precise moment of an upstroke of their collective bows, she was quickly hoisted back to her perch without missing a beat of the tune.[1,8–10]

But there were far more serious problems with *Allegro* than mere opening night jitters or mechanical mishaps. The critical responses ranged from laudatory to downright nasty. Brooks Atkinson, the *New York Times'* professorial theater czar, declared it to be "full of a kind of unexploited glory" and a "musical masterpiece."[15] Across the aisle, Woolcott Gibbs, the *New Yorker's* dour and frequently drunken drama critic, derided *Allegro* as a "shocking disappointment." Not content to merely tear apart Rodgers and Hammerstein, Gibbs even assailed Joe's wealthy patients as "suffering vividly from alcoholism, nymphomania, locomotor ataxia, and echolalia (compulsive repetition of idiotic lines)."[16]

Joseph Wood Krutch, writing for *The Nation*, called the production a "cross between Handel and Hollywood" swerving between "bastard oratorio" and "production numbers in a Technicolor movie."[17] In his influential column in *The Saturday Review of Literature*, John Mason Brown misinterpreted the musical as a flaming attack on the medical profession because it appeared to favor those who healed the poor and denigrate those who actually made a decent living at it. "According to Hammerstein," Brown groused, "[such a physician] has sold his soul; betrayed Aesclepius, and made a mockery of the Hippocratic Oath."[18]

Although there were several critics who praised *Allegro* for its innovative blend of story, song, and ballet, the majority consensus was that Rodgers telephoned in a rather uninspired score and Hammerstein's libretto and lyrics were simplistic, if not platitudinous and mawkish. Audience responses varied from "enthralled" to "mystified" and "bored."[1,10] In a very real sense, all these critiques were not exactly wrong, even if none were exactly right.

Today, only the rabid theater aficionado knows about this most experimental of Rodgers and Hammerstein's productions. Nearly three decades after *Allegro* ended its run on Broadway, Richard Rodgers admitted that the play was "too preachy" and questioned the wisdom of dramatizing the life of a physician with words and music.[9,10] Oscar Hammerstein was more pragmatic. "It's no use alibiing," Hammerstein told an oral historian in 1959, "if a horse throws you, he throws you—and apparently I didn't have a strong grip on the reins with the audience in that play."[7,19]

Ironically, a 17-year-old kid who Oscar Hammerstein II hired to be his "gofer" during the production of *Allegro* turned out to be Stephen Sondheim, the current dean of the American musical theater. *Allegro* taught Sondheim that a constellation of theatrical stars do not necessarily add up to a hit play. More cogently, Sondheim urges a second look at what he insists is so much more than just the story of a physician. "Oscar meant it to be a metaphor for what had happened to him," Sondheim told his biographer Meryl Secrest in 1998.[10]

Sondheim appears to have it exactly right. Rodgers and Hammerstein's seldom-sung medical masterpiece examines the exorbitant costs of blindly placing career advancement over the aims and the people in one's life. Hammerstein held the reins most tightly in his script when he dramatized a touching scene in which a seemingly successful Joe expresses remorse about a favorite patient he left behind in his hometown, a young man destined for the priesthood until stricken with incurable tuberculosis. "I guess I feel guilty about him," Joe explains to his nurse, "I can't get rid of the feeling that if I'd spent the last five years on one boy like Vincent, I'd have done the world more good than I could do in a lifetime here."[4] This poignant observation, it seems to me, contains the kernel of a tune that all in the healing arts ought to be whistling as they live their lives, ply their trades, dream of, and often misinterpret, their goals.

[Since writing this essay, there have been a few modern productions of the musical and cast recordings of those productions. This essay originally appeared as: Markel, H.: Gotta' Sing! Gotta' Diagnose!: A Postmortem Examination of Rodgers and Hammerstein's Medical Musical Allegro. Journal of the American Medical Association. 2007; 298 (13):1575–1577].

REFERENCES

1. Mordden, E. *Rodgers and Hammerstein*. (New York, NY: Abradale Press/Harry N. Abrams, 1992), pp. 86–105.
2. The careful dreamer. *Time*. October 22, 1947:66–72.
3. Allegro: Rodgers-Hammerstein have season's big opening. *Life*. October 12, 1947: 70–72.
4. Hammerstein O. *Allegro: A Musical Play*. [Libretto and Lyrics]. (New York, NY: Alfred A. Knopf, 1948).
5. Rodgers R, Hammerstein O. *The Theatre Guild Presents* Allegro: A Musical Play [Piano and vocal score edited by A. Sirmay]. (New York, NY: Williamson Music Co, 1995).
6. *Allegro: Original Cast Recording* [sound recording]. Music by Richard Rodgers; book and lyrics by Oscar Hammerstein II. (New York, NY: RCA Victor/BMG Music, 1993).
7. The Richard Rodgers Papers, 1914–1989. New York, NY: The New York Public Library for the Performing Arts. Series IV, Productions, 1943–1972; Series VIII, Photographs, 1931–1972; Sub-series 3, Productions.
8. Fordin H. *Getting to Know Him: A Biography of Oscar Hammerstein II*. (New York, NY: Da Capo Press, 1995), pp. 239–258.
9. Rodgers R. *Musical Stages: An Autobiography*. (New York, NY: Da Capo Press, 2002), pp. 246–253.
10. Secrest M. *Stephen Sondheim: A Life*. (New York, NY: Delta; 1998), pp. 53–56.
11. Secrest M. *Somewhere for Me: A Biography of Richard Rodgers*. (New York, NY: Applause Books, 2001), pp. 260–286.
12. Block G. *The Richard Rodgers Reader*. (New York, NY: Oxford University Press, 2002), pp. 309–311.

13. Green A., Laurie J. *Show Biz: From Vaude to Video*. (New York, NY: Henry Holt & Co., 1951), pp. 181, 562–564.

14. Phelan K. Allegro. *Commonweal*. October 31, 1947: 70–71.

15. Atkinson B. The New Play in Review: Allegro. *New York Times*. October 11, 1947: 10.

16. Gibbs W. And they still come. *New Yorker*. October 18, 1947: 55–61.

17. Krutch J.W. Allegro. *Nation*. November 22, 1947: 567–568.

18. Brown J.M. The patient's dilemma. *Saturday Review*. November 8, 1947: 30–33.

19. *Reminiscences of Oscar Hammerstein II*. (New York, NY: Oral History Collection of Columbia University, 1959), p. 1063.

CHAPTER 26

∽

Cole Porter's Eventful Nights and Days

Between the firestorms of World War I and the frosty exchanges of the Cold War, American popular music was ruled by names like Irving Berlin, Jerome Kern, Richard Rodgers, George Gershwin, Harry Warren, Harold Arlen, Frank Loesser, and Jules Styne. Their work constitutes what music historians have termed the "Great American Songbook" and includes many of the most-beloved songs of the 20th century. In almost every case, these gifted composers relegated the chores of lyric writing to a cadre of uniquely applied poets. Yet one man managed to combine both talents in a manner that will likely never be topped: Cole Porter (1891-1964).[1-3]

The composer and lyricist of dozens of landmark musical comedies including *Anything Goes, The Gay Divorce, Can-Can, Silk Stockings*, and his masterpiece, *Kiss Me Kate*, Cole Porter also gave birth to a canon of motion pictures, radio and television shows, and recordings. He convinced the world that "Anything Goes," "I Get a Kick Out of You," and "You're the Tops." He urged millions to "Begin the Beguine," "Let's Misbehave," and "Brush Up Your Shakespeare." Impeccably dressed, cigarette in hand, Porter was the avatar of high society. Appearances, of course, can be deceiving. In fact, much of his so-called charmed life transpired within a briar of physical pain.

Cole Albert Porter was born on June 9, 1891, in Peru, Indiana. The scion of a Baptist family, his domineering grandfather, J. O. Cole, was the richest man in the state thanks to investments in drugstores, coal, and timber. Young Cole loved poetry and playing the piano, and he began writing songs at age 10. Nascent talent aside, his family decreed that he become a lawyer and in 1909 sent him off to Yale. There, he distinguished himself by writing the music and lyrics of many Yale student productions, singing with the famed "Whiffenpoof" a cappella singers, and composing several football fight songs, including "Bulldog," a rousing march that

Literatim: Essays at the Intersections of Medicine and Culture. Howard Markel, Oxford University Press (2020).
© Oxford University Press.
DOI: 10.1093/oso/9780190087647.001.0001

continues to be played by the Yale Precision Marching Band every time the team scores a touchdown.

After graduating in 1913, Porter matriculated into the Harvard Law School. Realizing that his talents were best suited to a different type of bar, he soon transferred into Harvard's music school, where he perfected his knowledge of musical composition. His family's reaction was mixed. Cole's irate grandfather excised him from his will. Cole's mother, on the other hand, made certain to bequeath half of her $4 million inheritance to her son to ensure his artistic freedom.

In 1916, Porter saw his first Broadway musical, *See America First*, open and close within 14 days.[2,4] To salve his artistic wounds, he sailed for Europe in the winter of 1917 and pursued an alcohol- and drug-fueled grand tour of the continent, beginning with Paris. The following year, Porter married the wealthy socialite-divorcee Linda Lee Thomas. Although Cole and Linda loved each other deeply, theirs was not a physical relationship. Mrs. Porter accepted Cole's multiple affairs with men in exchange for his devoted companionship and elegant ways. Always a lavish spender, Porter enjoyed Linda's limitless wealth and, given the social taboos against openly declaring one's sexuality in that era, cast her as his wife in the double life he led.

On the afternoon of October 24, 1937, just as Cole's career was skyrocketing, infirmity struck with a resounding force. An accomplished equestrian, he was riding with the Countess Edith di Zoppola and the Duke de Verdura at the tony Piping Rock Club in Locust Valley, New York, when he found himself alone in the verdant woods. Cole's horse shied, stumbled, and rolled directly over the composer's legs. The half-ton horse's fall delivered compound fractures to both of Cole's femurs and provided the entryway for osteomyelitis, an especially daunting infection in the days before antibiotics.[2 (pp.210-224)] In later years, Porter claimed that during the hours he lay prostrate on the bridle path waiting for help, he took out his notebook and composed the opening refrain of a song called "At Long Last Love":

Is it an earthquake or simply a shock?

Is it the good turtle soup or merely the mock?

Is it a cocktail, this feeling of joy or is what I feel the real McCoy?

Have I the right hunch or have I the wrong?

Will it be Bach I shall hear or just a Cole Porter song?

Is it a fancy not worth thinking of or is it at long last love?[5]

Over the next 2 decades, Porter underwent a series of excruciating orthopedic operations. Porter rarely complained of his disabilities because, as he often explained, his mother taught him that "a gentleman never depresses his friends by relating his woes to them." Privately, however, he took to naming (and resenting) his lame legs: Josephine was the left and Geraldine—"a hellion, a bitch, a psychopath"—was the right leg. In 1945, for example, Porter described the details of his latest operation to a close associate. The surgeon began by rebreaking the femurs, followed by removal of the jagged ends, splicing of the Achilles tendons, and removal of 8 inches of tibial tissue for bone grafts over the primary fracture sites. Most vexing, however, was continued evidence of *staphylococcal* infection in the poorly healing bones and severe pain generated by scar tissue and nerve damage.[2(p 295)] Indeed, Cole's injuries transformed gentle touches to his limbs into a form of torture. Undaunted, he walked with canes, crutches, and cumbersome iron braces. In later years, he would rely on a burly valet to carry him into and out of theaters.

Porter's right leg—the psychopath Geraldine—was finally amputated, at mid-thigh, in 1958. Although he was fitted for a prosthetic leg and underwent rigorous physical therapy, any attempts at ambulation were painful and physically challenging. The man whose lyrics and melodies epitomized hope and joy suddenly had little to be hopeful about. Staring at the poorly healing wound where his leg used to be, Porter lamented, "I am only half a man now."[2 (pp. 383-387,394)]

After the amputation, Porter's world shrank drastically. No longer a habitué at Broadway openings or glamorous parties, he now hibernated in his plush apartment in the Waldorf Towers. His leg pains only increased despite an ever-increasing reliance on and addiction to alcohol and narcotic painkillers. During the last decade of his life, he also endured numerous bouts of pneumonia, bladder infections, kidney stones, clinical depression, and a recurring gastric ulcer that required surgical removal of part of his stomach.[6]

When Cole Porter died of kidney failure at age 73 on October 15, 1964, only his closest friends knew the extent of the physical and mental anguish he had endured for 27 years. Against all clinical odds, Porter managed to trip the light fantastic within his mind, occupying his best days and nights composing perfect songs like "Night and Day."

[*This essay originally appeared as: Markel, H. Cole Porter's Eventful Nights and Days. Journal of the American Medical Association. 2011; 305 (3): 310–311*].

REFERENCES

1. Cole Porter is dead. *New York Times.* October 16, 1964:1.
2. McBrien W. *Cole Porter: A Biography.* (New York, NY: Vintage, 2000).
3. Wilder A. *American Popular Song: The Great Innovators, 1900-1950.* (New York, NY: Oxford University Press, 1972), pp. 223–252.
4. Schwartz C. *Cole Porter: A Biography.* (New York, NY: The Dial Press, 1977).
5. Kimball R, ed. *The Complete Lyrics of Cole Porter.* (New York, NY: Da Capo Press, 1992), pp. 15, 229–230.
6. Lahr J. King Cole: The Not So Merry Soul of Cole Porter. *The New Yorker,* July 12, 2004; 80 (19): 100–104.

CHAPTER 27

༄

Physician, Heal Thyself

Arthur Miller, Henrik Ibsen, and
the Enemies of the People

L ike millions of others, I was introduced to Arthur Miller's work by one of my high school teachers. Enthralled by the raw realism of *Death of a Salesman*, I soon found myself running to the local library to plow through the rest of his literary oeuvre. A few years later, as an English literature major at the University of Michigan, I brazenly introduced myself to Arthur Miller, the man. A Michigan graduate (Class of 1938), Miller was a frequent visitor to Ann Arbor and was in town this particular afternoon in the spring of 1981 to deliver a major address.

After his lecture, in which he railed against the foes who controlled Broadway, I scurried up to the podium and offered one of his volumes for signature. Before uncapping his fountain pen, he asked the obligatory question adults pose to all college students: "What are you going to be when you grow up?" I replied that I hoped to enter medical school the next fall. This confession set Miller to reminiscing about the articles he wrote for the school newspaper, *The Michigan Daily*, about a now-forgotten internal medicine professor who locked human research participants into steam boxes and measured various metabolic components of their breath, sweat, urine, and feces.

As he inscribed my book, Mr. Miller inquired if I had ever read Ibsen's *An Enemy of the People*.[1] I admitted I had not. He gruffly rejoined in his thick Brooklyn accent, "Don't start studying medicine until you do. You will need it." This turned out to be remarkably astute advice, although neither of us recognized it at the time. Since 1989, I have read and taught Ibsen's medical masterpiece dozens of times to hundreds of students.

Literatim: Essays at the Intersections of Medicine and Culture. Howard Markel, Oxford University Press (2020).
© Oxford University Press.
DOI: 10.1093/oso/9780190087647.001.0001

The Norwegian poet and playwright Henrik Ibsen (1828-1906), of course, is widely regarded as the father of modern drama.[2,3] Perhaps the best one-line description of this revolutionary artist was offered by the Baltimore journalist H. L. Mencken: "[he was] the best [dramatist] to ever live" . . . [a man who was] "hymned and danced as anything and everything else: a symbolist, seer, prophet, necromancer, maker of riddles, rabble-rouse, cheap shocker, pornographer, spinner of gossamer nothings."[4]

One of Ibsen's most controversial works is *Ghosts*. Published in 1881, the play is centered on a rotting marriage plagued by philandering and syphilis; the latter is tragically passed onto the son, Oswald. Across the continent, bourgeois Europeans sniffed their patrician noses at Ibsen's outrageously bad taste. A smaller group of intellectuals, however, glowed with excitement when either reading translations or seeing productions of Ibsen's thought-provoking play.

Angered by critics calling him a dangerous radical ideologue, Ibsen looked forward to confronting his critics with another scathing commentary on Victorian morality, hypocrisy, and ignorance. He wrote *An Enemy of the People* in 1882, the year microbiologist Robert Koch discovered that the tubercle bacillus (*Mycobacterium tuberculosis*) causes tuberculosis. Koch's findings were widely reported in newspapers and magazines across the globe, and Ibsen certainly read about these exploits. There also exists some evidence that Ibsen took the plot from a news article about a Hungarian scientist who discovered that his town's water supply was tainted and who was pilloried for announcing that inconvenient truth.[5 (p.9)]

Regardless of the precise inspiration, *An Enemy of the People* is about courage, adhering to one's intellectual principles, and the importance of free thought. The play enacts events in the life of a physician named Thomas Stockmann who is hired to run a health spa by his brother Peter, the town's mayor. Unfortunately, the physician determines that pathogenic bacteria, originating from a tannery upstream owned by his wealthy father-in-law, contaminate the spa's waters. Dr. Stockmann relays this critical information to the mayor, but the latter refuses to believe the scientific evidence and urges the physician to delay making any sudden announcements lest it cost the town a fortune.

A simultaneously naive and arrogant Dr. Stockmann insists that it his duty to close the spa to protect the public's health. As a result, he demands a town meeting at which he expects to win the support and undying gratitude of the townspeople and the press—that is, until the men who run the town and its finances, including his brother, circumvent both his support and the veracity of the bacteriological report.

Railing against his political enemies and the mob of townspeople who take their side, Dr. Stockmann warns:

> The majority is never right. Never I tell you! That's one of these lies in society that no free and intelligent man can help rebelling against. Who are the people that make up the biggest proportion of the population—the intelligent ones or the fools? I think we

can agree it's the fools, no matter where you go in the world, it's the fools that form the overwhelming majority. But I'll be damned if that means it's right that the fools should dominate the intelligent.[1(p.76)]

Predictably, the townspeople attending the meeting object to being called fools, ridicule the report, and blame the messenger. Consequently, Dr. Stockmann, rather than the offending microorganisms, is declared an enemy of the people, his reputation is ruined, and no clear solution to cleaning up the polluted baths is in sight. Yet in a hopeful vein, the doctor declares a Pyrrhic victory at the final curtain. Telling his wife and children that truth will ultimately prevail, he reminds them that "the strongest man in the world is the man who stands alone."[1(p.106)]

Arthur Miller was being modest by not urging me that long-ago afternoon to consult his own "adaptation" of the play. Displeased with the stilted English translations then in print, in 1950 Miller worked from a "pidgin-English, word for word rendering of the Norwegian" that allowed him to "gather the meaning of each speech and scene without the obstruction of any kind of English construction."[5(p.11)] Miller's goal was to remind post–World War II theatergoers in the United States of what he believed was the play's central theme: "it is the question of whether the democratic guarantees protecting political minorities ought to be set aside in time of crisis. More personally, it is the question of whether one's vision of the truth ought to be a source of guilt at a time when the mass of men condemn it as a dangerous and devilish lie."[5(p.8)]

A sorry series of political events were likely the impetus for Miller's attraction to this text and the dramatic identification of enemies at this point in his life. As he wrote in his memoir *Timebends*, "At the same time that I was wrestling with this inner turmoil, rumors of weird games going on under HUAC [the U.S. House of Representatives Un-American Activities Committee] pressure were rocking the theatrical community."[6] It is well known that Miller was close to the Communist Party in the 1940s and 1950s, although he never admitted to being a card-carrying member, nor would he name the names of other Communist Party members. When Miller testified before HUAC on June 21, 1956, he was cited for contempt because of his lack of forthrightness. Miller received a 30-day suspended sentence and a $500 fine but in 1958 was exonerated by the courts.[7]

Unlike his 1952 allegory of McCarthyism, *The Crucible*, Miller's *An Enemy of the People* was hardly a commercial success. It ran on Broadway for less than a month, from December 28, 1950, to January 27, 1951, despite favorable reviews and a cast that included the great husband-and-wife team of Frederic March and Florence Eldridge as Dr. and Mrs. Stockmann.[8–10] It is only occasionally performed today.

Beside the clearly urban, North American cadences of the dialogue, Miller's version is true to the standard translations with one notable exception. Miller mutes key passages in which Stockmann asserts the primacy of his vision over the community's using the concepts and language also found in Nietzschean philosophy, fascist political tracts, and even the eugenics textbooks of Ibsen's era. In an essay published in the *New York Times* on December 24, 1950, Miller explains that Ibsen was writing in an era when the explanatory metaphor of social Darwinism was at its peak—an era when many intellectuals self-identified as being the type of human biologically endowed with "the natural right to lead, if not govern, the mass." Miller justifies his adaptation by insisting, without historical evidence, that Ibsen would never have made such statements in the post-Holocaust era: "the whole case of his thinking was that he could not have lived a day under an authoritative regime of any kind."[11] Nevertheless, in Ibsen's as well as Miller's versions, Dr. Stockmann makes a bumptious ass out of himself by refusing to listen to the ideas or thoughts of others and insisting that he, and he alone, knows how to solve the problem.

Both playwrights focused intensely on the power and virtue of the individual in their work: Ibsen upturned his social era by lobbying for the voice of the intellectual over the wealthy and inbred elite; Miller, who came of age during the radical movements of the Great Depression, argued in favor of the common man. For Ibsen and Miller, the sheep-like masses, cynical politicians, irresponsible journalists, and financiers who placed profit above health were all enemies of the people. Yet in the clinical dilemma they describe there exists another enemy who demands identification, if not help. Sometimes the physician can be wrong, too.

In Ibsen's as well as Miller's versions, Dr. Stockmann possesses information and expertise that can protect the lives of those in his community. Sadly, he negates his professional effectiveness by succumbing to his own anger and lashing out at the public. By misfiring his alienating tirades at those he most needs to convince, the doctor creates an insurmountable public health barrier: distrust of the very official the public needs to trust most.

Dr. Stockmann's expertise is thwarted by an excess of ego and pride. Even when one is certain that his plans and conclusions are correct, everyone has the singular power of arrogance to make a mess out of things.

Nearly a century after Ibsen wrote his brilliant play, the American cartoonist Walt Kelly composed an even more succinct means of identifying enemies—not only of society but, in essence, the planet. On the first proclaimed Earth Day in April 1970, Kelly had his swamp-dwelling character Pogo reflect on a polluted mess and exclaim: "I have seen the enemy and he is us."[12]

[*This essay originally appeared as: Markel, H.: Physician, Heal Thyself: Arthur Miller, Henrik Ibsen, and the Enemies of the People. Journal of the American Medical Association. 2009; 301 (23):2506–2507.*]

REFERENCES

1. Ibsen, H., *An Enemy of the People, The Wild Duck, Rosmersholm.* McFarlane J, trans. (Oxford, UK: Oxford University Press, 1999).
2. Matos T.C., Choleric fictions: epidemiology, medical authority, and *An Enemy of the People. Modern Drama.* 2008; 51(3): 353–368.
3. Meyer M., *Ibsen: A Biography.* (Garden City, NY: Doubleday, 1971), pp. 493–510.

4. Mencken H.L., Introduction. IN: *Eleven Plays of Henrik Ibsen*. (New York, NY: Modern Library, 1959), p. vii.
5. Miller, A. *An Enemy of the People: An Adaptation of the Play by Henrik Ibsen*. (New York, NY: Penguin Books, 1979).
6. Miller, A. *Timebends: A Life*. (New York, NY: Grove Press, 1987), p. 329.
7. Bentley E., ed. *Thirty Years of Treason: Excerpts from Hearings Before the House Committee on Un-American Activities, 1938–1968*. (New York, NY: Viking Press, 1971), pp. 789–825.
8. Zolotow S. Miller is revising "Enemy of the People." *New York Times*. August 28, 1950: 13.
9. Atkinson B. First night at the theatre: Frederic March in "An Enemy of the People" adapted by Arthur Miller. *New York Times*. December 29, 1950: 14.
10. Zolotow S. "Enemy of People" closes tomorrow. *New York Times*. January 26, 1951: 34.
11. Miller A. Ibsen's message for today's world. *New York Times*. December 24, 1950: 41.
12. Kelly W. *We Have Met the Enemy and He Is Us*. (New York, NY: Simon & Schuster, 1973).

PART IV

———∿———

"A Certain *PBS*-ness of the Soul"

CHAPTER 28

cVo

George Gershwin's Too-Short Life
Ended on a Blue Note

George Gershwin, the celebrated composer of *Rhapsody in Blue*, the opera *Porgy and Bess*, a long list of musical comedies, including the Pulitzer Prize-winning political satire, *Of Thee I Sing*, and hundreds of songs that continue to be sparkling examples of the Great American Songbook was born on September 26, 1898. During his 38-year-lifetime, Gershwin's jazz-inspired melodies transcended the stages of vaudeville and Broadway to the concert halls of New York, Europe and beyond. As the *New York Times* opined in his 1937 obituary, Gershwin "was a child of the Twenties. . . .he was to music what F. Scott Fitzgerald was to prose."

The cause of his untimely death was most likely glioblastoma, the same type of brain cancer that killed Senators Edward M. Kennedy (D-MA) in 2009 and John McCain (R-AZ) in 2018. Glioblastoma is one of the most common forms of brain cancer and its victims survive 15 to 18 months after their initial diagnosis and surgery. In 1937, however, there were relatively few imaging technologies available to detect brain tumors early enough, let alone effective chemotherapeutic or radiation treatments to halt the tumor's aggressive spread.

Gershwin's medical history during much of this ordeal was vague and frustrating. Beginning in 1936, he complained of headaches, stomach pain, irritability, worries over losing his hair, and outright depression. One cause of his sadness, incidentally, was an unrequited love affair with the film star (and wife of Charlie Chaplin) Paulette Goddard. Gershwin was said to have complained to one friend, "I am 38 years old, wealthy and famous, but I'm still deeply unhappy. How come?" His doctors were unable to find anything physically wrong with him and declared that George's ennui was "in his head."

On February 11, 1937, however, Gershwin lost consciousness for a period of 10 to 20 seconds while performing with the Los Angeles Symphony Orchestra.

Literatim: Essays at the Intersections of Medicine and Culture. Howard Markel, Oxford University Press (2020).
© Oxford University Press.
DOI: 10.1093/oso/9780190087647.001.0001

He was the solo pianist and the program featured his brilliant *Concerto in F*. While playing his part Gershwin experienced what neurologists now refer to as an absence seizure and missed playing several bars, as he sat erect at the grand piano. After the performance, he reported experiencing an olfactory hallucination—a doctor's term for smelling something that is not there. In George's case, it was the smell of burning rubber.

He experienced a second and equally brief loss of consciousness in April of 1937, accompanied by the smell of burning rubber and debilitating headaches. This constellation of symptoms was again misdiagnosed as psychosomatic and was felt to be caused by the stresses of overwork on his serious composing, performing, and the writing of Hollywood film scores. The spells continued to occur at unpredictable times, usually lasted about half a minute, and were all accompanied by the smell of burning rubber, dizziness, and worsening headaches. After consulting a psychiatrist in June of that year, Gershwin was finally referred to an internist to see if there was an organic cause for these problems.

Multiple visits to an internist failed to uncover physical abnormalities, even though the headaches worsened. Despite being admitted to the Cedars of Lebanon Hospital for a battery of tests on June 23, 1937, there still was no clear answer explaining his problems. On the list of possible diagnoses was some type of brain tumor but Gershwin refused a spinal tap, which might have revealed tumor cells in the cerebrospinal fluid, because he did not want to endure the pain of the procedure. He was discharged with a diagnosis of "hysteria."

A male nurse was hired to care for Gershwin at his home in Beverly Hills, but he only grew more ill, with constant and severe headaches, a loss of balance and coordination of his hands (something that would be easily recognized by a skilled pianist), and protracted episodes of irrational behavior. For example, he once tried to push his chauffeur out of a moving car and, in another instance, smeared chocolates all over his body.

He had to take time off from his composing chores for a film called *The Goldwyn Follies* (not surprisingly produced by Hollywood legend Samuel Goldwyn). He also complained of intolerable pain along the sides of his head at a dinner with composer Irving Berlin and, again, at luncheon with a gaggle of movie stars that included Goddard.

On the early evening of July 9, 1937, Ira Gershwin, George's brother and lyricist, came to visit him and discovered that George had been sleeping until 5:00 p.m. that day. When Ira tried to help George to the bathroom, he found his brother so feeble that he needed the help of the nurse in returning him to bed. George collapsed and lost consciousness. At the emergency room, doctors examined a comatose Gershwin, who was paralyzed on his left side and had swelling of the optic nerve (or papilledema, a sign of serious brain swelling).

The famed neurosurgeon Walter Dandy of the Johns Hopkins Hospital was summoned from a Chesapeake Bay cruise with the governor of Maryland, Harry Nice, to help with the procedure. After a long-distance telephone consultation with

Dandy, the physicians at Cedars of Lebanon performed a ventriculogram, a painful procedure where air is introduced into the spinal column via lumbar puncture, followed by X-raying the skull using the air as a contrast to assess the size of the brain's ventricles and space-occupying abnormalities, such as a tumor. The study revealed a large brain tumor in George's right temporal lobe.

At 3:00 on the morning of July 10, he was rushed into the operating room. When Dandy arrived in Newark, New Jersey, he was turned back by a telegram that said the operation was already underway. Despite four hours of valiant efforts by the neurosurgeons to debulk the huge tumor, Gershwin never regained consciousness. He died a few hours later, at 10:30 am. He was only 38 years of age.

Gershwin's final diagnosis was a malignant glioma. More recently, however, a few armchair diagnosticians have argued that the tumor was a pilocytic astrocytoma or even a benign tumor that was caught too late and far too big. Such cellular arguments are really all for naught. As Dandy concluded, given the aggressive growth of his malignancy, the late diagnosis, and the lack of any useful treatments beyond removing large parts of his brain meant that they would have only prolonged Gershwin's misery by a few months: "For a man as brilliant as he with a recurring tumor," Dandy said, "life would have been terrible; it would have been a slow death."

Our collective grief over Gershwin's tragically short life may be tempered by the rich melodic legacy he left behind. His operatic, symphonic and popular works continue to enrich the lives of the millions who listen to them. As but one lovely example of the lilting power of his songs, try to listen to his 1926 ballad, "Someone to Watch Over Me," without humming it over and over again during the course of your day.

CHAPTER 29

cℳↄ

Elvis' Addiction Was the Perfect Prescription for an Early Death

On August 16, 1977, millions of music lovers wept to the news that Elvis Presley, the King of Rock and Roll, was dead. He was only 42 years old and a bloated, fading version of the once-beautiful man whose rhythmic hip-swaying earned him the nickname "Elvis the Pelvis." His girlfriend, Ginger Alden, found Elvis unconscious, lying face down in the master suite bathroom on the second floor of his Memphis mansion, Graceland.

Presley was taken by ambulance to the Baptist Memorial Hospital, where the medical staff was known to be more discrete than the far-closer Methodist South Hospital. Once there, doctors struggled to revive him without success and the King was pronounced dead at 3:30 pm.

Later that afternoon, a team of pathologists, Drs. Eric Muirhead, Jerry Francisco, and Noel Florredo, conducted a two-hour post-mortem examination. At 8:00 pm, Dr. Francisco, who only witnessed the autopsy, acted without the consent or agreement of the other two pathologists in announcing to the press that "preliminary autopsy findings" indicated that Elvis's death was due to a "cardiac arrhythmia" and that drugs were not involved.

This statement was subsequently demonstrated not to be the case. Indeed, the other two pathologists later admitted that Francisco was covering up the real cause of death at the request of Elvis's mortified family who were concerned about the singer's reputation. After all, how would it look if the rock star who President Richard Nixon awarded a special badge from the Bureau of Narcotics and Dangerous Drugs had died of a drug overdose?

When the toxicology report came back several weeks later, however, Elvis' blood was found to contain very high levels of the opiates Dilaudid, Percodan, Demerol, and codeine—as well as Quaaludes. The other two pathologists Muirhead and

Literatim: Essays at the Intersections of Medicine and Culture. Howard Markel, Oxford University Press (2020).
© Oxford University Press.
DOI: 10.1093/oso/9780190087647.001.0001

Florredo eventually revealed they also had found evidence of severe and chronic constipation, diabetes, and glaucoma during their examination.

Elvis actually died a death that is quite common, albeit an embarrassing one. Elvis was sitting on the toilet, straining very hard to have a bowel movement— a maneuver that put a great amount of pressure on his heart and aorta. Thus, he likely died of a massive heart attack and keeled over onto the floor. But Elvis was not suffering from garden-variety constipation at the time of his death. Indeed, his medicine chest was filled with amber-colored, white-topped vials of medications, in doses no responsible doctor would have prescribed.

Presley was a long-time abuser of opiates, which not only kill pain but also cause savage constipation. He abused antihistamines, tranquilizers such as Valium, barbiturates, Quaaludes, sleeping pills, hormones—and laxatives, for the constipation.

Elvis' personal physician, George Nichopoulos, or "Dr. Nick," was at Elvis' beck and call for nearly a decade. He began treating "the King" for "saddle pain" in 1967 and all too soon Elvis turned into an opiate addict. Dr. Nick admitted at a hearing before the Tennessee Board of Health that he had prescribed thousands of doses of various addictive pills for Elvis but also claimed he often slipped him sugar pills, or placebos, to try to control his addictions. Dr. Nick testified he gave into all of Elvis's prescription requests because he wanted to keep Presley from seeking out these drugs "on the street."

The jury thought Dr. Nick was "acting in the best interests of the patient" (an extremely improbable conclusion, it seems to this doctor) and was acquitted. In 1980, the not-so-good doctor was indicted again for overprescribing to Presley as well as Jerry Lee Lewis, but was acquitted again. Nichopoulos, however, continued to over-prescribe to many other patients and in 1995, the Tennessee Board of Medical Examiners finally and permanently suspended his medical license.

Subsequent armchair diagnosticians (and a few geneticists who claimed to have a lock of Elvis's hair and performed a DNA analysis of it) have suggested Elvis had hypertrophic cardiomyopathy, a disease of the heart muscle in which there is thickening of the heart's walls, weakening and enlargement of the muscle itself, and, ultimately heart failure or sudden cardiac death. Some of the symptoms of this problem include fatigue, fainting spells and high blood pressure. Throw in the obesity Elvis suffered from near the end of his life, what appears to be type II diabetes, an enlarged heart, and a steady diet of unhealthy, fatty and fried foods, along with his notorious prescription pill consumption, and you have the perfect prescription for disaster.

Like so many rock stars, including Michael Jackson and Prince, Elvis employed an all-too-willing physician to feed his addiction and hasten his death. What a tragedy that this uniquely brilliant singer, musician, and popular cultural icon succumbed to such a sorry state. In the end, he died a lonely man whose ornate home became the embodiment of "Heartbreak Hotel."

CHAPTER 30

∽

How a Strange Rumor of Walt Disney's Death Became Legend

When hearing the phrase "Disney on Ice," many think of the wildly popular ice shows featuring Mickey and Minnie Mouse and other Disney characters skating in hockey arenas across the nation. But there's also the disturbing urban legend that Walt Disney's corpse was frozen in a cryonic chamber containing liquid nitrogen to be revived at a later date.

On December 15, 1966, television and radio broadcasts shared the news that Walter Elias Disney had died. The cartoon mogul who created Mickey Mouse and Donald Duck, produced some of Hollywood's greatest hits, and dreamed up Disneyland and Disney World, was one of world's most beloved storytellers. He was 65.

It is hard to pin down exactly when the rumors began. In early 1967, a few weeks after Disney's death, a reporter for a tabloid newspaper called *The National Spotlite* claimed he had snuck into St. Joseph's Hospital in Burbank, directly across the street from the Disney studios and where he was treated during his final illness. As the story went, the reporter disguised himself as an orderly, broke into a storage room, and saw the deceased Disney suspended in a cryogenic metal cylinder!

In 1969, the French magazine *Ici Paris* and, later still, *The National Tattler* in the U.S. advanced the rumors by predicting Disney would be thawed out in 1975. Some went as far as to claim that his burial spot was a freezer stored underneath the "Pirates of the Caribbean" ride at Disneyland. (It's not!)

And then there were several former Disney employees who continued to spread false stories about Disney's supposed "big freeze." During the 1990s, these now discredited legends were codified as "expert quotes" in a couple of less than reliable Disney biographies.

Literatim: Essays at the Intersections of Medicine and Culture. Howard Markel, Oxford University Press (2020).
© Oxford University Press.
DOI: 10.1093/oso/9780190087647.001.0001

To be sure, Disney was a science fiction fan who looked forward to future advances in science, technology and medicine. His creation of EPCOT, "Experimental Prototype Community of Tomorrow," (which his brother Roy later slashed into a quasi- world's fair), was originally designed to demonstrate how Americans would live, work and survive in the future.

And Walt couldn't help but raise some eyebrows with the last film he produced. Sensing his impending demise, he ordered the cameras to roll as he addressed his department heads one last time. Seated at his famous desk, just like he did during his television show that aired each Sunday evening, a smiling Walt Disney appeared to make laser-beam eye contact with each colleague as he told them what he expected of their performance in the future and that he hoped to see them soon.

Some have speculated that he had read, or heard of, Robert C.W. Ettinger's 1964 book, *The Prospect of Immortality*, which synthesized both believable and less likely ideas about cryonics. That book, and many others like it that appeared long after Disney's death, predicted a day when medical science advanced enough to repair the damage to the once disease-riddled person who was frozen, allowing cryonics experts to thaw them out and bring them back to life.

For the record, there is no solid evidence to suggest that Disney was frozen. Perhaps the most convincing conclusion comes from Disney's daughter Diane, who wrote in 1972, "There is absolutely no truth that my father, Walt Disney, wished to be frozen. I doubt that my father had ever heard of cryonics."

In truth, Walt Disney was cremated two days after his death and an urn containing his ashes were interred at the family mausoleum in the Forrest Lawn Cemetery of Glendale, California. It was a small, private service attended only by his wife, Lillian, his daughters and their husbands and children.

A chronic smoker, Disney's staff always knew when he was coming down the hall because of his hacking, dry cough. He had been in declining health for much of the last year of his life. Fans of the Sunday evening, NBC television show *Walt Disney's Wonderful World of Color* began to notice how haggard and exhausted he looked on the air and wrote concerned letters to him about how raspy his voice had become. He was a long-time sufferer of chronic-obstructive pulmonary disease and emphysema, as well as severe damage to his cervical spine from falling off a horse while playing in a Hollywood polo tournament in the 1930s.

In early November of 1966, Disney began to complain of severe neck and leg pain that interfered with his legendary ability to work and create. A chest X-ray uncovered a tumor the size of a walnut in his left lung and oncological surgeons recommended the immediate removal of a large portion of his left lung.

He cleared the most pressing things on his desk and was admitted to St. Joseph's for surgery on November 6. The surgeons found the tumor to be consistent with bronchogenic cancer. Disney's concern about this extensive surgery was how short of breath he was, but the real problem was that the lung cancer had already spread widely to his lymph nodes and elsewhere in his body.

The always energetic man struggled to go back to the Disney studios after the operation, but the chemotherapy and cobalt X-ray treatments drained him of both his creative and physical powers. He was rushed back to St. Joseph's Hospital two weeks later and died of "circulatory collapse" on the morning of December 15.

When contemplating his near-Himalayan shadow over popular culture, it's not hard to imagine why a "Disney on Ice" legend is so appealing. Americans never stopped loving good old Uncle Walt and all those wonderful stories, songs, and characters he introduced to the world. Our children and their children continue to thrill to the always familiar yet constantly expanding magical oeuvre that is Disney. Who among us wouldn't want to fantasize about the day he magically came back to life?

Alas, not even Walt's beloved "Imagineers" have the power to accomplish such a dream. Perhaps we ought to take some sage advice from the Disney cartoon *Frozen* and, simply, "Let It Go".

CHAPTER 31

ত৵৹

A Symphony of Second Opinions
on Mozart's Final Illness

For classical music lovers, December 5 may be the saddest day of the year. At 12:55 a.m., in 1791, Wolfgang Amadeus Mozart drew his last breath. Later, he was unceremoniously buried in a common grave—as was the custom of his era—in the St. Marx cemetery, just outside the Vienna city limits. Mozart was only 35.

Ever since, generations of doctors have been obsessed with figuring out what caused Mozart's premature death. At last count, there were more than 136 post-mortem diagnoses in the medical literature. This list is almost guaranteed to expand in the years to come.

During his last few months of life, the preternaturally prolific Wolfgang completed the score for *The Magic Flute* and conducted its premier and several subsequent performances. He also composed the lilting *Clarinet Concerto in A*, the *Masonic Cantata*, some new cadenzas for a few of his piano concerti, and began writing his haunting *Requiem in D minor*.

A week after Mozart's death, a Berlin newspaper falsely reported that the composer was poisoned to death. Fans of Peter Shaffer's 1979 stage play, and the 1984 Hollywood film, *Amadeus*, incorrectly believe his colleague and rival, Antonio Salieri, did the deed. Others went as far as to spread a false rumor that on his deathbed in May, 1825, Maestro Salieri confessed to the crime. (He didn't). Mozart added a bit of fuel to this fire: while composing the *Masonic Cantata*, he told his wife he felt ill, was likely to die, and that he must have been poisoned. Feeling a bit better by mid-November 1791, Mozart retracted claims to being poisoned and turned to writing his *Requiem*.

Diagnosing Mozart's final illness is complicated by the fact that the doctors who attended him at the close of the 18th century understood disease and practiced medicine in very different ways when compared to today. Mozart's personal

Literatim: Essays at the Intersections of Medicine and Culture. Howard Markel, Oxford University Press (2020).
© Oxford University Press.
DOI: 10.1093/oso/9780190087647.001.0001

physician, Thomas Franz Closset, concluded that the composer died of *hitziges Frieselfieber*, or acute miliary fever. The symptoms of this syndrome included a high fever and the eruption of tiny, millet-seed shaped (hence the name, miliary), red bumps that blistered the skin.

Mozart's sister-in-law, Sophie Haibel, provided the most detailed commentary of his final days and hours. Unfortunately, she gave this testimony some 33 years after the event, when her memory may have been less than reliable. During his last two weeks of life, Mozart developed severe edema (swelling of the hands, feet, legs, abdomen, arms and face due to retained body fluid). Mozart complained of pain all over his body, a fever, and a rash of some kind. The evening before his death, December 4, he was well enough to invite some friends to his bedside to sing parts of his *Requiem*. He was unlikely to have experienced shortness of breath on his last day of life because he was still singing parts of the *Requiem* to Franz Süssmayr, an Austrian composer and conductor who was serving as Mozart's copyist (rather than Salieri in the fictional *Amadeus*) and who, after Mozart's death, completed a commonly performed version of the *Requiem*. Sophie insisted that Mozart remained conscious until about two hours before his death.

The many modern medical diagnoses explaining Mozart's death include tuberculosis, mercury poisoning, syphilis, rheumatic fever, kidney failure due to chronic glomerulonephritis, Henoch–Schönlein purpura (a syndrome of bruising, arthritis, and abdominal pain, often accompanied by kidney problems), scarlet fever, and trichinosis from eating poorly cooked or raw pork.

Perhaps the most impressive retrospective diagnoses of the lot was a 2009 retrospective epidemiological study published in the *Annals of Internal Medicine* (2009; 151: 274-278). A team of intrepid scholars from Amsterdam, Vienna, and London collected reports of all the recorded deaths in Vienna between December 1791 and January 1792, as well as the corresponding periods from 1790 to 1791 and 1792 to 1793. They then studied the death patterns of 5,011 adults (3,442 men with a mean age of death at 45.5 years and 1,569 women with a mean age of death at 54.5 years).

The epidemiologists discovered a marked increase in the deaths of younger men in the weeks corresponding to Mozart's fatal illness when compared to the previous and following years. Also of import were reports of an epidemic in Vienna around the time of Mozart's death, where many people died of the same constellation of symptoms as he did.

All this data led the researchers to retrospectively diagnose a *streptococcal* infection, which virulently progressed to an acute nephritic syndrome (a swelling and dysfunction of the kidneys, hence Mozart's severe edema), caused by post-streptococcal glomerulonephritis (inflammation of the kidney cells after the infection).

The doctor in me is intrigued and muses, in *pianissimo*, "Maybe." Soon enough, however, another thought emerges, this time in *fortissimo*: "Does it really matter?" Speculating how the famous shuffled off this mortal coil is, of course, a fun parlor game for medical detectives. Nevertheless, I think December 5 is best spent celebrating the short life and enjoying the long-lived music of Wolfgang Amadeus Mozart.

CHAPTER 32

cᴧↄ

Marilyn Monroe and the Prescription Drugs That Killed Her

I f headlines could scream, then scream they did on August 5, 1962. According to nearly every newspaper, television, and radio broadcast in the world, Marilyn Monroe, Hollywood's brightest star, was found dead in the bedroom of her Brentwood, Los Angeles home. She was only 36.

Long before the opiate and opioid epidemics struck American life with such resounding force, there were plenty of other prescription drugs abused to excess with deadly results.

On Marilyn's bedside table was a virtual pharmacopoeia of sedatives, soporifics, tranquilizers, opiates, "speed pills," and sleeping pills. The vial containing the latter, a barbiturate known as Nembutal, was empty. In her last weeks to months, Marilyn was also consuming, if not abusing, a great deal of other barbiturates (amytal, sodium pentothal, seconal, phenobarbital), amphetamines (methamphetamine, Dexedrine, Benzedrine and dexamyl—a combination of barbiturates and amphetamines used for depression), opiates (morphine, codeine, Percodan), the sedative Librium, and alcohol (Champagne was a particular favorite, but she also imbibed a great deal of sherry, vermouth and vodka).

Her last two pictures, *Let's Make Love* (1960) and *The Misfits* (1961), were box office flops. The latter, written by her husband, the Pulitzer Prize-winning playwright Arthur Miller, served as the breaking point in their marriage and the two were divorced shortly after "wrapping" that film. During this period, Monroe suffered from several mental health problems, including substance abuse, depression, and, most likely, bipolar disorder, along with several physical ailments including endometriosis and gall bladder disease.

On June 8, 1962, the Hollywood film studio, 20th Century Fox, fired her while she was filming the ironically titled *Something's Gotta Give*, (which was intended

Literatim: Essays at the Intersections of Medicine and Culture. Howard Markel, Oxford University Press (2020).
© Oxford University Press.
DOI: 10.1093/oso/9780190087647.001.0001

to be a remake of the 1940 hit film *My Favorite Wife*). The studio claimed that the cause was her "unjustifiable absences." Marilyn protested she was too sick to work while the studio moguls complained she was apparently well enough to sing "Happy Birthday, Mr. President" at John F. Kennedy's famous soiree in New York's Madison Square Garden on May 19. This very public firing was an ignominious end for a superstar whose films had grossed more than $200 million during a relatively brief career.

Lonely and harassed, Marilyn found getting to sleep especially difficult. To counteract her insomnia, she often cracked open a Nembutal (pentobarbital) capsule (so that it would absorb faster into her bloodstream), added a chloral hydrate tablet (an old fashioned sedative better known in detective stories as a "Mickey Finn," or "knockout drops,"), and washed them both down with a tumbler of Champagne. This is a particularly lethal cocktail, not only because each of these drugs increase, or potentiate, the power of the other, but also because people who take this combination often forget how much they previously consumed, or whether they took them at all, and soon reach for another dose.

On her last day of life, Saturday, August 4, Marilyn lolled about her home in a drug and alcohol-fueled haze. Her publicist Patricia Newcomb, her housekeeper Eunice Murray, a photographer named Lawrence Schiller, and her psychiatrist Ralph Greenson were also present, off and on, for most of that day.

Before leaving for the night, Dr. Greenson asked Murray, who had lived with the movie star, to keep a close eye on Marilyn. Marilyn was last seen alive at 8 p.m., when she retired alone to her bedroom. At around 3:25 a.m., on August 5, Murray noticed that Monroe's lights were on but the bedroom door was locked and Marilyn did not respond to shouts to open it up.

Murray then walked outside the home and looked inside the bedroom's "French doors." She later recalled that Marilyn "looked peculiar. An arm was stretched across the bed and a hand hung limp on a telephone." Murray called Dr. Greenson, who, upon arrival, broke through the window door with a fireplace poker to get to Marilyn. Sadly, it was too late. Soon after, Monroe's personal physician, Hyman Engelberg, and the Los Angeles police arrived to the scene. As the entire world learned later that morning, Marilyn Monroe had died of an apparent, or accidental, suicide.

In the years since, Marilyn's legend and the details surrounding her tragic death and autopsy have transmogrified into a mountain of conspiracy theories and tall tales. Who was she trying to call just before she closed her eyes for the last time? Was she murdered? If so, who was involved? And what about those pesky and unsubstantiated rumors about the involvement of John and Bobby Kennedy, not to mention the Mafia, the CIA and even members of the Communist Party? On and on it goes, each theory seeming to be crazier or more far-fetched than the last. But because of the sequestered nature of her demise, we will likely never know the precise details.

What remains most cautionary to 21st century readers is that the majority of the substances Marilyn was abusing were prescribed to her by physicians, all of whom should have known better than to leave a mentally ill patient with such a large stash of deadly medications. The barbiturates that killed her are rarely, if ever prescribed, today. Nevertheless, Monroe, like Judy Garland, Michael Jackson, Prince, and so many other famous Hollywood stars who die of drug overdoses, was adept at manipulating her doctors to prescribe the drugs she craved and felt she needed to get through her tortured days and nights. This treacherous course worked, albeit haphazardly, until it didn't work anymore and resulted in a talented young woman dying far too young.

CHAPTER 33

∽

Did Lou Gehrig Actually Die
of Lou Gehrig's Disease?

O n the Fourth of July, 1939, 61,808 New York Yankees fans crowded into
the "House that Ruth Built." But they weren't there for the Bambino. Not
that day.

Instead, the afternoon marked a moment of appreciation and fond farewell for Lou Gehrig, the "Iron Horse," the first baseman who played in 2,130
consecutive games.

The tall, once-muscular ballplayer donned his flannel, pinstriped uniform one
last time on that hot July day in the Bronx. Just two weeks earlier, on June 19, he had
celebrated his 36th birthday.

On his back was the number 4, indicating his position in the batting order, right
after Ruth (#3); it was the first number to be "retired" in major league baseball. Lou
Gehrig approached the microphone, looked out at the vast crowd of fans, and said,
"For the past two weeks, you've been reading about a bad break. Today, I consider
myself the luckiest man on the face of the Earth . . . I may have had a tough break,
but I have an awful lot to live for."

Thanks to radio broadcasts, millions more heard what is, without doubt, the
most famous speech ever delivered from the diamond. And, of course, it was
reprised and immortalized for many millions more by Gary Cooper in the 1942
Hollywood motion picture, *The Pride of the Yankees*. The American Film Institute
later ranked "the luckiest man" speech the 38th best on its list of the 100 Greatest
Movie Quotes, but these were no scripted lines. Gehrig actually said them.

Virtually every American today, be they a baseball fan or not, knows Lou
Gehrig's "bad break" was his diagnosis with amyotrophic lateral sclerosis (ALS),
a fierce neurodegenerative disorder that robs one of muscle control, swallowing,
breathing, and ultimately, life.

Literatim: Essays at the Intersections of Medicine and Culture. Howard Markel, Oxford University Press (2020).
© Oxford University Press.
DOI: 10.1093/oso/9780190087647.001.0001

Two months earlier, on May 1, 1939, Gehrig gallantly took himself out of the lineup because he could no longer will his body to perform the athletic miracles that made him, arguably, the best baseball player ever to play the game. The Hall of Famer won the Triple Crown in 1934 and was the American League's Most Valuable Player twice, in 1927 and 1936. He was a member of six World Series Championship teams (1927, 1928, 1932, 1936, 1937, 1938) and during his 14-year career, he knocked out 493 homers and 2,721 hits, batted in 1,995 runs, and achieved a lifetime batting average of .340!

Gehrig began experiencing his first neurological symptoms in 1938, right around the time of his 35th birthday. Desperate to find out the cause of his problems, he and his wife visited the famed Mayo Clinic, from June 13 to June 19, 1939. On the 19th, Gehrig's 36th birthday, his internist, Dr. Harold Habein, certified his diagnosis of the poorly understood, rare and typically fatal ALS.

Today's medical consumer would be shocked to learn that Gehrig's doctors couched the prognosis in terms of a 50-50 chance of recovery, even though they knew this not to be so. Yet medical ethics and practice of this era often emboldened physicians to tell a patient partial truth about a lethal malady or, paternalistically, not to tell the patient at all, and, instead, only inform close relatives. Nevertheless, recovery was a belief Gehrig hung onto for the remaining two years of his life. In retirement, he took on an active role as a member of the New York City Parole Commission, but by spring 1941, he had lost too much strength to fulfill those duties. He died on June 3, 1941, just 16 days shy of 37 years of age.

Approximately 30,000 people living in the United States have the incurable and progressive ALS, most of them are men between the ages of 40 and 70 years. Many die within a few years of being diagnosed; others, such as the famed physicist Stephen Hawking, can live for years with their brains fully functioning even though their bodies and muscles have degenerated and wasted.

But was ALS the cause of Lou Gehrig's death?

Maybe not, say a group of neurologists, physicians and pathologists at the Boston University School of Medicine Center for the Study of Traumatic Encephalopathy. These doctors are presently conducting landmark research on the brains of deceased former NFL players. In 2010, they presented convincing pathological evidence that "repetitive head trauma experienced in collision sports" may be associated with the development of motor-neuron disease. In other words, repetitive head trauma, or chronic traumatic encephalopathy (CTE) may result in a syndrome that mimics ALS. (*Journal of Neuropathology and Experimental Neurology.* 2010; 69 (9): 918-929)

Lou Gehrig was called the Iron Horse not only for his incredible strength and speed, but also because he was always in the line-up, no matter what injury he incurred the day before. On numerous occasions, he was "beaned" by an errant pitch or hit in the face by ground balls, suffered repeated concussions, episodes of loss of consciousness, and other forms of head trauma, without the slightest protection, beyond wearing a woolen baseball cap. Gehrig collided with rapidly moving objects unrelated to the batter's box or first base, as well. In 1924, for example, during a post-game fight with the Detroit Tigers, Gehrig took a swing at Ty Cobb, missed, fell, and hit his head on concrete pavement, only to lose consciousness for a brief period of time.

It is unlikely that we will ever definitively prove whether Gehrig died of ALS or a trauma-related motor neuron disorder diagnosis. His remains were cremated and the Mayo Clinic has sealed his records. Without Gehrig's patient chart, it is impossible to even know if an autopsy was conducted. Yet his history of so many head injuries may well have played a role in his rapid decline and death.

The irony, of course, is that ALS is widely known and referred to as "Lou Gehrig's Disease."

It is only over the past several years that doctors (and athletes) have focused on the long-term effects of brain injuries associated with contact sports. With each passing year, the risks and dangers of these repetitive brain injuries have become abundantly clear. Indeed, they demand a slate of safety measures, especially for youngsters who engage in such activities.

Whatever Lou Gehrig's precise diagnosis was, what better way to celebrate his birthday than by fighting both amyotrophic lateral sclerosis *and* sports-related concussions? We can attack ALS by donating money to research about its cause and treatment; and we can begin to prevent chronic traumatic encephalopathy (CTE) by making certain the heads (and brains) of our children and loved ones are well protected whenever they engage in sporting events.

CHAPTER 34

cℳɔ

The "Home Run King"

How Babe Ruth Helped Pioneer
Modern Cancer Treatment

From a doctor's perspective, one of the most interesting scenes in the 1948 motion picture, *The Babe Ruth Story*, occurs at the film's end. The scene depicts Ruth's tragic death at 53 from a rare and deadly cancer of the nasopharynx (the air passages in the back of the nose and mouth).

"The Babe," bumptiously played by William Bendix, bravely volunteers to take an experimental drug. As Ruth explained in his 1948 autobiography of the same name: "I realized that if anything was learned about that type of treatment, whether good or bad, it would be of use in the future to the medical profession and maybe to a lot of people with my same trouble."

The audience watches Ruth's doctors wheel him down a darkened hospital corridor, and then the film cuts to dozens of boys playing on the sandlots while an orchestra breaks out into a rousing rendition of "Take Me Out to the Ball Game." An off-screen narrator confidently intones, "His name will live as long as there is a bat, a ball and a boy."

Babe Ruth was one of the first cancer patients to receive a combination of chemotherapy and radiation.

More than 50 years after Babe Ruth's death, the great medical journalist and doctor Lawrence Altman uncovered the Sultan of Swat's intricate medical history on the pages of the *New York Times*. Dr. Altman was reporting on a group of doctors who were retrospectively diagnosing Ruth (the common myth was that he had cancer of the throat or larynx, instead of nasopharyngeal cancer.) But Dr. Altman revealed an even greater truth in his elegant essay: Babe Ruth was one of the original

Literatim: Essays at the Intersections of Medicine and Culture. Howard Markel, Oxford University Press (2020).
© Oxford University Press.
DOI: 10.1093/oso/9780190087647.001.0001

cohort of cancer patients who were treated with combinations of chemotherapy and radiation, a protocol—while far improved from those long ago days—that is still employed in the treatment of a number of cancers.

During the fall of 1946, the "Sultan of Swat" noticed that his voice was growing increasingly hoarse. Soon after, he experienced excruciating pain behind his left eye. One doctor thought it was dental in origin and recommended that a dentist yank out three of Babe's teeth. Ruth only became more ill; he could barely speak or swallow. An X-ray revealed a large tumor at the base of the skull and his doctors prescribed an intensive round of radiation therapy, which did little to stem the malignancy or his painful symptoms.

In June of 1947, Dr. Richard Lewisohn and his team of researchers at the Mount Sinai Hospital of New York City were experimenting on rats with teropterin, an anti-cancer, folic acid antagonist drug extracted from brewer's yeast. (A similar drug amphothopterin, or methotrexate, is currently used to treat a variety of cancers and other diseases.) Dr. Lewisohn and his colleagues suggested a trial of teropterin for Ruth, even though it had never been used on human patients.

At first, the drug seemed miraculous. Ruth began to regain some of the 80 pounds he lost the prior year. On June 13, 1948, he felt well enough to don his old Yankee pinstripes, with the number 3 on the back, and play a starring role at the 25th anniversary of the opening of Yankee Stadium ("The House That Ruth Built").

His progress was short-lived, however, and a few days later he was admitted to Memorial Hospital (now Memorial-Sloan Kettering Hospital) in New York City. There remains some question over whether or not Babe Ruth was told he had terminal cancer, a diagnosis doctors often kept from their patients in that era.

Sadly, George Herman Ruth, perhaps the most beloved ballplayer ever to stand in the batter's box, died of pneumonia on Aug. 16, 1948. His autopsy revealed metastatic cancer originating from the nose and throat. His body lay in state at Yankee Stadium for two full days, where hundreds of thousands of fans paid their last respects; his funeral was held before a jam-packed crowd of dignitaries at St. Patrick's Cathedral on Fifth Avenue.

Who among us cannot cite at least one of Babe's athletic accomplishments? He hit 60 home runs in one season (1927)! His 714 dingers held the lifetime record for 52 years, 8 months and 21 days until Hank Aaron smashed it on April 8, 1974. The Babe was the guy who hit three homers in one World Series game (1926) for a little boy named Johnny Sylvester who was perilously ill. And in 1930, when his salary topped that of Herbert Hoover, the president of the United States, Ruth countered, "I know, but I had a better year than Hoover."

Babe Ruth was a hero to a legion of fans who followed his remarkable exploits on the diamond. But Babe Ruth was also a true Cancer hero. Today, thanks to the wonders of modern medicine, there are millions of cancer survivors—and many more millions of people who love those survivors.

As we mark the day Babe Ruth died, it seems appropriate that all of us take a moment of reflection for him and the thousands of selfless and dying patients who were "on first" when it came to trying chemotherapeutic therapies that became part of our arsenal against cancer. No one applauded their efforts, but they all hit the medical equivalent of a home run.

CHAPTER 35

༺༻

Remembering Ryan White, the Teen Who Fought Against the Stigma of AIDS

I t is high time we celebrate one of the great heroes in the war against AIDS: a quiet, unassuming and brave young man named Ryan White. He was only 18 when he died of the disease on April 8, 1990.

Ryan was born with hemophilia A, a rare, inherited disorder in which the blood system does not clot normally because of an inability to produce "Factor 8," a prosaically named protein related to this critical process. When a hemophiliac suffers a blunt or bruising injury to the body, internal bleeding often occurs, which causes damage to one's organs and can be life-threatening. Of particular risk is bleeding within the knee, ankle and elbow joints, which can be severely damaged over time.

Although there is no cure for hemophilia, doctors treat the bleeding episodes with injections of Factor 8 to help the clotting process along. But in the years before the threat of HIV/AIDS became widely understood, this substance was pooled and isolated from thousands of anonymous and untested blood donations. What no one knew back then was that every time a pediatrician administered this seemingly life-saving elixir (and I was one of those pediatricians), there was a real risk of administering an HIV-contaminated dose. Hence, many doctors were unknowingly infecting hemophiliac patients with the human immunodeficiency virus. Virtually every hemophiliac I treated in the mid-1980s has since died from AIDS. This was the way Ryan White became infected with HIV sometime in the late 1970s or early 1980s.

Ryan's path was not an easy one. Diagnosed in December of 1984, he was initially predicted to live only six more months. After he overcame his first serious bout of illness, however, Ryan wanted to return to the Western Middle School in Russiaville, Indiana. Sadly, the superintendent of the Western School Corporation (which included his town of Kokomo, Indiana) would not let him return and Ryan

Literatim: Essays at the Intersections of Medicine and Culture. Howard Markel, Oxford University Press (2020).
© Oxford University Press.
DOI: 10.1093/oso/9780190087647.001.0001

was forced to listen in on his seventh grade classes via the telephone. Several school officials, teachers, parents and students erroneously (and cruelly) insisted that Ryan might transmit his HIV by casual contact, such as a handshake, from using the public restrooms or even from handling the newspapers Ryan delivered on his paper route.

After winning a lengthy court case allowing him to return to his classes, Ryan was taunted and shunned by other students. Vandals broke the windows of the White's home, and cashiers refused to touch his mother's hands when making change at the supermarket. Not everyone in Kokomo was so vituperative, of course, and there were many families who supported Ryan's desire to attend school. Nevertheless, life there was a harrowing experience for the White family.

In 1987, the Whites moved to nearby Cicero, Indiana, and Ryan enrolled at Hamilton Heights High School. There, the principal welcomed him with a hand-shake and encouraged the student body to engage in accurate and informative discussions about HIV/AIDS.

When the nation was still grappling with homophobia, unsubstantiated fears of how the virus was transmitted, and a great deal of prejudice towards a growing number of terribly sick individuals, Ryan White's case became a national anti-dote. During this period, Ryan served as an eloquent spokesman about AIDS to his classmates, journalists and, through the wide reach of television, the American public. He valiantly fought against a battalion of bigots who saw AIDS as some kind of divine retribution against gay men and intravenous drug users (two of the largest groups stricken with AIDS during this time). He also demonstrated how the national blood supply needed to be fixed so that every donation was tested for evidence of HIV. AIDS, he declared, is an infectious disease, nothing more, and it has the power to harm anybody unfortunate enough to have contracted the human immunodeficieny virus. A television film was made about his life, *The Ryan White Story*, which aired nationally in 1989. Many celebrities and political leaders feted him, including Elton John, Michael Jackson, Nancy and Ronald Reagan, and Donald Trump. But Ryan often said he would gladly trade in his fame for a clean bill of health and that his greatest desire in life was "to be a regular kid."

By early 1990, his health plummeted. Ryan was able to attend the Academy Awards in Los Angeles in March of 1990 but a few days later, he developed diffi-culty swallowing and was rushed back to Indianapolis's Riley Children's Hospital. His respiratory condition worsened and he died on April 8, only one month before he would have graduated.

On August 18, 1990, President George H.W. Bush signed an important and bipartisan bill into law known as "The Ryan White CARE Act." This legislation provided more than $2 billion to help cities, states, and community-based organi-zations to develop and maintain coordinated and comprehensive systems of diag-nosis, care and treatment, especially for the poorest Americans contending with HIV/AIDS.

Today, modern medicine is making great strides in treating HIV/AIDS with a host of anti-retroviral drugs that allow patients to lead long and productive lives. Doctors and scientists are developing better means of diagnosis and the means for preventing infections. That said, there are about 1.2 million people in the United States infected with HIV and 1 out of 8 of them do not even know their HIV status.

More than 37,900,000 people around the globe are living with HIV. Since the global pandemic began, nearly 75 million people have contracted HIV and more than 32,000,000 died from AIDS. The awful fact of the matter is that AIDS remains one of the world's leading causes of death and, even at this late date, many AIDS patients still experience stigmatization and psychologically damaging bigotry.

That said, it is well worth taking some time to celebrate the life of a courageous young man who helped reduce such ugly impulses. Despite being dealt two bad hands—hemophilia and becoming infected with HIV from the very medication used to treat his blood disorder—Ryan White made a lasting and noble difference in the world.

CHAPTER 36

∽

The Day Judy Garland's Star Burned Out

On June 22, 1969, the music that was Judy Garland abruptly stopped. Her husband of only three months, a now forgotten fellow who called himself Mickey Deans (his real name was Michael De Vinko), broke open a locked bathroom door in her London flat only to find the singer and movie star slumped on the toilet with her hands still holding up her head. Although she looked well over 65, thanks to the ravages her body had endured for decades, Judy was only 47 years old at the time of her death.

A legion of fans from the 1940s to the present day have thrilled to Judy Garland's brilliant performances in such classics *The Wizard of Oz, Meet Me in St. Louis, Easter Parade, Babes in Arms*, several "Andy Hardy" films, *Strike Up the Band, Babes on Broadway, Meet Me in St. Louis, Easter Parade*, and her 1954 comeback film for the Warner Brothers, *A Star is Born* (for which she lost the 1955 Oscar for Best Actress to Grace Kelly, who starred with Bing Crosby in *The Country Girl*).

After Judy Garland's body was discovered, Scotland Yard was called and an autopsy was conducted by the London coroner Dr. Gavin Thurston. The cause of death was listed as "Barbiturate poisoning (quinabarbitone) incautious self-overdosage. Accidental." Dr. Thurston told the press, "This is quite clearly an accidental circumstance to a person who was accustomed to taking barbiturates over a very long time. She took more barbiturates than she could tolerate." Less surprising, given the amount of alcohol she routinely consumed, was evidence of cirrhosis of the liver, which may well have killed her had not the pills done the job first.

Accidental is not exactly the word I would have used to make the final diagnosis. Be it a predilection to alcohol, the now rarely prescribed barbiturates (then a common sleeping pill but extremely dangerous because of the risk of overdosing on them), "pep pills" (amphetamine), or the illicit drugs she was reported to have consumed while partying with musicians in swinging London of the late 1960s,

Literatim: Essays at the Intersections of Medicine and Culture. Howard Markel, Oxford University Press (2020).
© Oxford University Press.
DOI: 10.1093/oso/9780190087647.001.0001

active addiction is a slow but certain form of death. It is what one of my patients once called "a slow suicide for those too afraid to do it more quickly."

According to her obituary in the *New York Times*, Judy attempted suicide on, at least, 20 different occasions beginning at the age of 28. She was hospitalized many more times—for many different health crises ranging from "nervous breakdowns," injuries after, literally, falling down drunk, and laryngitis and vocal problems.

A singer of remarkable power and range, Judy Garland (born Francis Gumm on June 10, 1922 in Grand Rapids, Minnesota) was one of the brightest stars in the firmament that was the Metro-Goldwyn-Mayer film studio of the 1940s. She was abruptly fired in 1950 from playing Annie Oakley in the MGM production of *Annie Get Your Gun* for excessive tardiness, overweight, drunkenness, and "instability." Only one month into filming, *Annie Get Your Gun* Betty Hutton was hired to fill Judy's ruby slippers, so to speak.

Heavily drugged on a slurry of medications she had been legally prescribed by quack doctors since her earliest days at MGM, along with unhealthy doses of booze and opiates, she stumbled through her lines and songs. She also fought bitterly with the alcoholic and sadistic director Busby Berkeley, with whom she had a bitter history with, dating back to the 1942 film that introduced Gene Kelly to moviegoers, *For Me and My Gal*. The latter film is a stunningly terrific musical in glorious black and white. I challenge anyone to watch these two talented stars effortlessly sing and dance the title song without breaking into a warm smile.

After a lengthy hospitalization at the Peter Bent Brigham Hospital and the Austin Riggs Psychiatric Hospital, she was given another chance to work on the 1950 movie, *Summer Stock*, with her old pal, Gene Kelly. Judy's weight ballooned and dropped during the filming, which is evident from watching the different scenes, and her tardiness and absenteeism led to a final dismissal from MGM on June 17, 1950. Despondent and depressed, she attempted suicide by lightly grazing her throat with a shard of glass.

Long before those tough times, while filming all those wonderful movies at MGM with an impossibly young Mickey Rooney, Judy was prescribed stimulants and depressants, which she claimed was at the direct order of the studio mogul, Louis B. Mayer. Making matters worse, her adolescence was not spent in a high school like normal American teens but, instead, at the studio, film premiers and parties with the likes of Lana Turner and Clark Gable.

"They'd give us pep pills," she recalled, "then they'd take us to the studio hospital and knock us cold with sleeping pills...after four hours they'd wake us up and give us pep pills again...that's the way we worked, and that's the way we got thin. That's the way we got mixed up. And that's the way we lost contact." Mickey Rooney, incidentally, denied Judy's version, telling more than one journalist, "Judy Garland was never given any drugs by Metro-Goldwyn-Mayer. Mr. Mayer didn't sanction anything for Judy. No one on that lot was responsible for Judy Garland's death. Unfortunately, Judy chose that path."

Regardless of who gave who drugs, Judy was a full-blown alcoholic and drug addict long before she turned thirty, in an era when most Americans considered this rapacious killer to be a moral failing rather than a bona fide disease of the mind, body and soul.

As the *New York Times* opined, "perhaps the most remarkable thing about the career of Judy Garland was that she was able to continue as long as she did—long after her voice had failed and long after her physical reserves had been spent in various illnesses that might have left a less tenacious woman an invalid."

Several years ago, when writing my book *An Anatomy of Addiction*, I attempted to explain the risks of a disease that begins with a voluntary action but soon transmogrifies into a deadly obsession. I was reminded of those words while thinking and writing about the American icon that was Judy Garland:

"Addictive agents, when taken chronically and copiously, can transform anatomy. Like an overloaded power switch, an insurgency of bad judgment and risky behavior hijacks the brain's delicate circuitry, inducing temporary states of well-being and release from all inhibitions. Long after the high has disappeared, a neurologically mediated form of bondage forces the addict to pursue [her] own destruction. His body progressively demands greater amounts in exchange for briefer moments of escape amid a growing cascade of physical and mental health breakdowns. In the end, for the witness it is death at its most repellent and for the addict at its most seductive . . . Imagine this susceptibility as a wheel of misfortune that includes wedges depicting risks related to genetics, environment, mode of administration, and emotional or physical trauma. The addict's luck runs short when the wheel stops at the most harmful wedges."

Requiescat in pace, Miss Garland. Your luck ran out fifty years ago but the gifts you gave to the world, still available on film and recorded discs, remains our collective win.

CHAPTER 37

cʌɔ

How *A Raisin in the Sun* Author Lorraine Hansberry Defined What It Meant to Be "Young, Gifted and Black"

Lorraine Hansberry was the first African American woman playwright to have a play performed on Broadway. The play, of course, was the brilliant drama, *A Raisin in the Sun.*

Opening at the Ethel Barrymore Theatre on March 11, 1959, *A Raisin in the Sun* won Hansberry the New York Drama Critics' Circle Award for Best Play, garnered four Tony Awards (Best Play, Best Direction/Lloyd Richards, Best Actor/Sidney Poitier and Best Actress/Claudia McNeil), was translated in 35 different languages, and has been performed all over the world.

The play's title comes from a line of poetry by the great Harlem Renaissance poet Langston Hughes entitled "Harlem:" *What happens to a dream deferred? Does it dry up like a raisin in the sun?*

Hansberry's play tells the story of an African American family living in a cramped rental apartment in Chicago. The matriarch hopes to buy a house in a predominantly white neighborhood but cannot because of the racially restrictive home ownership covenants of the day.

The play was based on the experiences of Lorraine's father, Carl Augustus Hansberry, who was a successful real estate broker in Chicago. In 1938, he purchased a home in the predominantly white Washington Park subdivision of the Woodlawn section of Chicago's south side. Soon after, the Hansberry family was exposed to the rage of their white neighbors opposed to their moving in next to them.

Both Carl and his wife, Nannie Louise Hansberry, were active members of the Chicago chapters of the NAACP and Urban League (as well as the Republican Party, which was still known as the "party of Abraham Lincoln"). Carl challenged

Literatim: Essays at the Intersections of Medicine and Culture. Howard Markel, Oxford University Press (2020).
© Oxford University Press.
DOI: 10.1093/oso/9780190087647.001.0001

the racist notion of restrictive covenants in a long legal battle that went all the way to the U.S. Supreme Court (Hansberry v. Lee, 311 U.S. 32, 1940). The court found that Hansberry could sue over the covenant, but did not rule on the unconstitutionality of restrictive residential covenants in general. Carl later ran for U.S. Congress and lost.

In his final years, he grew increasingly frustrated over the raw racism in our nation. He hoped to move his family to Mexico but died prematurely in 1946 at age 51 of a cerebral hemorrhage.

Lorraine Hansberry was born on May 19, 1930, and grew up in an intellectual milieu where she had frequent contact with W.E.B. DuBois, Paul Robeson and other notable African American activist leaders.

One of her first jobs, after attending the University of Wisconsin and the New School in New York City, was working on *Freedom*, a black newspaper founded by Paul Robeson and Louis Burnham. She played many roles there: subscription clerk, receptionist, typist, editorial assistant, reporter and editorial writer.

She was active in the civil rights movement, as well as in campaigns for black Africans living under the yoke of colonialist rule, and the rights of Islamic women of Egypt. In 1952, she attended a peace conference in Montevideo, Uruguay, representing Robeson, whose passport had been revoked because of his Communist sympathies.

She was also active in the nascent gay rights movement in New York City. Recent biographical studies report Hansberry was a lesbian and closeted.

In 1953, Hansberry married Robert Nemiroff, a Jewish publisher, songwriter and activist. They lived in Greenwich Village. They divorced in 1962 but remained close friends and he became her literary executor until his death in 1991.

Hansberry wrote *Raisin in the Sun* between her 26th and 27th birthdays. When it was produced two years later, it was an immediate hit and, in 1961, a Golden Globe-nominated motion picture starring Sidney Poitier. In 1973, the play was transformed into a musical, "Raisin," which won the 1974 Tony for best musical. More recently, the play was performed on Broadway in 2004 and on television in 2008, starring Sean Combs, Audra McDonald and Phylicia Rashad.

While her most famous work has lived on in the 60 years since its debut, Hansberry died at the age of 34 of pancreatic cancer, currently the fourth-leading cause of cancer deaths in the U.S.

According to the American Cancer Society, in 2019 alone more than 56,000 people (nearly 30,000 men and 26,000 women) will be diagnosed with the disease. Roughly 45,000 people (nearly 24,000 men and more than 21,000 women) will die of the disease this year. The average lifetime risk of pancreatic cancer is one in 64, but there are risk factors that can increase those odds such as inherited genes, including BRCA2 and p16, the cause of Lynch syndrome;. Other risk factors include diabetes mellitus, family history of pancreatic cancer, pancreatitis, smoking, obesity and being over the age of 65.

Symptoms, which typically appear after the tumor has grown and spread, include pain in the upper abdomen that radiates to the back; loss of appetite or unintended weight loss; depression; new-onset diabetes; blood clots; fatigue; yellowing of the skin and the whites of the eyes (jaundice), which indicates liver involvement.

The diagnosis is most often made with imaging techniques, such as a CAT or MRI scans, but medical scientists are working on a series of blood and genetic tests to detect the disease before it has a chance to spread and kill.

Treatments include radiation, chemotherapy, and immune therapies, but the earlier the disease is caught, the better the chances one has of survival.

Hansberry was 32 when first stricken with pancreatic cancer and she was in and out of hospitals for the remainder of her life. She died at age 34 on January 12, 1965.

Her funeral was held at the Church of the Master in Harlem where she was eulogized by Robeson and the SNCC organizer James Forman; Langston Hughes read a poem; Reverend Martin Luther King Jr. and James Baldwin, a close friend, sent along written tributes.

After her death, Nemiroff created a play called *To Be Young, Gifted and Black*, based on Hansberry's writings, and which was later published as autobiographical collection.

The phrase comes from a speech Hansberry made to winners of a writing contest in 1964: "Though it is a thrilling and marvelous thing to be merely young and gifted in such times, it is doubly so, doubly dynamic—to be young, gifted and black."

When we celebrate Hansberry today, we can remember those who have fallen to pancreatic cancer, and cheer on those who have survived this terrible disease. Perhaps we ought to all listen to the 1969 civil rights song Nina Simone wrote in Lorraine's honor:

When you feel really low, Yeah, there's a great truth you should know,

When you're young, gifted and black, Your soul's intact

CHAPTER 38

༄

Edgar Allan Poe's Greatest Mystery Was His Death

Every January 19, mystery fans celebrate the birthday of one of America's most celebrated if also creepiest writers: Edgar Allan Poe.

I lived in Baltimore, Maryland in the late 1980s and early 1990s, during the years of my pediatrics and graduate school training. Whenever I drove to the airport, I always made sure to pass the Westminster Hall and Burying Ground at the southeast corner of West Fayette and North Greene Streets. It is there where Poe was buried, first in an unmarked grave in 1849, before being exhumed and reburied in 1875 under a monument (which erroneously lists his date of birth as January 20), paid for by a collection of pennies raised by Baltimore school children. (A penny went a lot further back then than it does today.)

For decades, an anonymous fan, dressed in black with a wide-brimmed hat, white scarf and a silver-tipped walking cane, has honored Poe's correct birthday by leaving a bottle of cognac and three long-stemmed roses at the foot of his monument.

My favorite tale about honoring Poe, however, is the probably apocryphal one in which controversial Baltimore satirist H. L. Mencken would conclude his drinking parties by walking over to the Westminster Burying Ground and urinating on Poe's grave out of respect.

Many medical fans of Edgar Allan Poe have shown their respect, too, but have done so in purely pathological contemplation on how (and why) the writer died so young.

As the story goes, one rainy, nasty night of October 3, 1849, Joseph Walker, a pressman for the *Baltimore Sun*, was making his way to Gunner's Hall. The occasion was election night and the hall was the polling place for Baltimore's old 4th Ward. On his way there, Walker found a man, lying in the gutter, confused, bedraggled, and under the influence of some type of intoxicant.

Literatim: Essays at the Intersections of Medicine and Culture. Howard Markel, Oxford University Press (2020).
© Oxford University Press.
DOI: 10.1093/oso/9780190087647.001.0001

Shabbily dressed (in someone else's clothing, as it turned out), Edgar Allan Poe was in dire need of medical assistance.

Poe was taken to the Washington Medical College. There, he spent the next four days chased by delirium, frightening hallucinations and incoherence, as he made repeated calls for someone named "Reynolds." The writer died at 5:00 a.m. on Sunday, October 7.

The attending physician, Dr. John J. Moran, reported the cause of death as phrenitis, an antiquated term for swelling or congestion of the brain. It was also a common way of politely referring to death by means of alcoholism. Sadly, none of Poe's medical records or even the actual death certificate survives. He was only 40 years old.

To this day, the cause of Poe's death or even how he came to die in Baltimore remains a mystery worthy of the man who invented the detective story. That story, of course, was *The Murders in Rue Morgue* (1841) and the detective was the extraordinary Monsieur C. Auguste Dupin. Forty-six years later, in the first Sherlock Holmes story (Arthur Conan Doyle's 1887 novel *A Study in Scarlet*), Holmes famously criticizes Dupin as "a very inferior fellow" after his roommate, John Watson, M.D., tells Holmes that he reminds him of Poe's character.

The mystery of Poe's death began on September 27, 1840, when he left Richmond, Virginia, bound for Philadelphia to help a now forgotten poet, Marguerite St. Leon Loud, prepare a collection of her poems for publication.

Poe never made it to the City of Brotherly Love and may have stopped over in Baltimore for a drinking spree with some old Army buddies he met while at West Point (from which he was dishonorably discharged in February, 1831 for disobedience, failure to follow orders and a decided refusal to attend classes, daily formations and chapel services).

A notorious drunk and opium addict, many historians have hypothesized that an inebriated Poe met up with some unsavory characters, was badly beaten, and left for dead in the street.

Other Poe-ologists insist he was a victim of "cooping," a form of voter fraud then practiced by political parties of the 19th century.

In short, cooping victims were basically kidnapped, beaten, disguised, and then forced to vote for the gang's candidate multiple times under different names. As a reward for each vote cast, victims were treated to a schooner of beer or a shot of rotgut whisky. This practice was especially popular in Baltimore during the mid-19th century and fits nicely with how Poe was found near a polling place, in another man's clothing, and, clearly, under the influence.

More creative post-mortems have suggested Poe died of carbon monoxide poisoning from spending too much time indoors and breathing in too much coal gas (tests on the writer's toenail clippings were inconclusive) or mercury poisoning, which Poe might have received as a treatment while in Philadelphia during a July, 1849 cholera epidemic. (Although Poe's hair did indicate exposure to mercury, a common medicinal of the day, it was 30 times less than the level seen with those suffering from true mercury poisoning).

And because doctors love to diagnose the diseases of long departed, famous people, the list of possible causes goes on and on (without any pathologic evidence or even common sense), including such widely various conditions as rabies, a brain tumor and influenza.

In the end, we'll probably never know what carted poor Edgar Allan Poe away (although I like the "cooping" explanation best). Oddly, for a poet whose most famous line is "Quoth the Raven, Nevermore," that ever-growing list is unlikely to die any time soon.

CHAPTER 39

ↈ

The Medical Mystery That Helped Make
Thomas Edison an Inventor

Thomas Edison often claimed that October 22, 1879 was the day of the first successful test of his famous light bulb and, hence, the true anniversary of its creation. It was on this date that his incandescent light bulb glowed for 13.5 hours.

In fact, dozens of scientists had worked on electric light sources since at least 1802, when Sir Humphrey Davy created an early form of the electric arc lamp by connecting a battery to a strip of platinum that subsequently glowed, albeit neither very brightly nor for very long.

What Edison did to best his competitors, and thus get credit for inventing the first economically practical light bulb, was to find an effective incandescent material (a carbonized filament); develop a far better vacuum in his bulbs; and create a high level of resistance (a measure of how a material reduces the electric current flow through it). He also figured out how to distribute electricity to people's homes and buildings from a centralized source—his dynamo-powered electric stations—which was affordable to consumers and profitable for him.

Tinkering with his bulb, he applied on November 4, 1879 for U.S. Patent # 223,898, for an electric lamp using "a carbon filament or strip coiled and connected to platinum contact wires." (Approved by the U.S. Patent office on January 27, 1880, this was, perhaps, the most famous of his 1,093 patents, along with those for the invention of the phonograph and a process for making motion pictures). Several months after the light bulb patent was filed, Edison developed a carbonized bamboo filament that allowed his bulbs to last more than 1,200 hours.

The world has never been quite as dark ever since.

One of the great medical mysteries surrounding Edison's genius, however, was his profound deafness, which he considered to be a blessing because it allowed him to think and read with total concentration. As a boy, Edison once noted, "my refuge

Literatim: Essays at the Intersections of Medicine and Culture. Howard Markel, Oxford University Press (2020).
© Oxford University Press.
DOI: 10.1093/oso/9780190087647.001.0001

was the Detroit Public Library. I started, it now seems to me, with the first book on the bottom shelf and I went through the lot, one by one. I didn't read a few books. I read the library."

But what caused his deafness is still debated by doctors and hearing experts to this day.

The romantic version, one that Edison told many times during his long life, occurred at the age of 12. Although a long time resident of Menlo Park, New Jersey, he was born in Milan, Ohio and grew up in Port Huron, Michigan. As a young boy, he took a job as a "news butcher" on the Grand Trunk Railway run between Port Huron and Detroit. He rode the rails selling sandwiches, candy, peanuts and newspapers to the passengers. For young children reading about the great man, Thomas Edison's account of the source of his hearing problems remains indelible:

> *I was trying to climb into the freight car with both arms full of heavy bundles of papers. I ran after it and caught the rear step, hardly able to lift myself. A trainman reached over and grabbed me by the ears and lifted me . . . I felt something snap inside my head and the deafness started from that time and has progressed ever since. . . .Earache came first, then a little deafness, and this deafness increased until at the theatre I could hear only a few words now and then.*

In another version, he told of being hit on the ears by a train conductor when his makeshift chemical laboratory in one of the boxcars caught fire. The pugilistic conductor then threw the young Edison off the speeding train, along with his chemicals and apparatus.

Years later, he told close friends that neither event actually occurred, but he held to the basic premise that his hearing loss began at age 12. If, indeed, these traumatic injuries had occurred, Edison may have developed a disruption of the delicate bones in the ear that might explain his deafness.

One of Edison's biographers, Paul Israel, who is also the director and general editor of the Thomas A. Edison Papers at Rutgers University, has suggested that Thomas suffered from numerous ear infections as a child (and, perhaps, a serious bout of scarlet fever) that may have caused or, at least, contributed to his deafness. A few ear surgeons have retrospectively diagnosed otosclerosis (abnormal growth and remodeling of the tiny bones in the middle ear) or cholesteoma (a destructive skin growth in the middle ear) as the cause of his bilateral conductive hearing loss.

While middle ear infections (or otitis media) remain a common bane of childhood, what has changed since Edison's era is that infections caused by bacteria can now be easily treated with a course of antibiotics. Back when Edison was a boy, these infections either resolved on their own or smoldered and raged within, causing worse infections of the middle ear, erosion of the ossicular bones, perforation of the ear drum, infections of the mastoid bone, just below the ear canal, and, in the worst cases, spread to the brain and caused meningitis. In 1905, for example, a 57-year-old Edison was rushed to the hospital for a mastoid abscess behind the ear that was "very close to the brain." He developed another mastoid abscess requiring surgical drainage in February of 1908.

Today, pediatricians are careful to point out that many ear infections are caused by viruses and, thus, antibiotics are not automatically prescribed as in years past. Nevertheless, the risk of developing mastoiditis and deafness, while thankfully rare today, remains a concern.

To this pediatrician, the history of frequent ear infections sounds about right as a cause for his deafness. The wonder of it all, however, is how Edison used it to his advantage. In an April, 1925 article that appeared in *Cosmopolitan* Magazine, Edison explained how his "deafness helped you to hear the phonograph:"

There were no great specialists, I presume, in that region at the time, but I had doctors. They could do nothing for me. I have been deaf ever since and the fact that I am getting deafer constantly, they tell me, doesn't bother me. I have been deaf enough for many years to know the worst, and my deafness has not been a handicap but a help to me.

Perhaps the greatest inventor of all time, Edison changed the world with his brilliance and love for creating new ways to improve our lives. For Edison, deafness allowed him to shut himself off from "the particular kind of social intercourse that is small talk . . . all the meaningless sound that normal people hear."

It also allowed him to embody his most famous observation that "genius is about 2 percent inspiration and 98 percent perspiration."

CHAPTER 40

cᐧᗶɔ

How a Hotel Convention Became
Ground Zero for This Deadly Bacteria

From July 21 to July 24, 1976, more than 2,000 members of the Pennsylvania chapters of the American Legion attended their annual state convention at the Bellevue Stratford Hotel on Philadelphia's Broad Street. In the days that followed, Dr. Sidney Franklin, a physician at the Philadelphia Veteran's Administration Hospital, began treating several retired servicemen for odd, or atypical, forms of pneumonia. Many of these cases were quite serious, with complaints of severe shortness of breath and excoriatingly high fevers. Worse, none of the laboratory tests Dr. Franklin ordered helped in making a definitive diagnosis of these cases and the antibiotics he had at his disposal did not seem to work all that well. By August 2, four of his patients had died.

Dr. Franklin next called the U.S. Centers for Disease Control and Prevention to help investigate this deadly pneumonia. Franklin was worried that his patients might be infected with a new strain of swine flu that had recently been diagnosed at Fort Dix in February of 1976. Indeed, it was precisely at this point in American history when the Gerald Ford administration was gearing up to deliver a mass immunization against "swine flu," a public health crisis some historians have referred to as "the epidemic that never was."

By August 15, 182 Legionnaires who attended the convention were ill with serious forms of atypical pneumonia, and 29 had died. There were also a few odd but clinically similar cases, such as a Philadelphia bus driver, some pedestrians who had merely passed by the hotel, and one hotel employee who was the air conditioner technician.

The biggest problem with figuring out this epidemic was that it was caused by a "new" bacterium that doctors had not yet recognized, let alone treated. Another issue was the public scrutiny this epidemic elicited.

Literatim: Essays at the Intersections of Medicine and Culture. Howard Markel, Oxford University Press (2020).
© Oxford University Press.
DOI: 10.1093/oso/9780190087647.001.0001

1976 marked the celebration of the nation's bicentennial and the lead up to that anniversary was filled with hoopla and cheers. Nowhere was it more intense than in the City of Brotherly Love. So, when it became known that former soldiers who had visited Philadelphia were now being struck by a deadly and unknown illness, the media spotlight on the epidemiologists struggling to figure it out was bright and harsh. Even the rock star (and now Nobel laureate) Bob Dylan added to the frenzy by writing a song about Legionnaires' disease:

> Some say it was radiation,
>
> Some say there was acid on the microphone.
>
> Some say a combination that turned their hearts to stone.
>
> But whatever it was, it drove them to their knees, Oh, Legionnaire's disease

The CDC task force rounded up all the usual suspects at the Bellevue Stratford Hotel, but kept coming up empty handed. They checked the cadmium content of pitchers used to serve the Vets their Bloody Marys, because cadmium poisoning sometimes resembles influenza. They checked the elevators, the carpets and wall paper for contaminants. They searched the rooms of shut-in residents for parakeets that might spread a flu-like, respiratory illness known as psittacosis.

On and on it went until after Christmas of 1976, when a CDC rickettsial diseases specialist named Joseph McDade holed himself up in the laboratory with a gaggle of guinea pigs and blood and tissue samples from those who became ill. He was still smarting over the criticism he received from a superior officer at a Christmas party for not yet finding the cause of the "Legionnaires' disease."

In one set of studies, Dr. McDade noted clusters of rod-shaped bacteria in the livers of guinea pigs after they were injected with lung tissue from the Legionnaire patients. He then requested some serum from the patients to see if there was an antibody reaction to be found and, indeed, there was.

McDade later recalled, "My hair bristled . . . I wasn't sure what I'd got there but I knew it was something."

After more tests and experiments, he and his colleague Charles Shepard discovered a new bacterium, *Legionella pneumophila*. Although several CDC investigators were concerned about leaky refrigeration units in the hotel basement as a possible source for the bacterial invitation, it was not until another outbreak in 1977 when they established that *Legionella* bacteria thrived in the cooling towers of large buildings which can be aerosolized and spread through air-conditioning systems. The bacterium is not spread by person-to-person contact but, instead, when breathed into one's lungs from a contaminated climate control system.

The Bellevue Stratford Hotel cases were probably the result of a temperature inversion on July 23 that produced an acute heating up of the ambient temperature. This set in motion a rapid cooling of the warm air by the hotel's water tower. Thus, the disease-causing bacteria were aerosolized or misted both within the building and along its exterior sides, leading to illnesses among those who inhaled large amounts of bacteria.

Today, Legionnaires' disease can be prevented with better scrutiny and maintenance of air-conditioning and climate control systems and the reduction of stagnant water in such systems. Thanks to better diagnostic practices and better antibiotics that can penetrate the cell walls of the *Legionella* microbe, the disease itself can be more easily treated. Although there is a milder form, known as Pontiac Fever (because this syndrome was first described in Pontiac, Michigan), the more serious Legionnaires' disease can lead to hospitalization and bumpy medical courses. The disease continues to be a public health risk wherever there are problems of maintenance of tall and extensive building complexes.

Although we have yet to vanquish this odd and serious infection, it may well represent the first illness to be named after an annual convention!

CHAPTER 41

༄

The Brilliant Brothers Behind
the Mayo Clinic

The 29th of June marks the birthdate of Dr. William (Will) Mayo, the elder half of one of American medicine's most dynamic duos. He is best known as one of the founders (with his brother Charles, better known as Charlie, and their father, William) of the storied Mayo Clinic in Rochester, Minnesota.

He was born in Le Sueur, Minnesota in 1861. Will's father, William Worrell Mayo, was a physician and general practitioner. In 1864, during the Civil War, W.W. Mayo (the father) was named an examining physician for the U.S. Army enrollment and recruitment board, which was based in Rochester. In 1865, when Charles was born, the family decided to stay in Rochester, where W.W. Mayo soon became one of the leading physicians in the region.

Even as young boys, the Mayo brothers were recruited into helping their father's practice. They took on all sorts of chores such as tending to and saddling up the doctor's horses, compounding pills and potions prescribed to the patients, and many basic tasks of patient care. Well-schooled in foreign languages and the sciences, young Will was a perfect candidate for the University of Michigan at Ann Arbor, which was home to one of the finest medical schools in the nation.

Passing his entrance examinations with flying colors, Will matriculated in 1880. Michigan offered a rigorous, graded three-year program featuring both didactic lecture courses and time spent caring for patients in a new university hospital. Ironically, time devoted to attending real patients was then a relatively new feature of American medical education.

Will Mayo rose to become an assistant in surgery and a demonstrator in anatomy at Michigan, but one of his professors told him he would never succeed in academic medicine. Undaunted, Will returned home to Rochester on June 28, 1883 to join his father's practice. A few years later, Charlie began medical school at Chicago's

Literatim: Essays at the Intersections of Medicine and Culture. Howard Markel, Oxford University Press (2020).
© Oxford University Press.
DOI: 10.1093/oso/9780190087647.001.0001

Northwestern University, from which he graduated in March of 1888, and he, too, joined the family practice.

Both Will and Charlie Mayo were gifted surgeons, always on the prowl for new techniques and procedures that would help their patients. They could not have found a better time during the 19th century to begin this task. For example, the benefits of antiseptic surgery, as prescribed by Dr. Joseph Lister of Edinburgh, were just beginning to be adopted by some of the most prominent and most forward-thinking surgeons in the United States.

To expand their medical horizons, the Mayo brothers traveled to New York City, then the nation's leading medical center, to learn how to reduce the incidence of post-operative infections with vigorous hand-washing and scrupulously sterilized instruments.

In subsequent years, they learned new techniques by traveling to the Johns Hopkins Hospital in Baltimore to observe master surgeons William Halsted and Howard Kelly and to many other leading hospitals in North America and Europe. By the early 1890s, they adopted William Halsted's practice of using rubber gloves during their operations and developed their own new methods of aseptic surgery.

Gradually, Will specialized in operations of the abdomen and pelvis, especially those surgical problems involving the gall bladder and the stomach, and Charlie focused on procedures of the head, neck, throat and brain.

Around the same time, the Sisters of St. Francis founded the St. Mary's Catholic Hospital in Rochester under the direction of Mother Superior Alfred Moes. Impressed by the Mayos' surgical skills, she recruited them to base their practice at St. Mary's and this was the genesis of what is now known as the Mayo Clinic. As news of the Mayo brothers' operative successes spread, more and more patients flocked to Rochester and the surgical facilities at St. Mary's grew by leaps and bounds.

Beyond their operative acuity, the Mayos hit on the brilliant (and then revolutionary) idea of hiring other doctors, not only to help in the operating room but also those who specialized in other area in order to build a large group practice under one roof. By 1905, they had developed laboratories for both diagnostic purposes and conducting research.

Although other doctors referring patients to the Mayos often called the practice "the Mayo Clinic," it was not until 1914, with the opening of new building to house all their medical and surgical staff and employees, when the name was formally adopted.

In the years that followed, the Mayo Clinic transformed into the Mayo Foundation for Medical Education and Research, which later became the Mayo Graduate School of Medicine and is now part of the University of Minnesota. The brothers endowed it with $2.5 million, a sum that represented their life savings.

Charlie and Will received some of the greatest honors in medicine. As brothers, they were so devoted to one another that in July 1939, only a few months after Charlie died in May 1939, Will passed away, too.

Perhaps the most endearing (and most likely apocryphal) anecdote about these two remarkable men involved a fabulously wealthy patient who approached Will with the headstrong query "Are you the head doctor here?" William Mayo responded without a hint of irony, "No, my brother is the head doctor. I'm the belly doctor."

CHAPTER 42

⌒⋎⌒

How Walter Reed Earned His Status as a Legend and Hospital Namesake

There was a time when almost every American could recite the tale of how Major Walter Reed proved the Cuban physician Carlos Finlay's theory that mosquitoes transmitted yellow fever to human beings.

From colonial days to the late 19th century, yellow fever plagued much of the United States. These epidemics were horrific events heralded by undertakers wheeling out large wagons in the streets, shouting, "Bring Out Your Dead!" But yellow fever was hardly unique to the United States. The virus causing it, *flativirus*, thrives and infects wherever the *Aedes aegypti* mosquito (and a few of its relatives) propagate and where swampy land abounds, including South and North America, Africa, southern Europe and much of Africa.

For some, a case with yellow fever is simply a self-limiting one of aches, pains, loss of appetite, headaches and fever. But in more severe cases (about 15 percent) it can cause abdominal pain, extensive liver damage, jaundice or yellow skin, bleeding, kidney damage and even death.

Born on September 13, 1851 in rural Virginia, Walter Reed was educated at the University of Virginia in Charlottesville, where he received his first medical degree in 1869 at the age of 18, and the Bellevue Hospital Medical College in New York City, where he earned a second medical degree in 1870. After interning at several New York City hospitals, he joined the New York City Health Department where he worked until 1875. That same year, he sat for a grueling examination that allowed him to join the Medical Department of the U.S. Army at the rank of first lieutenant.

In 1876, he married Emily Lawrence and he served in Arizona and other western posts, where he took care of Army personnel and Native Americans. After being promoted to the rank of captain, in 1880, he practiced at Fort McHenry in Baltimore. Subsequent posts took him to Nebraska and Alabama, but when Dr. Reed returned

Literatim: Essays at the Intersections of Medicine and Culture. Howard Markel, Oxford University Press (2020).
© Oxford University Press.
DOI: 10.1093/oso/9780190087647.001.0001

to Baltimore in 1890 he was caught up in the scientific sweep of a new science known as bacteriology. While there, he took courses in bacteriology and pathology at the newly created the Johns Hopkins University. Under the tutelage of the famed pathologist and bacteriologist William Henry Welch, Dr. Reed could not have found a better place to study.

From 1891 to 1893, Reed served at Fort Snelling, Minnesota, followed by a stint in Washington, D.C., under the command of the new Army Surgeon General George Sternberg, himself a prominent bacteriologist, at the Columbian University (now George Washington University) and the U.S. Army Medical School. But his most important assignment came with the Spanish-American War of 1898, first to combat epidemics of typhoid fever, and then to Cuba in 1900 to figure out the strange etiology and prevention of yellow fever.

It was a deadly pursuit. One of Reed's assistants, Dr. Jesse Lazear, succumbed to yellow fever in the experimental line of fire. Another, Dr. James Carroll, contracted the disease but fortunately survived. In 1901, on the basis of their meticulous findings, Dr. Reed prescribed aggressive mosquito-eradication procedures, involving the control of larvae and water-breeding spots, that sharply diminished the incidence of yellow fever in Cuba and, a few years later, in Panama, where 50,000 laborers were building the canal. In fact, the Panama Canal, one of humankind's greatest feats of engineering, could not have been completed if yellow fever was not outwitted first.

The yellow fever-Walter Reed legend was once the "poster child" of American contagion stories. So ubiquitous was this tale that it even served as the basis for best-selling books, a 1933 hit Broadway play, *Yellow Jack*, and the 1936 MGM motion picture of the same title, not to mention dozens of juvenile biographies and cartoons such as a March 1946 issue of *Science Comics* featuring a colorful account of "Walter Reed: The Man Who Conquered Yellow Fever." One of his biographers, Howard Kelly of Johns Hopkins, called Reed's work "the greatest American medical discovery." At the very least, it was the U.S. Army's greatest contribution to the nation's health and the reason why its premier military hospital in Washington, D.C., was named for Reed. The man behind the legend died in 1902, at the age of 51, of an abdominal infection after the removal of his appendix.

In recent historical accounts, much has been made of Walter Reed's insistence that the impoverished Spanish immigrants and the enlisted soldiers who "volunteered" for these human experiments were informed about the risks they were taking. Indeed, the bilingual consent form Reed created may well have set a precedent for all human experiments that followed. Yet the kudos afforded Reed are valid only to a point. This story demands a far more nuanced consideration than the common trope that Reed was "first" to develop what is now called informed consent. Enlisted soldiers who were asked to participate in a potentially deadly experiment by their superior officers may have interpreted such requests as orders; vulnerable, poor newcomers recruited with tempting offers of $200 in gold coins for participation and bonuses if they contracted the malady (a sum many times more than their annual incomes) were not exactly giving their consent freely either. Indeed, Dr. Reed's concept of informed consent contained a wide streak of coercion and imperialism.

Today, more than 30,000 deaths and 200,000 cases of yellow fever are reported per year, not to mention over 1,000,000 deaths and 300-500 million new cases of malaria per year, and 24,000 deaths and 20 million new cases of dengue fever per year. These are but a few of the mosquito-borne diseases stalking the planet. In recent years, we have witnessed "new epidemics" of the mosquito-borne spread of Zika virus and began learning about its destructive power on the brains of unborn children. Experts on vector-borne diseases predict that the deleterious effects of global warming could lead to more mosquitoes and still higher rates of these scourges, particularly in impoverished nations in Africa, Asia and South Africa.

Sadly, the story of mosquitoes and their carriage of deadly infectious diseases refuses to die with Walter Reed.

CHAPTER 43

∽

Dr. Alzheimer and the Patient Who Helped Reveal a Devastating Disease

I t is fitting that a disease of forgetting is named for a person who is all but forgotten. June 14, 1864 marks the birthday of Alois Alzheimer, the German psychiatrist who is often credited for first describing the clinical and micro-anatomic features of a brain disease that steals the memories of millions of people each year.

There are, of course, many causes of dementia, a term derived from the Latin word, *demens*, which means "without mind." (The prefix *de* connotes "off" or "not" and the noun *mens* refers to the mind).

Most commonly described among the elderly, the devastating loss of memory and other cognitive functions associated with dementia can result from traumatic injuries to the head and brain, cerebro-vascular events, or strokes, untreated metabolic and endocrine diseases, and many other maladies.

For centuries, doctors had no clue as to the cause or causes of dementia. Even when autopsies were conducted at various points of history, brain analyses were not always performed and when they were, poorly understood. By the mid-nineteenth century, however, more and more scientists began to search for the anatomical seat of specific diseases and this was especially so with the pathology of many entities all lumped together under the term "senile dementia."

Alois Alzheimer was born in the German village of Marktbreit am Main, in Bavaria. The second son of a notary, he attended the Royal Humanistic Gymnasium and proceeded to focus on medicine in Berlin (where he studied under the famed anatomist Heinrich Wilhelm Gottfried von Waldeyer), Tübingen, and Würzburg. In 1887, Alzheimer wrote his medical school thesis on the wax-producing ceruminal glands of the ear. He took his first professional post in December of 1888 as a clinical assistant at the Municipal Asylum for the Insane and Epileptics (*Städtischen Anstalt für Irre und Epileptische*) in Frankfurt am Main where he toiled for 14 years.

Literatim: Essays at the Intersections of Medicine and Culture. Howard Markel, Oxford University Press (2020).
© Oxford University Press.
DOI: 10.1093/oso/9780190087647.001.0001

Under the tutelage of the micro-anatomist Franz Nissel, Alois mastered the difficult tasks of preparing and staining microscopic specimens of brain and nervous tissue from his deceased psychiatric patients.

The patient who helped unlock the anatomical puzzle of Alzheimer's disease was named Auguste Deter. She came to Dr. Alzheimer's attention on November 26, 1901, the day after she was admitted to the municipal asylum. Alois found her sitting on the bed in her room with a helpless, if not befuddled, expression on her face. Although she had enjoyed a loving marriage for over 28 years, she began experiencing changes in her personality at the age of 51, expressed as jealously towards her husband, progressive memory loss, suicidal thoughts, paranoia, shouting spells, and the fear that others might try to kill her.

Confined to the asylum, Frau Deter's health deteriorated at a dizzying pace, much to the consternation of her doctors and family members. She lost the ability to speak and spent most of her last months in bed, depressed, indifferent, and balled up in a fetal position. On April 8, 1906, a little more than a month before her 56th birthday, she died of overwhelming sepsis, believed to have been caused by a nasty bed sore expanding from her sacral spine to the left hip.

By this time, Dr. Alzheimer was working at the Royal Psychiatric Clinic at the University of Munich. At Munich, he supervised the famed Anatomical Laboratory founded by Dr. Emil Kraepelin, who is often referred to as the father of scientific psychiatry and a strong proponent of linking psychiatry to the emerging science of neuropathology. Dr. Alzheimer joined Professor Kraepelin in 1902 when the latter was still at Heidelberg University, and then followed him to Munich in 1903.

Alzheimer continued to monitor Deter's disastrous progress from a distance and, after she died, he asked his colleagues in Frankfurt to send him her brain. After preparing a series of slides and studying them under the microscope, Alzheimer described the classic pathological features of the disease: a massive loss of neurons and the presence of amyloid plaques and neurofibrillary tangles.

Dr. Alzheimer presented his findings on November 3, 1906, at a meeting of the Southwest German Psychiatrists in Tübingen. After his presentation of "a peculiar disease of the cerebral cortex," the doctor was welcomed with a deafening silence. According to several accounts of the event, the audience exhibited far more interest in the next presentation on compulsive masturbation. The chairman of the session tried to ease the psychiatrist's embarrassment by stating, "So then, respected colleague Alzheimer, I thank you for your remarks, clearly there is no desire for discussion."

Alzheimer continued to toil in relative obscurity, under the guidance of Dr. Kraepelin, before developing bacterial endocarditis, a severe infection of the heart, and dying on December 19, 1915. He was only 51.

Today, Alzheimer's disease is the cause of some 60 to 70 percent of all cases of dementia and affects more than 30 million people around the globe. Although the majority of these people are over the age of 65, approximately 5 percent, like Frau Deter, develop the illness much earlier.

In the United States alone, more than 5.5 million people have Alzheimer's disease, and every 66 seconds someone develops it. The cost to care for these patients is more than $259 billion per year. By 2050, experts predict there will be more than 16 million Americans with Alzheimer's disease and the annual cost to care for them could be as high as $1.1 trillion. More than 15 million Americans currently provide care for people with Alzheimer's and other forms of dementia. In 2016, this added up to 18.2 billion hours, valued at over $230 billion. Although deaths from heart disease has decreased by 14 percent since 2000, deaths from Alzheimer's have increased by 89 percent, making it the sixth leading cause of death in the United States. It kills more Americans than breast cancer and prostate cancer combined. In fact, one out of 3 senior citizens dies with Alzheimer's or another dementia.

It is an odd quirk of the medical profession that so many physicians race to be the first to describe a particular illness. The goal, of course, is that their name might be forever linked to various wars of biological devastation taking place within the bodies of their patients. One can only wonder if Dr. Alois Alzheimer might have taken pride or experienced a deep-seated sense of horror at his name being so closely associated with one of the most devastating neurodegenerative disorders known to humankind.

CHAPTER 44

ഐ

Diagnosing Vincent Van Gogh

Everybody knows that Vincent Van Gogh cut off his ear. The bloody event occurred on December 23, 1888. But how much he sliced away (the entire ear, a chunk of his earlobe, or a mutilation in between) and why has been argued about ever since. An even hotter debate exists among medical sleuths: what was the cause of Van Gogh's mental health breakdowns, especially during the last few years of his life? And the corollary query: did his madness contribute to his magnificent artistic vision?

One is reminded of all these contretemps every March 30, Vincent Van Gogh's birthday. He was born in 1853.

Let's begin with the most famous ear in all of art history.

Doctors and historians have sparred over the "ear lobe vs. entire ear" question for more than a century. An art historian named Bernadette Murphy recently found a long lost diagram penned by one of Van Gogh's doctors, Felix Rey, which shows the mangled ear after the fact and demonstrates that the artist did lop off the entire ear with a razor. Yet the clinical notes of another doctor, Paul-Ferdinand Gachet (whose portrait Van Gogh famously painted in 1890) state that only the earlobe was gone. The injury was probably somewhere in between.

Less a topic for schoolchildren but certainly one that fascinates adults was Van Gogh's presentation of his bloody ear to a local prostitute. According to one contemporary local newspaper report, Van Gogh may have had visions of immortality in mind when he was said to have uttered, "Keep this object carefully." The prostitute (others have argued she was only a maid at the brothel) promptly fainted. The following day, the artist Paul Gauguin, who was living with Van Gogh at the time, but spent the previous night in a hotel to avoid his roommate's odd behavior, found the artist in bed, passed out and covered in blood. Gauguin took him to the hospital and telegraphed Van Gogh's brother, Theo, to come down from Paris immediately. The ever-loyal Theo was at Van Gogh's bedside by nightfall.

Literatim: Essays at the Intersections of Medicine and Culture. Howard Markel, Oxford University Press (2020).
© Oxford University Press.
DOI: 10.1093/oso/9780190087647.001.0001

Even before this act of madness—one that resulted in his being committed to an insane asylum—many people considered Van Gogh to be off the beam. As a young man, he was prone to spells of depression and obsession, especially on issues related to his religious faith, and may have exhibited a nervous tic. At 27, his parents practically begged him to seek mental health treatment, but he rejected this request—no doubt a response rooted in the denial of his problems and the sorry state of both psychiatry and asylums in the late 19th century.

Throughout his young adulthood, Van Gogh abused alcohol and other neurotoxic substances, such as absinthe. Ever the struggling artist, he also lived a chaotic and less than healthy life. Moreover, Van Gogh was a frequent customer at both the Parisian brothels and similar houses of ill repute in Arles, where he might have easily contracted syphilis. The sexually transmitted disease attacks the central nervous system in its end stages and can make one quite mad.

From July 15 to September 25, 2016, the Van Gogh Museum in Amsterdam mounted an exhibit entitled "On the Verge of Insanity: Van Gogh and His Illness." As part of the background materials for the exhibit, a researcher named Laura Prins collected the various armchair diagnoses offered by a slew of physicians in the medical literature. They range widely from epilepsy, schizophrenia, and bipolar disease to neurosyphilis, cycloid psychosis (a mixed bag of anxiety, elation, depression, hallucinations and schizophrenic and bipolar symptoms), and borderline personality. Because there is no way of proving any of these diagnoses, the "What Made Vincent Mad" industry is unlikely to end any time soon.

Another "medical argument" among Van Gogh aficionados concerns how Vincent actually died.

The long-held belief is that Van Gogh shot himself in the chest on July 27, 1890. After dragging himself back to the hotel he was living at in Auvers, he was treated by a local doctor named Felix Mazery and, later, his physician Paul-Ferdinand Gachet. The bullet, which deflected off of one of Vincent's ribs, was simply too deep for the medicos to remove. Van Gogh died of the wound two days later, on July 29, with his beloved brother Theo by his side. He was only 37.

In a superb, 2011 biography of Vincent Van Gogh, (*Van Gogh: The Life*), the Pulitzer Prize-winning authors Steven Naifeh and Gregory White Smith, raised several doubts of the conventional wisdom that the artist killed himself. "No physical evidence of the shooting was ever produced," the authors wrote. "No gun was ever found." The biographers insist that Van Gogh had no personal experience handling a gun, he left no suicide note, and the bullet entered his upper abdomen "from an unusual, oblique angle," rather than a straight-on path as one might expect when a person shoots himself.

Naifeh and Smith theorize that Vincent was accidentally shot by a friend's 16-year-old brother who carried a gun and often teased the artist to distraction, resulting in explosive episodes of anger on Van Gogh's part. The biographers further speculate that Van Gogh made "hesitant, halfhearted, and oddly hedged confessions" of an attempted suicide because he was depressed, eager to die, and did not want to incriminate the young man who did the deed.

Caught in the maelstrom of all these speculations, diagnoses, mental health mayhem, and, perhaps murder, we must appreciate that they all framed the stunning art we now treasure and adore. Madness, creativity, and masterpieces are all part of Vincent Van Gogh's legacy.

Perhaps, on the day of Vincent's birth, we might seek a bit of solace by quoting (or better still, singing) the final lines of Don McLean's 1971 hit ballad, "Starry, Starry Night":

> *Now I think I know*
>
> *What you tried to say to me*
>
> *And how you suffered for your sanity*
>
> *And how you tried to set them free*
>
> *They would not listen, they're not listening still*
>
> *Perhaps they never will.*

CHAPTER 45

ɔⱱɔ

How Poet John Keats Met
His Early End

February 23 marks the day in 1821 when John Keats, the Romantic poet who waxed on Grecian urns and nightingales, succumbed to tuberculosis. He was only 25. John was thought to have contracted the infection while taking care of his critically ill brother Tom, who died in 1819.

Born in 1795, John was the oldest of four boys (one who died as an infant) and one girl. His father, Thomas, ran a successful horse stable, which was owned by the father of Thomas's wife, Frances. On April 16, 1804, when John was only 9 years old, Thomas was thrown from a horse and killed. Frances left her children to marry again—a union that resulted in a legal separation only a few years later.

As a young boy, John was educated at the Enfield School, an institution known for providing a solid education in mathematics, science, literature, history, Greek, Latin and other sundry topics. Unlike the more prestigious Eton School, however, Enfield was did not prepare its students for going on to university. John was a voracious reader of the classics, history, mythology and even travel books, but in the classroom he was an indifferent student.

John's legal guardian, a tea merchant named Richard Abbey, convinced him to pursue a career in medicine. At age 15, he was apprenticed to work for Thomas Hammond, an apothecary-surgeon, for a period of five years at the cost of £210 (about $17,600 in 2016 U.S. dollars) for his room and board. Under Hammond's tutelage, John learned how to compound medicines, set fractured bones, deliver babies, pull teeth and, because the four body humors still reigned as the principal underpinning of disease causation, how to open veins, apply leeches and "blood-let."

At the time, the British medical field had a tripartite hierarchy of power.

Literatim: Essays at the Intersections of Medicine and Culture. Howard Markel, Oxford University Press (2020).
© Oxford University Press.
DOI: 10.1093/oso/9780190087647.001.0001

At the top of the pyramid were physicians who held medical degrees from Oxford, Cambridge or Edinburgh. They were considered to be the most learned, typically took care of well-heeled patients and, as a result, charged higher fees.

For the so-called "lower classes," both in the large cities and in the countryside, surgeons and apothecaries were consulted for health care. Surgeons were formally examined and held licenses to practice, but the snooty physicians considered them mere craftsmen. To this day, British surgeons are addressed with the title of "Mister" rather than "Doctor." These professionals were initially members of the Guild of Barbers and Surgeons but separated from the barbers in 1745 after forming the Corporation of Surgeons. In 1800, they established the Royal College of Surgeons.

Apothecaries, on the other hand, typically compounded and dispensed medications for physicians, surgeons and patients. After the passage of an Act of Parliament in 1815, however, apothecaries were licensed to diagnose and treat patients as a "general practitioner," upon completion of a compulsory apprenticeship and passing a set of formal examinations administered by the Society of Apothecaries.

An important part of Keats' medical training, aside from his apprenticeship with Hammond, was his work as a "house pupil" at the famed Guy's Hospital in London. There, he saw patients suffering from the worst maladies and assisted on horrific surgical operations, performed as quickly as possible not only to prevent massive bleeding, shock, and death, but also because ether anesthesia would not be introduced until 1846.

Keats' first surgical instructor was the famed Sir Astley Paston Cooper, one of Britain's leading surgeons. Sadly for Keats' education, he was soon yanked from Cooper's operating theatre and assigned to work under William Lucas Jr., a hack widely known as the worst surgeon in the hospital, if not all of London.

In 1816, Keats passed his apothecary's examinations and was licensed to practice. Before long, however, Keats told his guardian that he was abandoning medicine to pursue his poetic muse in earnest. Happily for English literature, he would never see a single patient as a doctor.

Struggling to survive as a poet, Keats competed with such marquee names as Percy Bysshe Shelley and Lord Byron (who once likened Keats' poems as a form of intellectual "Onanism," a Biblically polite way of referring to the poems as a form of mental masturbation). Keats also endured a slew of bad literary reviews in several high profile publications. Despite such sniping, Keats' poetry improved with each passing month. Unfortunately by 1820, Keats began to experience shortness of breath and lung hemorrhages, a result of his tuberculosis. His doctors advised him to take an ocean voyage (a common prescription doctors made for sickly, young men in the 19th century) and escape the dank, cold British winter.

On September 20, 1820, Keats and his close friend Joseph Severn sailed for Rome. It was a voyage plagued by rough waters and reports of a cholera outbreak in England. After spending 10 days in quarantine, he was placed under the care of a well-intentioned but incompetent physician named James Clark. Poor Dr. Clark has often been blamed for John Keats's early demise but given the state of medicine in this era, it mattered little who John consulted. That said, the therapy Keats endured remains shocking: starvation by means of a diet consisting of one anchovy and a piece of toast per day, multiple bleedings and too much laudanum (tincture of opium).

Some have claimed that John Keats died of disappointment over the poor literary reception his poems received. Indeed, upon learning of Keats' demise, the snobbish Lord Byron wrote his publisher John Murray in April of 1821:

> *Is it true, what Shelley writes me, that poor John Keats died at Rome of the* Quarterly Review?
> *[a dismissive 1818 review, written by John Wilson Croker, of Keats' Endymion] I am very
> sorry for it, though I think he took the wrong line as a poet, and was spoilt by Cockneyfying,
> and Suburbing, and versifying Tooke's Pantheon and Lempriere's Dictionary.–I know by ex-
> perience that a savage review is Hemlock to a sucking author—and the one on me (which
> produced the English bards &c.) knocked me down—but I got up again.—instead of bursting
> a blood-vessel—I drank three bottles of claret—and began an answer ...*

Poor reviews aside, Keats' consumption did what untreated, galloping tuberculosis often does: it consumed and destroyed his lungs. With respect to the bright red bleeding from his lungs, Keats observed, "I know the color of that blood. I cannot be deceived in that color. That drop of blood is my death warrant. I must die." As the young man hemorrhaged more and more arterial blood into his lungs, he basically suffocated and shuffled off this mortal coil on February 23, 1821. Although his corporeal life ended that day, his immortality as one of England's leading poets is extended every time a student reads and recites one of his beautiful odes.

Tragic though his premature death was, there can be no doubt that his choice to abandon clinical practice for poetry did not harm or hold back medical progress in the slightest degree. Any sawbones could open a vein or prescribe a powerful emetic. But only one man contained the literary power to compose a line like this:

> *Beauty is truth, truth beauty—that is all Ye know on earth, and all you need to know*

CHAPTER 46

ᴄᴧᴐ

The Infectious Disease That
Sprung Al Capone from Alcatraz

J anuary 25, 1947 marks the date of Al Capone's death. Better known as "Scarface Al" (a nickname Capone hated) or, as the FBI once referred to him, "Public Enemy No. 1," Capone is considered by many to be the most famous gangster in American history.

Yet after he was finally imprisoned for his life of crime, it was neither case law nor strong-armed tactics that set him free. It was, in fact, a tiny microbe called *Treponema pallidum*.

Capone's storied career included running gambling rings and bordellos, loan-sharking operations, protection services, murderous rampages, and a slew of other nefarious activities, all of which have served as the source for a multitude of motion pictures and television shows.

He was born in Brooklyn on January 17, 1899, and his parents, Gabriel Capone (a barber) and Teresa Raiola, were immigrants from Naples. True to form, Al was kicked out of public school at age 14 for hitting his teacher in the face. Shortly thereafter, he took to the streets as a low-ranking thug and gangster.

Sometime around 1920 (historians argue over the precise date), Capone stepped on the fast track to becoming a "made guy" when he was recruited by Johnny Torrio (whom Capone considered his mentor) to join "Big Jim" Colosimo's crew in Chicago. The two later colluded to murder Big Jim so that Torrio could take over the Colosimo's business.

It was Al Capone's first job in Chicago, as a bouncer in one of Colosimo's bordellos, where our medical story begins. Eager to partake in the business's offerings, Capone sampled many of the prostitutes working there and, soon enough, contracted syphilis. Capone was too ashamed to seek out medical attention for his "venereal disease." As a result, his disease was allowed to fester and progress in an unchecked manner. Yet at

Literatim: Essays at the Intersections of Medicine and Culture. Howard Markel, Oxford University Press (2020).
© Oxford University Press.
DOI: 10.1093/oso/9780190087647.001.0001

this point in medical history, even if he had consulted a physician, there was no guarantee of cure. Salvarsan, or arsphenamine, the medication developed by Paul Ehrlich, who won the 1908 Nobel Prize for Physiology or Medicine, was a fairly good treatment for what was once known as "the Great Pox." That said, it was hardly perfect. Indeed, syphilis remained a major cause of death in the United States until after World War II when the real magic bullet, penicillin, became widely available.

Syphilis has three major stages. The primary stage is heralded by a painless sore, or chancre. Because the infection is typically transmitted sexually, that sore is most commonly found on the genitals and appears anywhere from three to 90 days after exposure. After the chancre heals, the infected person then experiences a rash over all or much of the body. This secondary stage occurs four to 10 weeks after exposure. And then the infection goes quiet—without any symptoms or problems for years. But syphilis is merely fooling the infected individual that all is well. Over the next several years, the syphilis microbes are pathologically boring their way into various organs of the body, especially the liver, the heart and the brain. When the symptoms of this damage do appear (the third stage of syphilis), a decade or more after infection, it is typically too late to change the disease's march toward killing the infected person.

Al Capone, of course, graduated to terrorizing Chicago and beyond. It took dozens of years of criminal mayhem before the U.S. federal government finally nailed him in 1931 for, of all things, tax evasion. He was sentenced to 11 years, first at a federal penitentiary in Atlanta and, soon after it opened in 1934, Alcatraz Island, the famed prison in the middle of San Francisco Bay.

"The Rock," as Alcatraz was nicknamed, was widely heralded to be inescapable. Not so for Al Capone whose unchecked syphilis destroyed his brain while he was an inmate there, confined to Cell No. 181.

Neurosyphilis has many manifestations along the central and peripheral nervous system but Capone's case was notable for making him certifiably insane. He often failed to follow the guards' orders even at the penalty of severe punishment, less out of defiance than out of an inability to intellectually process them. Occasionally, he wore a "strange grin" on his face and even dressed up in his winter coat, hat and gloves while sitting quietly in his heated cell. At other times, he was somewhat lucid.

His wife, Mae, seized on Al's increasingly odd behavior and petitioned the warden to release him from Alcatraz. The "fact" that cinched the deal was a formal diagnosis of syphilis of the brain made in February of 1938. Capone was released on November 16, 1939 on the grounds of "good behavior" and, more cogently, his medical condition.

Capone's life back "on the outside" was hardly a picnic. His physical and mental health continued to deteriorate and his syphilis worsened with each passing year until his death in Florida, of heart failure, on January 25, 1947. He was only 48.

Yet how ironic, despite all the "tommy guns" Capone shot at others, it was "a shot of syphilis"—as the vernacular of the day referred to such infections—that served as his "get out of jail free" card.

CHAPTER 47

∽

Dr. Albert Schweitzer, a Renowned Medical Missionary with a Complicated History

Dr. Albert Schweitzer was born on January 14, 1875. Today, he may be a somewhat forgotten, or even a controversial, figure but a half a century or more ago, the mere mention of the name Schweitzer instantly conjured up images of selflessness, heroism and the very model of a modern, humane physician.

Among his many charitable works, Dr. Schweitzer founded a hospital in Lambaréné, which was situated in what was then known as French Equatorial Africa, and is today the capital of the province of Moyen-Ogooué in the nation of Gabon. His 1931 autobiography, *Out of My Life and Thought*, describing much of his work in Africa, was an international best-selling book. In 1952, he won the Nobel Peace Prize.

Albert was born in 1875 in Kaysersberg (Alsace-Lorraine), Germany, (now Haut-Rhin, France), only two months after Germany annexed that province from France, as a result of winning the Franco-Prussian war. His father, a Lutheran pastor, moved the family to a nearby town, Gunsbach, which was situated in the foothills of the Vosges mountain range. It was a beautiful locale that Albert would often return to for the rest of his life, especially when he was weary from his many medical and missionary responsibilities.

As a boy, Albert was frail in health but robust in intellect and talent. He took to playing the organ as soon as he was big enough to reach the pedals and amazed all who listened to him. The doctor never entirely left the pursuit of music and became well known as a virtuoso on the keyboard and pipes, especially when he played the works of Bach.

Literatim: Essays at the Intersections of Medicine and Culture. Howard Markel, Oxford University Press (2020).
© Oxford University Press.
DOI: 10.1093/oso/9780190087647.001.0001

Albert entered the Kaiser Wilhelm University of Strasbourg at age 18. There he studied theology, philology, and the theory of music. He progressed to studying for his Ph.D. in theology in 1899 at the Sorbonne, where he focused on the religious philosophy of Immanuel Kant. The University of Tübingen published the dissertation that resulted in 1899.

During his compulsory military service in 1894, Schweitzer had an epiphany of sorts while reading the *Book of Matthew*, Chapters 10 and 11 (in Greek, no less). The passage that appears to have directed his professional life describes Jesus exhorting his followers to "Heal the Sick, cleanse the lepers, raise the dead, cast out devils: freely ye have received, freely give." (*Matthew*, 10:8) In 1896, at the age 21, he decided to devote a period of time studying science and the arts and then to dedicate the rest of his life to helping the suffering.

Ever the autodidact, during this period Albert also served as curate for the church Saint-Nicolas in Strasbourg. At the same time he gave organ concerts, delivered lectures and wrote books about theology. The latter activity resulted in several volumes over the years that made his reputation as a major, albeit somewhat controversial, theologian.

In 1905, he decided to take up a call from the Society of Evangelist Missions of Paris to become a physician and help them advance their cause and work. The following year, 1906, (and despite pleas from his family to pursue his religious studies) a 31-year-old Albert began medical school. He received his M.D. in 1913 with specialization qualifications in tropical medicine and surgery. His medical dissertation was titled, "The Psychiatric Study of Jesus."

In June of 1912, he married Helene Bresslau (the daughter of a professor of history at Strasbourg). Helene took up nursing to help her husband in his pursuits; later, she became skilled at delivering anesthesia to the patients on whom Albert would operate. On Good Friday of 1913, the couple set sail, at their own expense, from Bordeaux to Africa. Once in Lambaréné, he established a small hospital at a station set up by the Paris Missionary Society. It was about 200 miles away from the mouth of the Ogooué River at Port Gentil (now Cape Lopez).

The maladies the Schweitzers treated were both horrific and deadly. They ranged from leprosy, dysentery, elephantiasis, sleeping sickness, malaria, yellow fever, to wounds incurred by encounters with wild animals and many common health problems to which the human body is subject. The living conditions, too, were horrid with makeshift huts for shelter and medical care, hot, steamy tropical days, cold nights, and huge gusts of wind and rainfall.

Schweitzer and his wife did the best they could. In their first nine months in Africa, they treated more than 2,000 patients. In the years that followed, the hospital grew by leaps and bounds, not only in terms of bricks and mortar but also in its delivery of comprehensive and modern health care. By the 1950s, 3 unpaid physicians, 7 nurses and 13 volunteer aides staffed the Schweitzer Hospital. At the time of Dr. Schweitzer's death, at age 90 in 1965, the compound comprised 70 buildings, 350 beds and a leper colony for 200.

Dr. Schweitzer became especially famous for giving benefit concerts and lectures in Europe as a means of fundraising for his hospital back in Africa. His philosophy, he often stated, was built upon the principle of a "reverence for life" and the religious and ethical imperatives of helping others.

In the early 1950s, as the horrors of Hiroshima and Nagasaki finally settled into the world's conscience, he joined forces with Albert Einstein, Otto Hahn, Bertrand Russell, and others to urge social responsibility and a ban on the use of nuclear weapons. Lecturing widely on "the problems of peace," Dr. Schweitzer told his wide audience, "The end of further experiments with atom bombs would be like the early sunrays of hope which suffering humanity is longing for."

Not all was sunny with Schweitzer's social commentary. In recent years, many have taken him to task for decidedly paternalistic and racist descriptions of his African patients that would offend many a 21st century observer. For example, he once said, "The African is indeed my brother, but my junior brother." On other occasions, he opined, "I let the Africans pick all the fruit they want. You see, the Good Lord has protected the trees. He made the Africans too lazy to pick them bare."

The list, alas, goes on and his prejudices are difficult, if not impossible, to ignore.

Although unacceptable in today's culture, Dr. Schweitzer's comments about those he treated were, sadly, all too common during his era, one marked by colonialism, paternalism and racist views. Such comments were, at the very least, a contradiction of his worldview of showing reverence for all human life in both deeds and words.

That said, Dr. Schweitzer did devote more than half a century to practicing medicine in a remote location where few of his colleagues would dare to visit and for people who desperately needed medical care.

A complex man, to be sure, but his humanitarianism did affect the lives of many patients in desperate need of attention and, for the most part, he positively influenced the world in which he inhabited.

CHAPTER 48

ᖌᖕ

How Playing with Dangerous X-Rays Led to the Discovery of Radiation Treatment for Cancer

When the German physicist Wilhelm Conrad Röntgen's announced his discovery of X-rays in December of 1895, he lauded on the front page of just about every newspaper in the world. Indeed, many journalists called this phenomenon "X-Ray Mania."

In the months and years that followed, inventors like Thomas Edison set out to manufacturing X-ray fluoroscopes, shoe stores used X-rays to measure the size of their customers' feet, and carnival barkers hawked them as novelties for fairgoers who eagerly purchased "radiographs" of their bones. Most importantly, physicians began to figure out ways to apply this earthshaking discovery to the diagnosis and treatment of a host of serious illnesses that had long plagued humankind.

One of the first Americans to use X-ray radiation to treat cancer was a Chicago chemist and homeopathic physician named Émil Grubbé (1875–1960). The patient, Rose Lee, was a 55-year old woman suffering from the recurrence of inoperable breast cancer.

Grubbé graduated from the Hahnemann Medical College, a homeopathic medical school, in 1898. But in 1896, he was earning his living as a chemist and assayer. As part of his work, he often tinkered with the latest electronic gadgets of the day, such as Crookes tubes, induction coils, electric generators and fluorescent and photographic chemicals and plates. Included in many of the newspaper accounts of the discovery of X-rays were precise drawings of Röntgen's apparatus. Grubbé had all of these devices, including the important Crookes tube, on his workbench. As a result, he was able to reproduce Röntgen's work and set out to make his own "radiographs," or X-rays, on photographic plates.

Literatim: Essays at the Intersections of Medicine and Culture. Howard Markel, Oxford University Press (2020).
© Oxford University Press.
DOI: 10.1093/oso/9780190087647.001.0001

Like many a scientific investigator of this era, Grubbé was his own "guinea pig." Every day for two weeks, he took numerous x-rays of his left hand. At this point in time, however, no one yet understood just how dangerous the overexposure to X-rays was—and is—to human tissue.

As a result of his experiments, Grubbé developed severe burns on the back of his hand. On January 27, 1896, he consulted his medical professors at Hahnemann. The homeopathic doctors were astounded by the physical damage the X-rays caused to Grubbé's hand. But Grubbé's greatest insight came when J.E. Gilman, one of the doctors he consulted that day, observed: "any physical agent capable of doing so much damage to normal cells and tissues might offer possibilities, if used as a therapeutic agent, in the treatment of pathologic conditions in which irritative, blistering, or even destructive effects might be desirable".

According to Grubbé's memoirs, one of the other professors present was Dr. Reuben Ludlam. He was the doctor of record treating Rose Lee. She was suffering from a recurrence of her breast cancer after a radical mastectomy. A metastatic tumor had developed within her chest wall. At this point in medical history, long before effective radiation therapies and anticancer drugs, cases like Mrs. Lee's were horrible affairs, accompanied by bleeding, foul-smelling, painful ulcers and festering infections.

Desperate for a cure or, at least, an extension of her imperiled life, Lee agreed to Grubbé's suggestion of radiation therapy and the first treatment commenced at 10 a.m. on January 28. Placing lead sheets around the breast to shield the rest of her chest, Grubbé suspended a Crookes tube three inches above the malignant tumor. The X-rays were administered for about an hour—a shockingly long time compared to modern day radiation oncology protocols. Grubbé repeated this therapy several more times over the next 17 days.

On January 29, Grubbé later claimed to apply the new radiation therapy to a man named "Mr. A. Carr" who suffered from ulcerous lupus vulgaris (a tuberculosis infection of the skin) on his face and neck. Carr underwent several one-hour exposure treatments through mid-February.

Both patients are believed to have died within a month of their treatments. Rose Lee died of malignant cancer. Carr was said to have died after falling off an elevated sidewalk in Chicago.

But here is where historical matters become interesting if not downright muddled. Grubbé did not publish these accounts or claim credit for his medical accomplishments until the early 1900s. And when he finally did announce it, members of the medical community heatedly contested Grubbé's assertions. Moreover, a number of other doctors claimed they deserved the credit for discovering "radiation therapy." When asked what took him so long, Grubbé explained that he did not report these patients in the medical literature earlier because he was not yet a doctor when the treatments occurred. But this hardly explains why he did not publish the cases immediately after he received his homeopathic degree in 1898, unless, as he sometimes added, he was worried about the criticism he might receive from "regular," or allopathic, medical doctors. Yet given how many homeopathic physicians were in active practice in the United States at this time, this exculpatory explanation seems a bit hard to swallow.

No historian has yet been able to find a death certificate for either Lee or Carr, despite extensive searches in the warehouse containing the Cook County death certificates for 1896 and 1897. On the other hand, an FBI analysis determined that the patient notes on their cases, which Grubbé discovered among his papers in the early 1930s, appear to have been written at the turn of the 19th century.

That said, Dr. Grubbé did develop a large and successful X-ray clinic in Chicago, and enjoyed a hugely successful, albeit contentious, career. Sadly, his frequent unshielded exposures to radiation left him with a number of health problems requiring more than 100 surgical operations and amputations.

Recalled by some as flamboyant and colorful and by others mean-spirited and bitter, Grubbé spent a great deal of time and money seeking credit as the "father of radiation therapy." When Dr. Grubbé died, he bequeathed his fortune and medical library to the University of Chicago with the stipulation that someone there write his biography and memorialize his career. The chairman of radiology at the university, a distinguished and judicious physician named Paul Hodges, dutifully took on the task and discovered that the more he learned about Grubbé, the less he liked him. The result is a balanced but often critical tome published by the University of Chicago Press in 1966. Dr. Hodges later advised a historian interested in Grubbé's work: "if you're going to be fool enough to leave your money to have your biography written, then try to lead an exemplary life. Failing that, for God's sake, remember to tell your lawyer to stipulate that it be a positive biography."

To this day, Grubbé's place in medical history is often challenged, if not outright ignored.

Was Émil Grubbé the first doctor to employ radiation therapy? This, alas, is a difficult question to definitively answer and it seems unlikely we will ever have the precise answer with respect to his claims of primacy.

One thing that has become all too clear during my too many years of practice as a historian of medicine, is that whenever someone claims to be first to do anything, there is always another person who has evidence or a claim that he or she was "firster." Perhaps the better part of valor is to say that if Grubbé was not the first doctor to employ radiation therapy for cancer, he was, at least, among the first.

CHAPTER 49

cᐢ

How Medicare Came to Be, Thanks to Harry S. Truman

On July 30, 1965, President Lyndon B. Johnson found himself in Independence, Missouri. Although he was surrounded by a gaggle of politicians, distinguished guests and Secret Service agents, the president was armed only with a fountain pen, a bottle of ink and a sheath of papers. Seated directly beside him, so as to accommodate the newspaper photographers and the television cameras, was Independence's favorite son, the 33rd president of the United States, Harry S. Truman.

LBJ had traveled to the "Show-Me-State" to sign the Medicare Act of 1965 into law and to praise the 81-year-old Truman who, as Johnson drawled in his thick Texas accent, was "the real daddy of Medicare."

Designed to provide health insurance for Americans aged 65 and older as well as younger citizens with specific medical conditions or disabilities, Medicare was originally divided into two categories prosaically named "Part A" and "Part B."

Part A covered hospitalization with payroll taxes and Part B was an optional health insurance program requiring a monthly premium to cover specific outpatient services, medical tests and equipment, among other things. Back in 1965, the payroll deduction for Part A was about $40 per year and Part B cost only $3 a month!

President Johnson was hardly stretching the truth by honoring President Truman at the signing ceremony. During his administration, President Truman called for the institution of a federally funded health insurance program in 1945 and again in 1947 and 1949. Each presidential plea, however, was thwarted or ignored by the U.S. Congress, aided and abetted by powerful medical lobbies such as the American Medical Association and the American Hospital Association, which denigrated such efforts as a descent into "socialized medicine." Harry Truman's devotion to this cause was, in a sense, a means of honoring his former boss, Franklin

Literatim: Essays at the Intersections of Medicine and Culture. Howard Markel, Oxford University Press (2020).
© Oxford University Press.
DOI: 10.1093/oso/9780190087647.001.0001

D. Roosevelt who, for political reasons, was forced to remove an extensive health benefit plan from what became the Social Security Act of 1935. Parenthetically, another Roosevelt—Theodore Roosevelt—included a government-backed health plan on the platform of his failed presidential run in 1912 on the Progressive ("Bull Moose") ticket.

There was some movement towards developing a national health care program during the Eisenhower years and even more so during John F. Kennedy's far too brief presidency. But it was the powerful and politically savvy LBJ and the Democrats' landslide victory in 1964 giving them control of both houses of the U.S. Congress that pushed Medicare across the federal finish line.

Today, Medicare is much more complicated and expensive as it funds a medical-industrial complex featuring a great many medical miracles that could only be imagined in 1965 as well as a great deal of spending that requires scrutiny, better evidence of efficacy and, ultimately, reduction. Part C (or Medicare Advantage) was instituted during the Clinton administration in 1997 to allow beneficiaries to choose a health maintenance program (HMO) instead of traditional fee for service. In 2003, George W. Bush signed Medicare Part D into law, which asks beneficiaries to pay an additional premium in order to receive prescription drug benefits. The passage of the Patient Protection and Affordable Care Act of 2010, during the Obama administration, allowed for Medicare beneficiaries to receive a wide menu of preventive health care services and health screens and seeks to reduce the out-of-pocket expenses of Part D beneficiaries.

Today, more than 49 million Americans enjoy the benefits of Medicare; by 2030, experts estimate that number will balloon to 70 million. Health economists project a cost of more than $1 trillion a year to fund Medicare by 2022, thanks to the increase in the average American's lifespan, the ever-rising costs of medical care and new medical technologies, and the aging of the Baby Boom generation. And while these rising costs are cause for concern for those who worry about the health of our nation's future economy, polling data consistently note that Medicare remains one of the most popular federal government programs. For example, a conducted by the Henry J. Kaiser Foundation in February of 2012 reported that 70 percent of Americans believed Medicare "should continue as it is today with the government guaranteeing seniors health benefits and making sure that everyone gets the same defined set of benefits."

Back in July of 1965, President Johnson predicted that Medicare would be a vital protection for elderly Americans from the "hopeless despair" of not being able to afford health care. So in a very real sense, Harry Truman had a far more compelling reason beyond the merely political or presidential when he accepted Lyndon Johnson's invitation to sit beside him 49 years ago: the first Medicare card issued was presented to "Give 'Em Hell Harry," making Truman the nation's first Medicare beneficiary, and the second Medicare card was presented to his loving wife Bess.

CHAPTER 50

ᴄᴧᴐ

How to Save a Dying Heart

December 3, 1967 is a red-letter day in the history of medicine. It was also an important date in the personal history of Dr. Christiaan Barnard.

The South African surgeon made international headlines by successfully removing the dying heart of a 54-year-old grocer named Louis Washkansky and replacing it with a healthy heart. The donor, a 25-year-old woman named Denise Darvall, was in a car accident the day before. While still technically alive, Darvall was diagnosed by her physicians as "brain-dead." The operation, at Cape Town's Groote Schuur Hospital, lasted nine hours and required a team of 30 people, including Dr. Barnard's brother Marius, who was also a surgeon.

Louis Washkansky emigrated from Lithuania to South Africa in 1922 and built a thriving grocery business in Cape Town. A decorated World War II veteran who saw action in Africa and Italy, Louis was once an avid athlete who excelled in swimming, football and weightlifting.

Unfortunately, Washkansky was also a diabetic who developed a progressive and incurable form of congestive heart failure. Unresponsive to medications and rest, Washkansky's cardiologist referred him to Dr. Barnard, who had been hard at work experimenting with heart transplants in animals.

Although the kidney transplant was still a relatively new but successful procedure, having been developed in the early 1950s, heart transplantation was a far more difficult problem both in terms of surgical procedure and in effectively turning off a patient's immune system to prevent the rejection of another person's heart. There was also the issue of finding suitable organ donors—a concept now well-known and acceptable to most people, was once a disturbing, ethical dilemma.

Dr. Barnard was hardly the only surgeon interested in heart transplantation during this period. He had active competition from Dr. Adrian Kantrowitz and his surgical team at Brooklyn's Maimonides Medical Center, where the world's second (and the United States' first) heart transplant was performed on December 6,

Literatim: Essays at the Intersections of Medicine and Culture. Howard Markel, Oxford University Press (2020).
© Oxford University Press.
DOI: 10.1093/oso/9780190087647.001.0001

1967. Two other surgeons who performed the controversial procedure soon after Barnard were Drs. Norman Shumway of Stanford University, on January 6, 1968, and Richard Lower of the Medical College of Virginia in May of 1968.

As Dr. Barnard later wrote in his memoir, *One Life*, it was relatively easy to convince Louis Washkansky to undergo the novel operation: "For a dying man, it is not a difficult decision because he knows he is at the end. If a lion chases you to the bank of a river filled with crocodiles, you will leap into the water, convinced you have a chance to swim to the other side."

Getting a suitable heart to replace Washkansky's damaged one was a bit more difficult. Brain death was a controversial diagnosis back in 1967 and several judges around the globe threatened to arrest and jail surgeons who took organs from such afflicted individuals. Nevertheless, Dr. Barnard secured permission from Denise Darvall's father and commenced with the operation.

Recalling these historic moments years later, Dr. Barnard explained, "as soon as the donor died, we opened her chest and connected her to a heart-lung machine, suffusing her body so that we could keep the heart alive. I cut out the heart. We examined it, and as soon as we found it was normal, we put it in a dish containing solution at 10 degrees Centigrade to cool it down further. We then transferred this heart to the operating room, where we had the patient and we connected it to the heart-lung machine. From the time we cut out the heart, it was four minutes until we had oxygenated blood going back to the heart muscle from the donor's heart lung machine. We then excised the patient's heart."

After suturing the donor heart into Washkansky's chest cavity, it was gently warmed up to body temperature and began to beat with a lively vigor. The procedure worked!

Sadly, Washkansky lived only 18 more days. The massive doses of immuno-suppressive drugs (azathioprine and hydrocortisone), along with the radiation treatments he received in order to prevent a rejection response, left the grocer wide open to contracting life-threatening infections. The all-but-forgotten medical hero died of pneumonia on December 21, 1967.

A few weeks later, on January 2, 1968, Christiaan Barnard again made global headlines by transplanting the heart of a bi-racial young man into the body of a retired, white dentist named Philip Blaiberg. This was especially controversial not only because of that era's vastly different views on race and integration, but also because of South Africa's racist apartheid policies. Blaiberg survived 19 months and 15 days, probably due to organ rejection after an attempt to markedly reduce the strong immunosuppressive drugs he was taking.

Today, nearly half a century after the first heart transplant, organ transplantation medicine has advanced by leaps and bounds and has prolonged and improved the lives of countless people with failing kidneys, hearts, livers, lungs and other organs. Better drugs, better procedures, more advanced technologies, and modern systems of organ donation have all made this once-shocking surgical approach a common means of saving lives in the 21st century.

CHAPTER 51

∽

C. Everett Koop's Rise
from "Dr. Unqualified"
to Surgeon-in-Chief

On November 16, 1981, the U.S. Senate confirmed Dr. C. Everett Koop, in a vote of 60 to 24, as the 13th Surgeon General of the United States. He was sworn into office on January 21, 1982, by the president who appointed him to the post, Ronald Reagan.

Although the physician and surgeon had never served in a public office before assuming this role, Dr. Koop's character, forthright determination to serve the health needs of all Americans, and his stern, bearded visage helped make him the most influential and powerful surgeon general in American history. By the time he stepped down from his office in 1989, Koop was a household name.

Koop's tenure as surgeon general was filled with many public health triumphs. For example, Dr. Koop took strong stands on the dangers of tobacco and smoking.

He also was the nation's most visible health official during the early years of the AIDS pandemic.

Finally, despite his strong religious, moral and philosophical opposition to abortion, Dr. Koop refused to allow the office of the Surgeon General get drawn into the cultural wars of pro-choice/pro-life politics.

His work won supporters among those who opposed his nomination, specifically, the pro-choice movement and the gay community and, in turn, made enemies out of those in the tobacco industry, the conservative politicians who represented tobacco-growing states, the religious right, and members of the pro-life movement.

With his bushy white-gray beard (sans mustache), a 6 foot, 1 inch erect frame and the blue-black, gold festooned uniform of a vice admiral in the United States Public Health Service, Dr. Koop was a major leader in getting Americans to "kick

Literatim: Essays at the Intersections of Medicine and Culture. Howard Markel, Oxford University Press (2020).
© Oxford University Press.
DOI: 10.1093/oso/9780190087647.001.0001

the habit" of cigarette smoking—one of the leading killers of people around the globe, both then and today. Thirty three percent of all Americans smoked when he took office and that number fell to 26 percent by the time he returned to private life.

Moreover, by 1987 there were 40 states in the union that had completely banned smoking in public places; 33 had banned it on public transportation; and 17 had prohibited it in the workplace. His term witnessed the passage of over 800 local anti-smoking laws and the federal government banned the practice in 6,800 federal buildings.

More than any other federal official at the time, Dr. Koop immediately understood the import of the early reports of acquired immunodeficiency syndrome, or AIDS, that were appearing among gay men living in San Francisco, Los Angeles and New York during the early 1980s, as well as intravenous drug users, sex workers, hemophiliacs, and Haitians.

Although he later lamented that he was not able to interest either President Reagan or his successor, George H.W. Bush in making health in general and AIDS in particular a major emphasis of their administrations, Dr. Koop served as a superb role model for physicians and health professionals around the nation to become involved in the battle against AIDS, especially after its etiologic cause, the Human Immunodeficiency Virus, or HIV, was discovered and a blood test to detect it was developed.

He insisted on public health programs that taught adults and youngsters on the precise ways one contracted HIV and methods of safer sexual activity to lower one's risk, no matter how uncomfortable these messages may have been to the majority of Americans at the time. He also helped oversee a major effort at improving the nation's blood banks so that virus-tainted blood products were quickly removed from the blood donor pool.

Before he became Surgeon General, Dr. Koop was a prominent pediatric surgeon at the University of Pennsylvania. A graduate of Dartmouth College and the Cornell University Medical School, he specialized in correcting severe congenital birth defects, such as esophageal atresia (the incomplete formation of the esophagus, which is the tube that delivers food into the stomach).

In the years before his surgeon generalship, Dr. Koop was a well-known and fervent anti-abortion activist, who collaborated with Francis Schaeffer, a Christian evangelical pastor well known for his anti-abortion views. Koop was also a strong supporter of the rights of infants with severe birth defects to receive life-saving medical care. In the early 1980s, there was great debate over whether such infants should be allowed to die without extraordinary efforts to save their lives, especially when most of the medical and surgical interventions available were not yet as miraculous as they are today. At the time, Dr. Koop insisted that the medical and legal system had an absolute duty to protect all citizens, regardless of age, against neglect or discrimination—even if that went against parental wishes.

It was these associations that garnered the angriest comments directed at him during his confirmation process, a vitriolic set of events led by the powerful

Democratic U.S. Senator from Massachusetts, Edward M. Kennedy, who claimed that Koop's beliefs indicated a "cruel, outdated and patronizing stereotype of women." The *New York Times* castigated him as "Dr. Unqualified."

Still, it was Dr. Koop's unimpeachable integrity that both won the day in terms of his being confirmed as surgeon general and during his entire term in office. As he told his wife, Elizabeth, while traveling to Washington D.C. to testify at his confirmation hearing: "If I ever have to say anything I don't believe or shouldn't be said, we'll go home." His detractors had little to worry about, regardless of Dr. Koop's religious or moral views; to the end, he served as physician, not as an activist, and stuck to the medical facts for guidance.

Dr. Koop was a stellar physician, a superb advocate for the nation's health, and a role model for those who care for patients as well as those seeking out healthy lives. His death, at 96, on February 24, 2013 made the front pages of virtually every newspaper in the country and evoked sympathy among every American whose lives he so valiantly improved.

Even the *New York Times*, which initially opposed Dr. Koop's confirmation in 1981, admitted its errors in judging the doctor too quickly and too harshly. A 1989 editorial opined: "Throughout he has put medical integrity above personal value judgments and has been, indeed, the nation's First Doctor."

It took the editorialists eight years to do it, but they finally got the story right.

CHAPTER 52

cᴧɔ

A Hormonal Happy Birthday

The word hormone has long been a familiar part of the English vernacular. It can refer to a wide variety of things from the life-saving medications, such as insulin and epinephrine, to the biological and psychological maelstrom of adolescence.

The study of internal secretions, or what we now call endocrinology (a word coined in 1904, by Maurice-Adolphe Limon) was one of the major intellectual avenues of medical science during the late 19th and early 20th centuries. But the actual word, hormone, did not make its scientific debut until the great British physiologist Ernest H. Starling slipped it into his prestigious Croonian lecture, delivered to the Royal Society of Physicians in London on June 20, 1905.

The concept of a hormone was probably first posed sometime earlier when the distinguished biochemist Joseph Needham invited Starling to dine with him at the high table of Gonville and Caius College, Cambridge. The topic of the evening was Starling's 1902 discovery of secretin, a protein that is considered by many to be the first isolated hormone.

Secretin is synthesized by the inner lining of the duodenum, a portion of the small intestines, and stimulates the pancreas to release a watery load of bicarbonate. This process of alkalization neutralizes the highly acidic stomach contents and facilitates the small intestine's digestion of food. Upon hearing about this incredible chemical messenger, the classicist W.T. Vesey suggested calling it and kindred agents "hormones," from the Greek root for "to set in motion, to excite, or arouse."

Tall, impeccably dressed and quiet in tone, Professor Starling began his formal Croonian address to the British Empire's best medical minds with a boldly accurate declaration:

> From the remotest ages, the existence of a profession of medicine, the practice of its art and its acceptance as a necessary part of every community have been founded on

Literatim: Essays at the Intersections of Medicine and Culture. Howard Markel, Oxford University Press (2020).
© Oxford University Press.
DOI: 10.1093/oso/9780190087647.001.0001

a tacit assumption that the function of the body, whether of growth or activity of the organs, can be controlled by chemical means; and research by observation or accident or by experiment for such means has resulted in the huge array of drugs which from the pharmacopeias of various civilized countries and the common armamentarium of the medical profession throughout the world.

Starling went on to define hormones as "chemical messengers," which are "carried from the organ where they are produced to the organ which they affect by means of the blood stream and the continually recurring physiological needs of the organism must determine their repeated production and circulation from the body."

The first of four articles transcribing his momentous medical announcements about secretin and hormones appeared in print in the venerable medical journal, *The Lancet*, on August 5, 1905.

Interestingly, Starling's assertion contradicted the opinion of the leading and most powerful physiologist of the day, Ivan Pavlov of St. Petersburg. Conducting an enormous laboratory staffed by dozens of eager students and assistants, Pavlov developed a theory called nervism, which ascribed the control of the body's chemical messengers to the central nervous system. It was a view that many physiologists subscribed to and one that Pavlov believed was inviolable.

Starling and his brother-in-law, William M. Bayliss, repeatedly tried to reproduce Pavlov's experimental findings that neural reflexes controlled the acid-base content of food as it passed from the stomach to the duodenum but they could not.

Although Starling and Bayless acknowledged that neural reflexes might play a role in the digestive process, their experiments led them to isolate and identify secretin. It was a discovery that spawned a revolution of biomedical thought and, as Starling boasted in his 1905 Croonian lecture, successful treatments for a long list of endocrine diseases.

Back in St. Petersburg, Pavlov ordered several of his acolytes to replicate Bayless and Starling's experiments. Secretin's importance—and Starling's correctness— soon became obvious. Retreating to his study for an hour or more, the great Pavlov emerged to tell his students and colleagues, "Of course, they are right. It is clear that we did not take out an exclusive patent for the discovery of the truth."

CHAPTER 53

cﾟﾚ

For Dostoevsky, Epilepsy Was a Matter
of Both Life and Literature

November 11, 1821 is the birthday of Fyodor Dostoevsky, one of Russia's greatest novelists. The author of such classics as *The Brothers Karamazov*, *The Idiot*, and *Crime and Punishment*, Dostoevsky was also one of the most famous epileptics in literary history.

In his biography, *Dostoevsky, 1821-1881*, E.H. Carr uncovered a doctor's treasure trove of evidence documenting Dostoevsky's epileptic seizures as a young man, especially during his student years, 1838 to 1843. One of these episodes included a rather serious, generalized tonic-clonic (or grand mal) seizure in 1844, which was observed and described by several of Dostoevsky's friends. During his 20s, the novelist recorded several "journal descriptions" of what appear to be simple partial seizures. He also described how certain triggers, such as the lack of sleep, alcohol consumption or overwork, brought on his seizures.

Contemporary observers recorded more episodes during the 1840s, when Fyodor appears to have been stricken by several seizures of different types. Most famously, in 1849, he was diagnosed with epilepsy shortly before being taken to a Siberian prison in Omsk. He was sentenced there to four years of forced labor for espousing Socialist beliefs. His seizure activity only worsened during his imprisonment, and by 1853, he was quite debilitated from epilepsy as well as a series of mental health and physical ailments.

During his last decades of life, epilepsy continued to affect his life, work and output. Fortunately for literature lovers, in 1880, he was able to finish his masterpiece, *The Brothers Karamazov*. He died in 1881 after multiple bouts of bleeding from his lungs, most likely caused by tuberculosis.

Interestingly, not every doctor has agreed that the novelist suffered from epilepsy. For example, in 1928, Sigmund Freud, the famed psychoanalyst and neurologist,

Literatim: Essays at the Intersections of Medicine and Culture. Howard Markel, Oxford University Press (2020).
© Oxford University Press.
DOI: 10.1093/oso/9780190087647.001.0001

penned an essay, "Dostoevsky and Parricide," in which he argued that the novelist's seizure disorder was merely a symptom of "his neurosis," which "must be accordingly classified as hystero-epilepsy—that is severe hysteria."

Today, many neurologists have refuted Freud's psychogenic claim and have retrospectively diagnosed Dostoevsky with cryptogenic (of no clear cause) epilepsy of probable temporal lobe origin (the region of the brain where his seizures seemed to originate; temporal lobe epilepsy is one of the most frequently diagnosed forms of epilepsy and is notable for frequent, unprovoked focal or complex-partial seizures).

Like many great writers, Dostoevsky wrote about what he knew and how he experienced the world. Not surprisingly, many of his characters suffered from epileptic seizures. For example, he mentions the disease in his 1847 story, "The Landlady," where an old man named Murin experiences a seizure when he attacks the story's protagonist, Ordynov.

What is interesting about this description and those that follow is that they do more than merely note a trembling of the body or a loss of consciousness. Dostoevsky describes many of the cardinal symptoms of various types of seizures even down to the sensory auras and the sense of *déjà vu* many epileptics experience before a seizure and the intense fatigue they often feel after one.

Like Charles Dickens, Dostoevsky (who was a huge Dickens fan) eschewed cliché descriptions of diseases for his fictional world and worked hard to make sure he got the symptoms and disease patterns correct before committing them to the written page.

Epilepsy and seizures appear elsewhere in his work including his 1861 serial story "Insulted and Injured," which features an abused orphan girl with violent epileptic seizures or "fits." Dostoevsky also describes characters with seizures in his novels *The Idiot* (1868) and *Demons* (1872).

But the Russian novelist made the most famous use of his neurological illness when creating the illegitimate son Smerdyakov in *The Brothers Karamazov*. Smerdyakov, it may be remembered, suffers from epileptic seizures for most of his life. He murders his father Fyodor Pavlovich Karamazov and creates a series of alibis that he ties to several imagined seizures. Smerdyakov later commits suicide but not before framing his brother Dimitri for the father's death.

There were points in his life when Dostoevsky wrote he was grateful for his seizure disorder because of the "abnormal tension" the episodes created in his brain, which allowed him to experience "unbounded joy and rapture, ecstatic devotion and completest life." At other times, the author regretted the disability because he thought it had wreaked havoc with his memory.

Good or bad, useful or not, epilepsy shaped Dostoevsky's life as tightly as the "Superman" or *Ubermensch* philosophy seemed to frame the life of *Crime and Punishment* main character Raskolnikov. What remains so remarkable about this 19th century writer is that he was able to create such great art out of his disability rather than allow his disability to define or defeat him.

CHAPTER 54

ฝฆ

The Death of Oscar Wilde

The Wittiest Man Who Ever Lived

O scar Wilde uttered his last words in Room 16 of the dingy Hôtel d'Alsace
in Saint-Germain-des-Prés, Paris. The wittiest man of his epoch was said to
have exclaimed, "My wallpaper and I are fighting a duel to the death. One or the
other of us must go."

True or no, it was Oscar who went first. The great playwright, poet, novelist, and
essayist, Oscar Wilde drew his last, labored breath on November 30, 1900. He was
only 46 years old.

Ever since that moment, literary scholars, doctors, and Wilde fans have argued
about the precise cause of his death.

The long-held theory was that Oscar Wilde succumbed to the ravages of tertiary,
or end-stage, syphilis. Oscar told intimate friends that he initially contracted the
sexually transmitted disease in 1878, while still an undergraduate at Oxford, after a
brief liaison with a prostitute named "Old Jess."

For decades after Wilde's death, the common wisdom was that his syphilis
progressed into a serious brain infection during and after the time he was imprisoned in Pentonville Prison, Wandsworth Prison, and finally, Reading Gaol (Jail) for
"gross indecency" and sodomy. In the hushed parlance of Victorian England, Wilde
was a "practicing homosexual." This tragic series of events began when John Sholto
Douglas, the Marquess of Queensbury, accused Wilde of committing sodomy with
his son, Lord Alfred "Bosie" Douglas, and several other young men. The confrontation set in motion a travesty of justice that culminated with Oscar being sentenced,
on May 25, 1895, to two years of "hard labor, hard fare and a hard bed."

The British journalist and author, Arthur Ransome first publicly posited
syphilis as the cause of Oscar's death in a biography he published in 1912. This

Literatim: Essays at the Intersections of Medicine and Culture. Howard Markel, Oxford University Press (2020).
© Oxford University Press.
DOI: 10.1093/oso/9780190087647.001.0001

was a somewhat suspect conclusion given that none of Wilde's doctors recorded this malady as a cause of his death. In subsequent editions of the book, however, Ransome deleted this assertion. Nevertheless, the syphilis theory kept gathering steam and reached its zenith of credibility 76 years later, in 1988, with the publication of Richard Ellmann's magisterial and Pulitzer Prize-winning biography of Oscar Wilde. It was a diagnosis that left many uncomfortable, especially Oscar's grandson, Merlin Holland.

Fortunately, a London neurologist named MacDonald Critchley and two ear surgeons from South Africa, Ashley H. Robins and Sean L. Sellars, have spent considerable time poring over Wilde's medical and prison records to propose an entirely different, and far more credible, diagnosis. Critchley published his account in a 1990 *Medical and Health Annual* supplement to the *Encyclopedia Britannica* and Robins and Sellars published their findings in *The Lancet* (2000; 356: 1841-43).

To begin, there is no definitive proof that Wilde was infected with syphilis from the Oxford prostitute, even though he believed he was. Before marrying Constance Mary Lloyd in 1884, for example, he underwent a medical examination, in which his doctor found no overt signs of the disease. This, in itself, is not conclusive because the microbe that causes syphilis (*Treponema palladium*) had not yet been discovered; there existed no blood test to definitively prove infection; and even with the best of medical examinations at that time, he could have been entirely asymptomatic and still infected or entirely normal and falsely diagnosed earlier. In favor of a false diagnosis is the fact that Constance was never infected and Oscar and Constance had two sons Cyril (b. 1885) and Vyvyan (b. 1886) who were entirely syphilis-free. (They later changed their surname to Holland after their father's conviction in order to escape the maelstrom of notoriety that surrounded poor Oscar's final years).

When reviewing Oscar's prison medical records, Drs. Critchley, Robins, and Sellars found no evidence of syphilis recorded by the seven different doctors (two of them psychiatrists) who examined him. In fact, Oscar showed none of the signs of the chronic form of the disease: he had none of the neurological or cardiac complications associated with tertiary syphilis, and his mental faculties remained in fine fettle as he laboriously composed what became *The Ballad of Reading Goal*. More germane, Oscar Wilde did have a long history of progressive deafness in the right ear with a chronic aural discharge that refused to yield. Sadly, his prison doctors did little to treat or ameliorate this painful condition.

In retrospect, Robbins and Sellars suggest that Oscar Wilde was suffering from a cholesteotoma, a tumor in the middle ear that destroys normal tissue and yields a chronic infection of the ear, with significant discharge or drainage of pus and fluid. Along with Critchley (who did not retrospectively diagnose a cholsteotoma in his report), all three doctors assert that it was an out of control middle ear infection that killed Oscar Wilde.

Oscar's ear infection and discharge appeared to resolve upon his release from prison. It returned with a vengeance, a few years later, especially toward the end of

September, 1900 while he was living at the Hôtel d'Alsace. He was attended to by several ear surgeons and physicians but the infection soon spread into the mastoid bone, which in the days before antibiotics was a harbinger of a much worse infection of the brain and its lining (the meninges) called meningoencephalitis. Wilde underwent an operation on October 10, 1900 (most likely a mastoidectomy) but, thereafter, suffered terrible pain and required a great deal of oral opium and the sedative, chloral hydrate. His infection raged during the second week of November and by the 25th he was racked with fever, pain, and delirium. On the 29th, he fell into a coma, most likely from the brain infection; his magnificent voice was permanently silenced at 1:50 p.m., the following day.

More than a century later, the present-day observer can only shake his head at the many layers of terrible tragedy surrounding Oscar Wilde's death. First, Wilde would never have been tried, let alone convicted and publicly humiliated, in today's Great Britain for simply expressing his sexuality. Second, the modern medical intervention of prescribing antibiotics, early and, perhaps, often, would have probably prevented the middle ear infection from fatally spreading to his brain.

Perhaps most interesting is the fact that Oscar's father, Sir William R.W. Wilde was one of Ireland's most eminent ear surgeons and who often treated ear infections like the one that killed his son. In his well-received 1853 textbook, *Practical Observations on Aural Surgery and the Nature and Treatment of the Diseases of the Ear*, Sir William warned of the infectious and deadly power of discharges from the ear: " . . . so long as otorrhoea [ear discharge] is present, we never can tell how, when, or what it may lead to." His son's course of illness proves this morbid observation all too well.

A middle ear infection and its subsequent spread to his brain appears to be the best medical explanation for Oscar Wilde's death. Others less medically inclined might say with equal conviction that he died of a broken heart and spirit.

Regardless of the precise cause of his premature death, we ought to praise "the Importance of Being Oscar." Every Oscar Wilde admirer has his or her favorite "Wilde witticism." One of his most enduring lines, however, might well serve as his credo:

"Be yourself; everyone else is already taken".

CHAPTER 55

∽

April 23, 1616

The Day William Shakespeare Died

"To be or not to be," Hamlet famously soliloquized.

But his maker William Shakespeare added, only a few stanzas later, that once one ceases to be, or

dies, no one knows to where that soul may go:

"The undiscovered country from whose bourn

No traveler returns…"

A nd the same might be said for the final days and hours of the immortal Bard
of Stratford upon Avon. We do know that his remains are most certainly
buried at the chancel of the Holy Trinity Church, there. The date of his death was
probably April 23, (which was also his likely birthday) and his funeral, which is
listed in the Stratford parish register, appears to have been held on April 25, 1616.
Upon reading Shakespeare's gravestone epitaph, Mark Twain cracked wise, "He was
probably dead when he wrote them." That said, it is worth quoting:

> Good friend for Jesus sake forbeare
>
> To digg the dust encloased heare,
>
> Blest by man that spares these stones
>
> And curse be he that moves my bones.

William was only 52 when he died, an age that might seem extraordinarily young
to modern-day readers. But the Elizabethan Age was a perilous time, fraught with
epidemics, deadly assaults, and dangerous medical treatments for all that ailed the

Literatim: Essays at the Intersections of Medicine and Culture. Howard Markel, Oxford University Press (2020).
© Oxford University Press.
DOI: 10.1093/oso/9780190087647.001.0001

nation; indeed, the average life span of men living in England at the time was about 42 years of age and much younger among the urban poor. Conversely, there were many who did live to the riper ages of 70 to 80 years. Childbearing, on the other hand, was especially dangerous and was the cause of many deaths among women in their 20s and 30s.

In his last few years of life, Shakespeare wrote very little and, of course, anyone who has passed their 40th birthday can tell you, he may have experienced more fatigue at activities he once dominated while in his twenties. Indeed, he moved back to Stratford, from London, with the intention of retiring from the stage. We do know that Shakespeare either wrote or revised a draft of his last will and testament on March 25, 1616, one month before his demise. An earlier draft was probably written in January of 1615. Some scholars have speculated that the Bard wanted to revise his will because of his daughter Judith's marriage to Thomas Quiney. Although the union was a happy one, Thomas got involved in a bit of a scandal prior to marrying Judith by impregnating an already-married woman named Margaret Wheeler. Both the woman and the baby died in childbirth but the gossiping tongues wagged for much longer. Others have pointed out that many people of his era tended to write their wills when they felt the end was near—and who better to understand the timing of a *grand finale* than William Shakespeare. Still, this is not the precise evidence we need to answer our primary question of how did Shakespeare die? Indeed, in the will, Shakespeare described himself *"in perfect health & memorie, God be praysed."*

Legends, tales and convoluted theories abound about Shakespeare's death. The most common version is that he went out on a drinking binge with some theatrical buddies, the playwright Ben Jonson, a friend and rival, who traveled from London to Stratford, and the poet-playwright Michael Drayton who lived in nearby Clifton Chambers. By the next day, he was dead. John Ward, the vicar of the Holy Trinity Church wrote in his diary, for example, "Shakespeare, Drayton and Ben Jonson had a merry meeting and it seems drank too hard, for Shakespeare died of a fever there contracted." But Vicar Ward wrote that entry some fifty years after Shakespeare died and death by acute alcohol poisoning, while certainly possible, is not all that common among experienced drinkers—which Shakespeare likely was.

The fever issue is more vexing. There, was, indeed typhus, or "new fever" brewing about Stratford but because it has so many distinct symptoms (e.g., scorching high fevers, mania and incoherence, and a distinct mulberry rash all over the body, caused by broken blood vessels) it would be helpful if there was some record of these findings in the Bard's case, but, alas and alack, there are none.

To thicken this fatal plot, Shakespeare's son-in-law, John Hall, was a prominent physician who enjoyed a close relationship with his father-in-law and travelled to London with him in 1614. Hall was reported to be the only physician in Stratford and, one assumes, must have been called in to examine the ailing William. In 1654, 22 years after Hall died, his clinical notes (which included his treatment of his wife, Susanna Shakespeare Hall) were published under the title: *Select observations on*

English bodies, or Cures both empericall and historicall performed upon very eminent persons in desperate diseases. Oddly, Dr. Hall left no information about the demise of his famous father-in-law.

More likely, Shakespeare probably experienced an acute cerebral hemorrhage, (also known in those days as "apoplexy" and today as a stroke) or a sudden myocardial infarction (heart attack). In the end, we will never know. But we can be thankful to John Heminge and Henry Condell, two actors of "the King's Men" (formerly "the Lord Chamberlain's Men" during Elizabeth I's reign and the playing company Shakespeare belonged to and wrote for most of his career). They compiled the Bard's 36 plays, which had up until then not been formally published and were only printed on flimsy sheets of paper for the actors' use, and published them as *Shakespeare's Comedies, Histories and Tragedies*. We know this volume as "the First Folio" and it preserved such theatrical gems as *Macbeth* and *Julius Caesar*, which might have otherwise been soon destroyed and forgotten. In fact, William Shakespeare has never really died. He lives on in theatres, books, films, broadcasts, and the hearts of every well-read man, woman, and child in the world. He is, just as he hoped in his lovely *Sonnets*, immortal as long as someone, somewhere utters one of his lyrical lines or swoons to his brilliant storytelling.

CHAPTER 56

cᐱ⌒ᐱ

But What Caused Houdini's
Mysterious Death?

Nearly a century after his death in Detroit, Michigan made international
headlines, the name Harry Houdini still conjures up images of great escapes
from impossible situations.

His real name was Erik Weisz and he was born on March 24, 1874 in Budapest.
The Weisz family immigrated to the United States in 1878 when Erik was only
4 years old. He grew up in Appleton, Wisconsin, where his father was the rabbi for
the Zion Reform Jewish Congregation. There, the family surname was changed to
the German spelling of Weiss and Erik became Ehrich, a boy better known for his
talent at acrobatic feats and picking locks than rabbinical piety.

It was show biz, and not the Talmud, that captured Ehrich's attention. At the age
of 9, he ran away to join the circus as a trapeze artist and contortionist. Fascinated
by conjuring of all kinds, especially that enacted by the great 19th century French
magician Jean-Eugène Robert-Houdin, Ehrich later took the name Harry Houdini,
thinking that the additional "I" meant "like" in French. The climax of his act in these
early days of his remarkable career was when he invited anyone in the audience
to tie him up and he would free himself, inside a locked cabinet. As the *New York
Times* reported in its obituary of Houdini, one night in Coffeyville, Kansas the local
sheriff baited him with his handcuffs, bellowing to the audience, "If I put these on,
you'll never get loose." It was a challenge that changed the young performer's life.
He emerged *sans* shackles and was soon riding the rails and, billed as "the Handcuff
King," performed at vaudeville houses across the nation.

Ever the scintillating showman, Houdini kept developing new tricks and escape
techniques beyond merely wiggling out of a cop's manacles. In 1900, he made his
first European tour and conducted sensational escapes from Scotland Yard and
dozens of other famous prisons. In 1902, he had himself locked into Cell No. 2 of the

Literatim: Essays at the Intersections of Medicine and Culture. Howard Markel, Oxford University Press (2020).
© Oxford University Press.
DOI: 10.1093/oso/9780190087647.001.0001

Washington D.C. federal prison, the same cell that once housed Charles Guiteau, the man who assassinated President James Garfield. Soon enough, Houdini got out of jail free.

By 1908, Houdini graduated to far more dangerous and daring escapes from air tight vessels filled with water as well as being completely tied up and chained, while hanging off of a skyscraper or being thrown from a bridge into an icy river, always reappearing unrestricted within minutes.

It was Houdini's death that has remained a source of conjecture among magicians and surgeons. Houdini never told anyone, save his wife and assistant, Bess, the secret of his great escapes. On the other hand, he was proud enough of his superb musculature and toned body to allow the audience to feel his biceps or punch him in his ripped abdomen.

As the story goes, a few medical students from McGill University visited Houdini in his dressing room at 5 pm on October 22, 1926, after his matinee show at the Princess Theatre in Montreal. A few days earlier, Houdini had lectured at McGill about his work in exposing fake mediums and spiritualists. One student, Joselyn Gordon Whitehead, asked if he could take a punch and immediately Houdini nodded an assent. The student hit the great magician twice but before he had a chance to tighten his abdominal muscles and brace himself. The "hammer-like" punches caused visible pain and Houdini stopped Whitehead in mid-blow on the third attempt to punch his gut. The pain failed to abate as Houdini travelled by train, more than 15 hours, to his next performance in Detroit. He was also suffering from a recently broken bone in the foot, so Houdini was experiencing a great deal of pain during the trip that he blamed solely on the fractured foot and the belly punches.

By the time Houdini got to the Garrick Theatre in Detroit, his temperature was 104 degrees Fahrenheit. A physician was called to his dressing room and diagnosed Harry with acute appendicitis. The doctor ordered an ambulance to take Houdini immediately to the hospital but Harry was schooled on the old adage that "the show must go on!" He declined the medico's help, declaring, "I'll do this show if it's my last." The performance was not his best but did not include him collapsing on the stage or having to be rescued from the water torture chamber by an ax-wielding assistant as many apocryphal tales and motion pictures have claimed.

After the performance, Houdini checked into his hotel. He still refused medical treatment but the pain was so great that his wife, Bess demanded he be rushed to the nearby Grace Hospital. There, on October 24, he underwent an emergency operation to remove his appendix, which had already ruptured and caused severe peritonitis, a raging and difficult to treat infection of the abdominal cavity. After a second operation on October 28, and the introduction of a new anti-streptococcal serum, the great Houdini succumbed to overwhelming sepsis. He died on October 31, 1926 at the age of 52. His last words, reportedly, were "I'm tired of fighting."

The doctors at the time concurred that the appendicitis was likely caused by the blunt force of the medical student's blows, which burst and then caused Houdini's fatal infection. But a 2013 literature review published in the World Journal of

Emergency Surgery (2013; 8:31) concludes that as a cause of acute appendicitis, "blunt abdominal trauma is rare and, occasionally, appendicitis and trauma exist together, which causes an interesting debate whether trauma has led to appendicitis."

The poor medical student probably went to his grave thinking he had deprived the world of the great Harry Houdini. Fans still concoct conspiracy theories of Whitehead's intentions of causing harm. It is possible that the blows caused Houdini's appendicitis, but it also more than quite possible that the blows and the appendicitis were coincidental rather than causal and that the muscular pain from Whitehead's wallops gave Houdini a false explanation for his abdominal pain. Harry may have simply ignored the fire brewing in his belly and chalked it up to a punch in the gut, which delayed him seeing a doctor, having his appendix removed before it ruptured, and recovering—all reasonable outcomes in 1926, provided there was no peritonitis.

Always interested in the possibility that spiritualism might be real, Houdini promised to send his wife a message from beyond, if he died first. The message never came.

Just as with Houdini's spectacular escapes on stage, we will never really know how he escaped from this life or if he was able to escape into the next.

CHAPTER 57

cᐯᗞ

September 29

The Tylenol Murders of 1982

E arly on the morning of September 29, 1982, a tragic, medical mystery began
with a sore throat and a runny nose. It was then that Mary Kellerman, a 12-
year-old girl from Elk Grove Village, a suburb of Chicago, told her mother and father about her symptoms. They gave her one extra-strength Tylenol capsule that,
unbeknownst to them, was laced with the highly poisonous potassium cyanide.
Mary was dead by 7 am. Within a week, her death would panic the entire nation.
And only months later, it changed the way we purchase and consume over-the-
counter medications.

That same day, a 27-year-old postal worker named Adam Janus of Arlington
Heights, Illinois died of what was initially thought to be a massive heart attack but
turned out to be cyanide poisoning as well. His brother and sister in law, Stanley,
age 25, and Theresa, age 19, of Lisle, Illinois, rushed to his home to console their
loved ones. Both experienced throbbing headaches, a not uncommon response to
a death in the family and each took a Tylenol extra-strength capsule or two from
the same bottle Adam had used earlier in the day. Stanley died that very day while
Theresa died two days later.

Over the next few days, there occurred three more strange deaths: 35-year-old
Mary McFarland of Elmhurst, Illinois, 35-year-old Paula Prince of Chicago, and 27-
year-old Mary Weiner of Winfield, Illinois. All of them, it turned out, took Tylenol
shortly before they died.

It was at this point, early October of 1982, that investigators made the connection between the poisoning deaths and Tylenol, the best-selling, non-prescription
pain reliever sold in the United States at that time. The gelatin-based capsules were
especially popular because they were slick and easy to swallow. Unfortunately, each

Literatim: Essays at the Intersections of Medicine and Culture. Howard Markel, Oxford University Press (2020).
© Oxford University Press.
DOI: 10.1093/oso/9780190087647.001.0001

victim swallowed a Tylenol capsule laced with 65 mg of cyanide, an amount 10,000 times greater than the lethal dose.

McNeil Consumer Products, a subsidiary of the health care giant, Johnson and Johnson, manufactured Tylenol. To its credit, the company took an active role with the media in issuing mass warning communications and immediately called for a massive recall of the more than 31 million bottles of Tylenol then out in circulation. Tainted capsules were discovered in early October in a few other grocery stores and drug stores in the Chicago area, but, fortunately, they had not yet been sold or con-sumed. McNeill/Johnson and Johnson offered replacement capsules to those who turned in pills already purchased and a reward for anyone with information leading to the apprehension of the individual or people involved in these random murders.

The case continued to be confusing to the police, the drug maker, and the public at large. For example, Johnson and Johnson quickly established that the cyanide lacing occurred after cases of Tylenol left the factory. Someone, police hypothe-sized, must have taken bottles off the shelves of local grocers and drug stores in the Chicago area, laced the capsules with poison, and then returned the restored packages to the shelves to be purchased by the unknowing victims.

To this day, however, the perpetrators of these murders have never been found.

One man, James Lewis, claiming to be the Tylenol killer, wrote a "ransom" letter to Johnson and Johnson demanding $1,000,000 in exchange for stopping the poisonings. After a lengthy cat and mouse game, police and federal investigators determined that Lewis lived in New York and had no demonstrable links to the Chicago events. That said, he was charged with extortion and sentenced to 20 years in prison. He was released in 1995 after serving only 13 years.

Other "copy-cat" poisonings, involving Tylenol and other over-the-counter medications, cropped up again in the 1980s and early 1990s but these events were never as dramatic or as deadly as the 1982 Chicago-area deaths. Conspiracy theo-ries about motives and suspects for all these heinous acts continue to be bandied about on the Internet to this day.

Before the 1982 crisis, Tylenol controlled more than 35 percent of the over-the-counter pain reliever market; only a few weeks after the murders, that number plummeted to less than 8 percent. The dire situation, both in terms of human life and business, made it imperative that the Johnson and Johnson executives respond swiftly and authoritatively.

For example, Johnson and Johnson developed new product protection methods and ironclad pledges to do better in protecting their consumers in the future. Working with FDA officials, they introduced a new tamper-proof packaging, which included foil seals and other features that made it obvious to a consumer if foul play had transpired. These packaging protections soon became the industry standard for all over-the-counter medications. The company also introduced price reductions and a new version of their pills—called the "caplet—a tablet coated with slick, easy-to-swallow gelatin but far harder to tamper with than the older capsules, which could be easily opened, laced with a contaminant, and then placed back in the older non-tamper-proof bottle.

Within a year, and after an investment of more than $100 million, Tylenol's sales rebounded to its healthy past and it became, once again, the nation's favorite over-the-counter pain reliever. Critics who had prematurely announced the death of the brand Tylenol were now praising the company's handling of the matter. Indeed, the Johnson and Johnson's recall became a classic case study in business schools across the nation.

In 1983, the U.S. Congress passed what was called "the Tylenol bill", making it a federal offense to tamper with consumer products. In 1989, the FDA established federal guidelines for manufacturers to make all such products tamper-proof.

Sadly, the tragedies that resulted from the Tylenol poisonings can never be undone. But their deaths did inspire a series of important moves to make over-the-counter medications safer (albeit never 100 percent safe) for the hundreds of millions of people who buy them every year.

CHAPTER 58

ⲟⲭⲟ

The Day Doctors Began
to Conquer Smallpox

One of the most celebrated medical anniversaries concerns a country doctor named Edward Jenner (1749-1823) who lived in the tiny village of Berkeley in Gloucestershire, Great Britain. Like every general practitioner of his day, Dr. Jenner attended to too many patients struck down by smallpox. For millennia, it was humankind's deadliest foe—that is, until Jenner figured out a means of preventing it entirely.

As with any great medical discovery, Jenner was hardly alone in his quest for a safe smallpox vaccine. For centuries, healers around the globe introduced their patients to a technique called inoculation (from the Latin *inoculare*, to graft; its other name was variolation, from the Latin for *variola*, the scientific name of the smallpox virus). The procedure entails lancing open a wound and implanting dried scabs or fresh pus containing variola under the skin of a healthy, uninfected person.

Said to have originated in China, smallpox inoculation was commonly practiced across the Orient and Ottoman Empire. It typically caused a milder form of smallpox but conferred lifelong immunity. Still, inoculation had the power to make many people incredibly ill and some died as a result of it. Fueling the debate were fears that those inoculated would infect and harm others.

What especially made Dr. Jenner the right man at the right moment was his passion for natural history. His acclaimed studies, ranging from the habitats of cuckoo birds to the dormouse, as well as a deep appreciation of the intersecting lives (and ills) of humans and animals, led him to contemplate how infectious diseases traveled among and between species.

As the story goes, sometime in the 1770s, Dr. Jenner was making his appointed rounds when he came across a loquacious milkmaid. Jenner reported an outbreak of

Literatim: Essays at the Intersections of Medicine and Culture. Howard Markel, Oxford University Press (2020).
DOI: 10.1093/oso/9780190087647.001.0001

smallpox along the countryside and the milkmaid boastingly replied: "I shall never have smallpox for I have had cowpox. I shall never have an ugly pockmarked face."

Jenner thought long and hard about that woman's observation during every case of smallpox—and cowpox—he saw thereafter. He hypothesized that the pus in the milkmaid's cowpox blisters were the result of an infection that was similar to smallpox. This infection, he believed, may have originated in horses before spreading to cows and humans but appeared far less virulent and dangerous to human beings when compared with smallpox. Over the years, Jenner observed that people who encountered cowpox became immune to future encounters with the smallpox virus. But how to scientifically prove such a claim without causing any harm?

On May 14, 1796, Dr. Jenner finally found his chance. That morning, a milkmaid named Sarah Nelmes consulted him about a rash of blisters that suddenly appeared on her arms. Jenner was certain he was examining a case of cowpox and drained some of the pus collecting in Sarah's blisters. Legend has it that Sarah contracted cowpox from a proper Gloucester dairy cow named Blossom, whose leathery hide hangs in the library of the St. George's Medical School of London (Jenner's *alma mater*) to this very day.

Armed with the miraculous elixir, Jenner wanted to try it out on an 8-year-old Berkeley boy named James Phipps. An Institutional Review Board would never approve such a potentially perilous experiment today. Yet in the late 1700s, smallpox represented a clear and present danger. So when Dr. Jenner promised the boy's parents that the risks were minimal compared to the powerful gift of immunity to the dreaded smallpox, they readily agreed.

Taking no chances, Jenner made inoculation scars on each of Jimmy Phipps' arms and, the next day, nursed the boy through a course of mild fever and some generalized discomfort. Six weeks later, Jenner exposed Phipps to the real smallpox virus and . . . nothing happened! As Jenner later declared, "the cowpox protects the human constitution from the infection of smallpox." The Latin word for cow is *vacca*, hence the Latin name for cowpox virus, *vaccinia*, and, more famously, the English word "vaccine".

Jenner combined his collection of patients who had contracted cowpox and developed immunity to smallpox as well as those he vaccinated with cowpox to form the body of his 1798 treatise, *An Inquiry into the Cause and Effects of the Variolae Vaccinae, a Disease Discovered in Some of the Western Counties of England, Particularly Gloucestershire, and Known by the Name of the Cow-Pox*. And because Jenner's vaccine has prevented hundreds of millions of deaths over the past 217 years, his *Inquiry* may well be one of the most important books in the history of medicine.

Within months of publication, Jenner's cowpox vaccine became the major means of preventing smallpox, especially across Europe and in the United States. In 1801, President Thomas Jefferson declared vaccination one of the nation's first public health priorities. Two years later, he instructed Meriwether Lewis and William Clark to bring vaccine on their expedition to the Pacific and encourage those they met "in the use of it." In 1806, Jefferson predicted to Jenner that smallpox would be someday eliminated from human experience. Jefferson was right, of course, but that noble goal was not accomplished until 1979.

In recent years, several armchair historians have questioned the primacy of Edward Jenner's discovery. To be sure, the inoculation of *variola*, or smallpox, virus predates Jenner by centuries and was famously recommended on both sides of the Atlantic by such luminaries as Cotton Mather, during the Boston smallpox epidemic of 1721, and Lady Mary Wortley Montague who imported the technique from Istanbul to London that same year. During the late 18th century, several people considered cowpox as a means of preventing smallpox, including John Fewster, a London physician, in 1765, and Benjamin Justy, a remarkably observant farmer from Dorset, in 1774. Nevertheless, it was Edward Jenner who published the most authoritative medical investigation first and it is Jenner who we most consistently celebrate as the smallpox vaccine's parent.

Alas, such contretemps over "who was first" is a common one in the history of science and medicine. When attempting to accommodate the long list of others who contributed to Jenner's historical victory, one is reminded of that great line from John Ford's 1962 film, *The Man Who Shot Liberty Valance*: "When the legend becomes fact, print the legend."

CHAPTER 59

ᘒᕤ

In 1850, Ignaz Semmelweis Saved Lives with Three Words

Wash Your Hands

On May 15, 1850, a prickly Hungarian obstetrician named Ignaz Semmelweis stepped up to the podium of the Vienna Medical Society's lecture hall. It was a grand and ornately decorated room where some of medicine's greatest discoveries were first announced. The evening of May 15 would hardly be different—even if those present (and many more who merely read about it) did not acknowledge Semmelweis's marvelous discovery for several decades.

What, exactly, was the doctor's advice to his colleagues on that long ago night? It could be summed up in three little words: wash your hands!

At this late date, we all expect our doctors to wash their hands before examining us or performing an operation in order to prevent the spread of infection. Surprisingly, physicians did not begin to acknowledge the lifesaving power of this simple act until 1847.

It was then that Dr. Semmelweis began exhorting his fellow physicians at the famed Vienna General Hospital (*Allgemeines Krankenhaus*) to wash up before examining women about to deliver babies. His plea was far more than aesthetic; it was a matter of life and death and helped to prevent a deadly malady known as "childbed" or puerperal (from the Latin words for child and parent) fever.

In the mid-19th century, about five women in 1,000 died in deliveries performed by midwives or at home. Yet when doctors working in the best maternity hospitals in Europe and America performed deliveries, the maternal death rate was often 10 to 20 times greater. The cause was, invariably, childbed fever. And a miserable end it was: raging fevers, putrid pus emanating from the birth canal, painful abscesses in

Literatim: Essays at the Intersections of Medicine and Culture. Howard Markel, Oxford University Press (2020).
© Oxford University Press.
DOI: 10.1093/oso/9780190087647.001.0001

the abdomen and chest, and an irreversible descent into an absolute hell of sepsis and death—all within 24 hours of the baby's birth.

The reason seems readily apparent today, if not back then. Medical students and their professors at the elite teaching hospitals of this era typically began their day performing barehanded autopsies on the women who had died the day before of childbed fever. They then proceeded to the wards to examine the laboring women about to deliver their babies.

Dr. Semmelweis was brilliant but had two strikes against him when applying for a position at the Vienna General Hospital in 1846: he was Hungarian and Jewish. Medicine and surgery were considered to be the premier specialties in Vienna but because of his background and religion Semmelweis was relegated to running the less desirable division of obstetrics. Nevertheless, his claim to immortality was the result of an obsession with finding the means to end the childbed fever epidemics that were killing nearly a third of his patients. (The hospital ward run by midwives, without autopsy duties, had far better outcomes with their deliveries).

Every day he heard the heart-rending pleas of women assigned to his care begging to be discharged because they believed these doctors to be the harbingers of death. Fortunately, Dr. Semmelweis was smart enough to listen to his patients.

The obstetrician made the vital connection that puerperal fever was caused by the doctors transferring some type of "morbid poison" from the dissected corpses in the autopsy suite to the women laboring in the delivery room. That morbid poison is now known as the bacteria called Group A hemolytic *streptococcus*.

Historians are quick to remind that Semmelweis was not the first physician to make this clinical connection, one that many expectant mothers of the era called "the doctors' plague." For example, the obstetrician Alexander Gordon of Aberdeen, Scotland, suggested in his 1795 *Treatise on the Epidemic of Puerperal Fever* that midwives and doctors who had recently treated women for puerperal fever spread the malady to other women. More famously, in 1843 Oliver Wendell Holmes, the Harvard anatomist and self-proclaimed "autocrat of the breakfast table," published an essay in the *New England Quarterly Journal of Medicine* entitled, "The Contagiousness of Puerperal Fever," in which he discerned that the disease was spread by physicians and recommended that actively practicing obstetricians abstain from performing autopsies on women who died of puerperal fever as one of their "paramount obligations to society."

That said, it was Dr. Semmelweis who ordered his medical students and junior physicians to wash their hands in a chlorinated lime solution until the smell of the putrid bodies they dissected in the autopsy suite was no longer detectable. Soon after instituting this protocol in 1847, the mortality rates on the doctor-dominated obstetrics service plummeted.

Unfortunately, Semmelweis's ideas were not accepted by all of his colleagues. Indeed, many were outraged at the suggestion that they were the cause of their patients' miserable deaths. Consequently, Semmelweis met with enormous resistance and criticism.

A remarkably difficult man, Semmelweis refused to publish his "self-evident" findings until 13 years after making them despite being urged to do so repeatedly by those who supported him. To make matters worse, he hurled outrageously rude insults to some of the hospital's most powerful doctors who deigned to question his ideas. Such outbursts, no matter how well deserved, never go unnoticed, let alone unpunished, in the staid halls of academic medicine.

Becoming shriller and angrier at each detractor's critique, Semmelweis lost his clinical appointment at the Vienna General Hospital and in 1850 abruptly left for his native Budapest without even telling his closest colleagues. In 1861, he finally published his work, *Die Aetiologie, der Begriff und die Prophylaxis des Kindbettfiebers* (*The Etiology, the Concept, and the Prophylaxis of Childbed Fever*), in which he explained his theories on childbed fever, the ways to avoid spreading it by means of vigorous hand-washing and an attack on every one of his critics with a vitriol that still leaps off the page.

Dr. Semmelweis's behavior became more and more erratic and he was finally committed to an insane asylum on July 30, 1865. He died there, two weeks later, on August 13, 1865, at the age of 47. Historians still argue over what caused Semmelweis's mental health breakdown and subsequent death. Some point to an operation Semmelweis performed, wherein he infected himself with syphilis, which may also explain his insanity. Others believe he developed blood poisoning and sepsis while imprisoned in the asylum for what may have been an unbridled case of bipolar disease. More recently, some have claimed that the obstetrician had an early variant of Alzheimer's disease and was beaten to death in the asylum by his keepers.

Semmelweis's professional timing could not have been worse. He made his landmark discovery between 1846 and 1861, long before the medical profession was ready to accept it.

Although Louis Pasteur began exploring the role of bacteria and fermentation in spoiling wine during the late 1850s, much of his most important work initiating the germ theory of disease occurred between 1860 and 1865. A few years later, in 1867, the Scottish surgeon Joseph Lister, who apparently had never heard of Semmelweis, elaborated the theory and practice of antiseptic surgery, which included washing the hands with carbolic acid to prevent infection. And in 1876, the German physician successfully linked a germ, *Bacillus anthracis*, to a specific infectious disease, anthrax.

Since the early 1900's, however, physicians and historians have heaped up high praise for Semmelweis's work and expressed sympathy for his emotional troubles and premature death. Today, in every school of medicine and public health, his name is uttered with great reverence whenever the critical topic of hand washing is taught. Sadly, in real time, he was derided as eccentric at best and, at worst, as an angry, unstable man who ought to be drummed out of the profession.

The real truth of the matter is that his detractors were wrong and he was right. Dr. Semmelweis paid a heavy price as he devoted his short, troubled life to pushing the boundaries of knowledge in the noble quest to save lives.

When contemplating his landmark medical discovery, it seems fitting that we pay grand tribute to the great Dr. Semmelweis. Perhaps the gesture he might appreciate the most, however, is for us all to simply wash our hands often and well.

CHAPTER 60

∽

"Goodbye, Farewell and Amen"

The Final Episode of M*A*S*H, February 28, 1983

For many Americans, some who weren't even alive for the real event, the Korean War did not really end until February 28, 1983. That's the date when 121.6 million viewers watched the final episode of *M*A*S*H*, making it the most watched television broadcast in American history. No scripted show has come close. It was not until February, 2010 when the Super Bowl XLIV surpassed the number of total viewers, but not in ratings or share. For the 1983 finale of *M*A*S*H*, the CBS television network charged sponsors $450,000 for each 30-second block of commercial time, a sum worth more than $1,000,000 today.

The hit television show *M*A*S*H* was loosely based on the 1970 Robert Altman film of the same name and even more loosely on a 1968 novel, *M*A*S*H: A Novel About Three Army Doctors*, by former U.S. Army surgeon H. Richard Hornberger, who wrote under the pen name of Richard Hooker.

The Mobile Army Surgical Hospital, or MASH, concept was first deployed by the U.S. Army during World War II. They were initially called Auxiliary Surgical Groups and were an attempt to move surgical care closer to wounded soldiers than the fixed-in-place field hospitals then in existence. These units were based on a concept dating back to the Napoleonic wars, when doctors struggled to save the lives of soldiers wasted by cannons, muskets, buckshot, and shrapnel. Some were mortally wounded, others just needed to be patched up and sent back into the fray. In the midst of battle, these doctors were forced to develop a system of setting priorities in their gory duties. They called it *triage*, from the French word *trier*, which means to sort out.

The MASH units of the Korean war were located close enough to the front that wounded soldiers might be more expeditiously treated, but were distant enough

Literatim: Essays at the Intersections of Medicine and Culture. Howard Markel, Oxford University Press (2020).
© Oxford University Press.
DOI: 10.1093/oso/9780190087647.001.0001

so that the surgeons, nurses, and other personnel would not be exposed to direct combat. Tent-based, the people in MASH units worked long hours and endured horrific stresses of warfare. The key word, of course, was mobile and they moved from location to location on, at least, a monthly basis. (In the final episode of M*A*S*H, the fictional 4077th does move to a different location but only rarely did so in previous episodes).

In 1951, Dr. Hornberger was drafted out of his surgical internship, inducted into the U.S. Army, and assigned to the 8055th MASH, which traveled along the 38th parallel, the now infamous demilitarized zone dividing the Korean peninsula into North and South Korea. The 8055th was one of 10 fully-functioning mobile hospitals operating during the Korean War.

Dr. Hornberger, who created Hawkeye to represent his own audacious surgical exploits, pioneered in the use of arterial repairs on the frontlines of war. This was still a relatively new procedure, time-consuming, and then forbidden by the U.S. Army. The surgeons at the 8055th flouted such rules because they felt that not to repair such injuries, and prevent needless amputations of countless limbs, would be to disobey their Hippocratic Oath, a far more important bond than the oath they took upon induction into the military.

It required more than a decade for Dr. Hornberger to write his novel, something he began to help him deal with the trauma he saw and experienced in Korea. It took another five years before he finally secured a publisher, William Morrow and Company. After the war, he returned to his native Maine and practiced as a thoracic surgeon there. He died in 1997 at the age of 73. Ironically, for all the money the television show made for its producers, writers, developers, actors and the CBS Television Network, Hornberger sold the rights for a ridiculously low amount and only earned $500 per episode!

There are, of course many similarities to Hornberger's novel to the film and television show, but none more critical to the success of all three than the sarcastic surgeon with the heart of gold, Benjamin Franklin "Hawkeye" Pierce. In Alan Alda's memorable performances, there was always a healthy dose of Groucho Marx thrown in to carry off more than a decade of terrific one-liners mixed with the character's heartfelt empathy for his patients.

The television series, which ran from 1972 to 1983, increasingly articulated the nation's growing disillusionment with the terrible human costs of the Vietnam War. Dr. Hornberger rarely watched the show and resented the character based on his own life being tied to such sentiments. In an interview with *Newsweek* Magazine he said that while the show accurately portrayed what a MASH unit looked like during the Korean conflict, the show "tramples on my memories." Later, in the doctor's obituary for the *New York Times*, his son William Hornberger said:

> He liked the movie because he thought it followed his original intent very closely, but my father was a political conservative, and he did not like the liberal tendencies that Alan Alda portrayed Hawkeye Pierce as having. My father didn't write an anti-war book. It

was a humorous account of his work, with serious parts thrown in about the awful kind of work it was, and how difficult and challenging it was.

For my generation of doctors, who came of age in the 1970s and graduated from medical school and trained in the 1980s, M*A*S*H was vitally important influence on our choice of medicine as a career, even for those of us who decidedly were not surgeons. Every time I crab-walked across a hospital heli-pad to meet a helicopter-ambulance carrying an acutely ill patient, I replayed the opening scene of all 256 episodes of *M*A*S*H* in their minds, hoping to emulate Hawkeye Pierce and the rest of his goofy gang of medics.

Re-watching that last episode the other week, I was startled to find tears in my eyes as the cast said goodbye to one another and to the American public. That is, until Hawkeye and Margaret "Hotlips" Houlihan, the doctor and nurse who antagonized each other longer than the Chinese, Korean and U.S. armies by five-fold, embraced and locked lips for a 36 second long kiss (a veritable eternity on television). It was then that I recalled how much the 4077th Mobile Army Surgical Hospital made a gawky, teenaged boy from Southfield, Michigan laugh, think, and aspire to become a doctor just like Hawkeye Pierce.

CHAPTER 61

ᥫᩚ

Louis Pasteur's Risky Move to Save a Boy from Almost Certain Death

arly in the morning of July 4, 1885, a "mad dog" attacked a 9-year-old boy from Alsace, France. His name was Joseph Meister. The vicious and crazed dog proceeded to throw the boy to the ground and bite him in 14 places, including the hand, legs and thighs. Some of the wounds were so deep that he could hardly walk. Twelve hours later, at 8:00 in the evening, a local doctor named Weber treated Joseph's most serious wounds by cauterizing, or sealing them, with searing doses of carbolic acid, in and of itself a horribly painful process.

Beyond the bites themselves, the boy's mother feared her child had contracted rabies, which was widely feared as a near certain path to death. Despite the relative rarity of rabies in 19th century France, the shocking symptoms and grisly power to kill captured that nation's attention, just as many newly emerging contagious events—such as SARS, Ebola and Zika—have done in the United States today.

Mrs. Meister took Joseph straight to Paris because she heard that a scientist there was working on a cure for rabies. Once there, she made inquiries on how to find this man and was told to go directly to the laboratory of the famous microbiologist, Louis Pasteur.

Pasteur was, indeed, hard at work developing a rabies vaccine, using dogs as his experimental subjects. Up until now, however, he had not administered the vaccine to a human being. In reality, he could not do so legally because he was not a medical doctor; his doctorate was awarded for dissertations in chemistry and physics. More importantly, he could not yet prove that his rabies vaccine was effective—as opposed to useless or even harmful—for humans.

Pasteur was so taken by the boy's plight that he consulted two physicians, Alfred Vulpain and Jacques Grancher at a weekly meeting of the French Academy of Sciences. They, too, were struck by the need to do something, and to do it fast.

Literatim: Essays at the Intersections of Medicine and Culture. Howard Markel, Oxford University Press (2020).
© Oxford University Press.
DOI: 10.1093/oso/9780190087647.001.0001

Pasteur later reported, "Since the death of the child appeared inevitable, I resolved, though not without great anxiety, to try the method which had proved consistently successful on the dogs."

Pasteur escaped the medical license dilemma by having his medical colleagues present when the vaccine was first administered on July 6, 1885, some 60 hours after the initial dog attack. Mrs. Meister expressed little concern over the potential dangers of the experimental vaccine because she was so fearful that her son would die. She readily gave Pasteur her consent.

The first injection was made in a fold of skin covering the boy's right upper abdomen. Over a period of three weeks, Joseph was given 13 such inoculations. Pasteur monitored the virulence of each dose by first injecting them in healthy rabbits to insure the vaccine did not cause rabies. Each dose came from progressively more rabid rabbits. At the end of the treatment course, Joseph was inoculated with an especially virulent rabies virus from a mad dog. Nothing happened! Pasteur was pleased to announce, thanks to his vaccine, Meister had developed an immunity to rabies virus.

The rest of Louis Pasteur's remarkable career as a world-changing scientist has been well documented in a shelf of books and articles about him.

But whatever happened to Joseph Meister?

He fully recovered from the dog attack, for starters. Louis Pasteur later hired him to work as a concierge at the *Institut Pasteur*, his deluxe laboratory where some of the most important discoveries elucidating infectious diseases were made. There Meister happily worked for several decades until the second World War broke out.

On June 24, 1940, 10 days after the German army conquered Paris, a 64-year-old Meister took his own life. For many years, the popular legend of Meister's death was that he committed suicide rather than allow (or watch) the Nazi invaders to pillage Pasteur's crypt.

Recently, however, this story had been debunked, or at least augmented with more accurate facts, thanks to two intrepid researchers named Héloïse Dufour and Sean Carroll.

Using the diary of Eugene Wollman, the head of the institute's bacteriophage laboratory at this time, other archival sources, and interviews with Meister's granddaughter, Dufour and Carroll discovered that Meister killed himself by turning on a gas stove, rather than a self-inflicted gunshot as has often been reported. In fact, he did not take his life out of an obligation to protect Pasteur's remains. Instead, he was despondent over his wife and children. They had fled Paris a few weeks earlier to escape the Nazi bombing, and Meister somehow got it into his head that the Germans had killed them.

Here's the most striking irony of this tragedy: His very much alive wife and daughters returned to Paris later that day only to find Joseph dead.

The story of Meister standing guard over the coffin of the man who saved his life is just a myth, but a heroic myth, nevertheless. What has never been in doubt, however, is the fact that on July 6, 1885, Joseph Meister made medical history.

CHAPTER 62

⤮

"I Have Seen My Death"

How the World Discovered the X-Ray

In November of 1895, the phenomenon of electricity and electrons was all the rage. It was around this time that a physics professor at the University of Würzberg named William Röntgen began playing with a cathode tube featuring a thin aluminum window that allowed some of the electromagnetic rays to escape.

He covered the tube with black cardboard to shield its fluorescent glow, and, shortly after, noticed beams escaping several feet to a nearby plate made of barium platino-cyanide. Secreted in his lab for six weeks, pausing only to take meals, he experimented with other fluorescent screens and photographic paper, the latter a common item in laboratories for purposes of documentation and illustration.

Röntgen's great discovery arrived shortly after noticing that his newly discovered beams passed through opaque objects and affected the film beneath. The results included shadowy radiographs of a set of weights, a piece of metal, and, most famously, the bones of his wife's hand and her wedding ring. When she underwent the world's first X-ray on a human, on December 22, 1895, Mrs. Röntgen exclaimed, "I have seen my death."

Because he did not know the precise physical nature of these electromagnetic beams, Röntgen referred to them as "X-rays." Röntgen published his initial findings in late December of 1895. It took a matter of weeks before such news spread around the world and X-rays became the media sensation of the day.

Thomas Edison and others manufactured commercial fluoroscopes, carnivals employed them as novelties for fair-goers wanting a radiograph of their bones, and shoe stores used them to measure the size of feet.

Eventually, physicians, surgeons and dentists learned to employ them widely as central tools in their diagnostic arsenal. X-rays, and their progeny such as CT scans,

Literatim: Essays at the Intersections of Medicine and Culture. Howard Markel, Oxford University Press (2020).
© Oxford University Press.
DOI: 10.1093/oso/9780190087647.001.0001

MRIs, and ultrasound, allowed the doctor to check a running engine, so to speak, without ever opening the hood.

In 1901, Röntgen was awarded the first Nobel Prize in Physics. It is no understatement that his discovery revolutionized the modern practice of medicine in ways the physicist could have never imagined.

CHAPTER 63

cℵɔ

How a Boy Became the First to Beat Back Diabetes

On January 11, 1922, a 14-year-old boy hovered between life and death. His name was Leonard Thompson and he was suffering the end stages of diabetes mellitus.

Because the only treatment available was a starvation diet, the boy weighed a mere 65 pounds when he was admitted to the Toronto General Hospital. Worse, Leonard was drifting in and out of a diabetic coma. His father was so desperate to save the boy that he agreed to let the doctors inject Leonard with a newly discovered wonder drug that had never been tried on another human being. The doctors called it insulin.

Insulin was discovered a year earlier by Frederick Banting, a tenacious, young surgeon from London, Ontario. During the fall of 1920, Dr. Banting became fascinated by studies on the role of the pancreas in regulating the metabolism of sugar and carbohydrates.

Soon enough, he hit upon the idea of ligating, or tying off, the pancreatic duct in order to isolate the gland's "internal secretion," a yet-to-be-identified biological substance which facilitated this critical metabolic process. Soon after, Banting took his idea to a world-renowned University of Toronto physiologist named J.J.R. Macleod.

Initially skeptical of the young surgeon's idea, Macleod eventually and somewhat begrudgingly lent Banting a makeshift laboratory for his use during the summer of 1921. Macleod also provided some dogs for Banting to experiment upon and assigned an eager medical student named Charles Best to help Dr. Banting with the necessary chemical analyses. Later that year, a University of Toronto biochemist named James Collip helped purify the "extract" into a form of insulin that could be administered to human beings.

Literatim: Essays at the Intersections of Medicine and Culture. Howard Markel, Oxford University Press (2020).
© Oxford University Press.
DOI: 10.1093/oso/9780190087647.001.0001

On January 23, 1922, Leonard underwent a second series of insulin injections and the results were stunning. His life was, literally, saved by insulin and he became the poster boy of the now commonplace medical miracle.

Banting and Best wrote these results up for the February 1922 issue of the *Journal of Laboratory and Clinical Medicine*. No stuffy medical paper, the discovery of insulin and its application to human beings made front-page news around the world.

By 1923, insulin was produced in seemingly unlimited quantities by the Eli Lilly Company of Indianapolis. It was a blockbuster drug of gargantuan proportions and a reprieve from certain death for tens of thousands of diabetics that year, and millions in the years since.

Later, in 1923, Banting and Macleod (but neither Best nor Collip) received the Nobel Prize for Medicine or Physiology. Banting magnanimously shared his prize money with Best; Macleod followed suit by sharing his prize money with Collip. Leonard lived another 13 years, thanks to insulin, before succumbing to pneumonia, most likely a complication of his diabetes, at the age of 27 in 1935.

Insulin opened the door for a series of discoveries on hormones and a slew of other "wonder drugs" that continue to improve and save the lives of billions of people around the world.

A quintessential great moment of 20th century medical science, the discovery of insulin by a determined surgeon assisted by a mere medical student continues to inspire a legion of scientists working in 21st century laboratories. And it all began with a borrowed laboratory, a few experimental dogs, a desperate patient, and an inspired surgeon with an extremely good idea.

CHAPTER 64

cVo

Alfred Nobel's Spirit of Discovery

Every December 10, since 1901, the eyes of the world have turned to Stockholm, Sweden, where the Nobel Prizes are formally awarded to the brilliant men and women who have made exemplary inroads in Physiology or Medicine, Physics, Chemistry, and Literature. The "Prize in Economic Sciences in Memory of Alfred Nobel" is a separate award founded by the Sveriges Riksbank (the Swedish National Bank) and the Nobel Peace Prize is awarded in Oslo, Norway.

The first Nobel Prize for Physiology or Medicine was awarded in 1901 to Emil Adolf von Behring for his discovery of diphtheria antitoxin. William Röntgen, the man who discovered X-rays, won the first prize awarded for Physics.

Although everyone seems to know something about the Nobel Prize, few recall the man who created them, Alfred Bernhard Nobel. During his working life, Alfred Nobel earned a huge fortune as an inventor and industrialist. His most profitable creation was dynamite. Upon his death on December 10, 1896, Nobel devoted his wealth to funding his eponymous awards. His last will and testament ordered the accrued interest to be "annually distributed in the form of prizes to those who, during the preceding year, shall have conferred the greatest benefit on mankind." Although Alfred Nobel never gave a public explanation for why he decided to create the awards, many have speculated that it emerged from his remorse over inventing a slew of agents used to such lethal effect in the wars and various national aggressions of his age.

The endowment he left was worth more than 31 million Swedish Krona (SEK), which, according to the Nobel Prize official website, is worth over 1.7 billion SEK today, nearly $200 million U.S. dollars. The amount of money awarded this year for each of the Nobel Prizes is set at 8 million Swedish Krona, or about $940,000, depending on the daily exchange rate of SEK to U.S. dollars.

Alfred Nobel was born in Stockholm in 1833. His family moved to St. Petersburg in 1837 where his father owned a mechanical workshop that made explosive

Literatim: Essays at the Intersections of Medicine and Culture. Howard Markel, Oxford University Press (2020).
© Oxford University Press.
DOI: 10.1093/oso/9780190087647.001.0001

naval mines (wooden barrels filled with gun powder). His biggest client was Czar Nicholas I of Russia who needed the mines to block enemy naval ships from entry. After the Crimean War ended in 1856, Mr. Nobel's factory became less and less profitable and by 1859 he declared bankruptcy. That same year the Nobels moved back to Sweden. There, Alfred, who trained as a chemical engineer in St. Petersburg, buttressed by post-graduate work in Sweden, Germany, France and the United States, opened his own laboratory to develop a series of more reliable explosives.

Alfred's first breakthrough in 1863 involved mastering the means to detonate the highly volatile and dangerous liquid, nitroglycerin. In 1864, Alfred's nitroglycerin factory exploded killing his younger brother, Emil, and many of his workers. As a result he had to move his workshop from populous Stockholm to a barge on Lake Mälaren, outside of town.

Over the next three years Nobel searched for a safer means of manufacturing nitroglycerine-based explosive devices, including the development of a detonator or blasting cap. *The Dictionary of Scientific Biography* cites his company, Nitroglycerine Ltd., established outside of Stockholm in 1865, as "the world's first true factory for producing nitroglycerin. In 1867, Alfred figured out a means of combining nitro-glycerine with a substance called *kieselguhr*, a porous form of diatomite. By mixing the two, he turned the liquid nitroglycerine into a paste that he then molded into rods and cylinders. He called his new invention "dynamite," after the Greek word *dynamis*, or power.

In the years that followed, he founded a laboratory in San Remo, Italy, where he discovered the chemical means to make dynamite an even more powerful weapon as well as for blasting rock and construction work. He held the patents for dynamite in Sweden, Great Britain and the United States. All told, he held more than 355 patents in several different countries.

Less well-known, Nobel also conducted experiments in the fields of electro-chemistry, optics, biology and physiology. Among his researches were techniques later applied to manufacturing artificial versions of silk, leather and rubber. He also became interested in the international peace movement of his era, which may explain his establishment of a Peace Prize.

The impressive and long list of life-saving work honored by the Nobel Prize committee would, undoubtedly, please the man who endowed their magnificent award.

CHAPTER 65

༄

The Real Story Behind Penicillin

The discovery of penicillin, one of the world's first antibiotics, marks a true turning point in human history—when doctors finally had a tool that could completely cure their patients of deadly infectious diseases.

Many students can still recite the basic facts of the story. Penicillin was discovered in London in September of 1928 when Dr. Alexander Fleming, the bacteriologist on duty at St. Mary's Hospital of London, returned from a summer vacation in Scotland to find a messy lab bench and a good deal more.

Upon examining some colonies of *Staphylococcus aureus*, Dr. Fleming noted that a mold called *Penicillium notatum* had contaminated his Petri dishes. After carefully placing the dishes under his microscope, he was amazed to find that the mold prevented the normal growth of the *staphylococci*.

It took Fleming a few more weeks to grow enough of the persnickety mold so that he was able to confirm his findings. His conclusions turned out to be phenomenal: there was some factor in the *Penicillium* mold that not only inhibited the growth of the bacteria but, more important, might be harnessed to combat infectious diseases.

As Dr. Fleming famously wrote about that red-letter date: "When I woke up just after dawn on September 28, 1928, I certainly didn't plan to revolutionize all medicine by discovering the world's first antibiotic, or bacteria killer. But I guess that was exactly what I did."

Fourteen years later, in March 1942, Anne Miller became the first civilian patient to be successfully treated with penicillin, lying near death at the New Haven Hospital in Connecticut, after miscarrying and developing an infection that led to blood poisoning.

But there is much more to this historic sequence of events.

Actually, Fleming had neither the laboratory resources at St. Mary's Hospital nor the chemistry background to take the next giant steps of isolating the active

Literatim: Essays at the Intersections of Medicine and Culture. Howard Markel, Oxford University Press (2020).
© Oxford University Press.
DOI: 10.1093/oso/9780190087647.001.0001

ingredient of the *penicillium* mold juice, purifying it, figuring out which germs it was effective against, and how to use it. That task fell to Dr. Howard Florey, a professor of pathology who was director of the Sir William Dunn School of Pathology at Oxford University. He was a master at extracting research grants from tight-fisted bureaucrats and an absolute wizard at administering a large laboratory filled with talented but quirky scientists.

This landmark work began in 1938 when Florey, who had long been interested in the ways that bacteria and mold naturally kill each other, came across Fleming's paper on the *Penicillium* mold while leafing through some back issues of *The British Journal of Experimental Pathology*. Soon after, Florey and his colleagues assembled in his well-stocked laboratory. They decided to unravel the science beneath what Fleming called *Penicillium*'s "antibacterial action."

One of Florey's brightest employees was a biochemist, Dr. Ernst Chain, a Jewish German émigré. Chain was an abrupt, abrasive and acutely sensitive man who fought constantly with Florey over who deserved credit for developing penicillin. Despite their battles, they produced a series of crude *Penicillium*-mold culture fluid extracts.

During the summer of 1940, their experiments centered on a group of 50 mice that they had infected with deadly *streptococcus*. Half the mice died miserable deaths from overwhelming sepsis. The others, which received penicillin injections, survived.

It was at that point that Florey realized that he had enough promising information to test the drug on people. But the problem remained: how to produce enough pure penicillin to treat people. In spite of efforts to increase the yield from the mold cultures, it took 2,000 liters of mold culture fluid to obtain enough pure penicillin to treat a single case of sepsis in a person.

In September 1940, an Oxford police constable, Albert Alexander, 48, provided the first test case. Alexander nicked his face working in his rose garden. The scratch was infected with *streptococci* and *staphylococci* and the germs spread to his eyes and scalp. Although Alexander was admitted to the Radcliffe Infirmary and treated with doses of sulfa drugs, the infection worsened and resulted in smoldering abscesses in the eye, lungs and shoulder. Florey and Chain heard about the horrible case at high table one evening and, immediately, asked the Radcliffe physicians if they could try their "purified" penicillin.

After five days of injections, Alexander began to recover. But Chain and Florey did not have enough pure penicillin to eradicate the infection, and Alexander ultimately died.

Another vital figure in the lab was a biochemist, Dr. Norman Heatley, who used every available container, bottle and bedpan to grow vats of the *Penicillium* mold, suction off the fluid and develop ways to purify the antibiotic. The makeshift mold factory he put together was about as far removed as one could get from the enormous fermentation tanks and sophisticated chemical engineering that characterize modern antibiotic production today.

In the summer of 1941, shortly before the United States entered World War II, Florey and Heatley flew to the United States, where they worked with American scientists in Peoria, Illinois, to develop a means of mass producing what became known as the wonder drug.

Aware that the *Penicillium notatum* would never yield enough penicillin to treat people reliably, Florey and Heatley searched for a more productive species.

One hot summer day, a laboratory assistant, Mary Hunt, arrived with a cantaloupe that she had picked up at the market and that was covered with a "pretty, golden mold."

Serendipitously, the mold turned out to be the fungus *Penicillium chrysogeum*, and it yielded 200 times the amount of penicillin as the species that Fleming had described. Yet even that species required enhancing with mutation-causing X-rays and filtration, ultimately producing 1,000 times as much penicillin as the first batches from *Penicillium notatum*.

In the war, penicillin proved its worth. Throughout history, the major killer in wars had been infection rather than battle injuries. In World War I, the death rate from bacterial pneumonia was 18 percent; in World War II, it fell to less than 1 percent.

From January to May in 1942, 400 million units of pure penicillin were manufactured. By the end of the war, American pharmaceutical companies were producing 650 billion units a month.

Fleming did little work on penicillin after his initial observations in 1928. Beginning in 1941, after news reporters began to cover the early trials of the antibiotic on people, however, the unprepossessing and gentle Fleming was lionized as "the discoverer of penicillin." And much to the quiet consternation of Florey, the Oxford group's contributions were virtually ignored.

That problem was partially corrected in 1945, when Fleming, Florey, and Chain—but not Heatley—were awarded the Nobel Prize in Physiology or Medicine. In his acceptance speech, Fleming presciently warned that the overuse of penicillin might lead to bacterial resistance.

In 1990, Oxford made up for the Nobel committee's oversight by awarding Heatley the first honorary doctorate of medicine in its 800-year history. Maybe this September 28, as we celebrate Alexander Fleming's great accomplishment, we will recall that penicillin also required the midwifery of Florey, Chain and Heatley, as well as an army of laboratory workers.

CHAPTER 66

⚭

The Day Scientists Discovered
the "Secret of Life"

The place: The Eagle, a genial pub and favorite luncheon spot for the staff, students and researchers working at the University of Cambridge's Cavendish laboratory on nearby Free School Lane.
The date: Feb. 28, 1953, a day when real, honest-to-goodness history was made.
The time: 12 noon.

Two men entered the noisy pub to create even more noise. The first was a tall, gangly, 25-year-old American bacteriologist with uncombed hair named James Watson. The second, Francis Crick, was a 37-year-old British physicist who, according to one of his scientific rivals, looked like "a bookmaker's rout."

With booming voices and youthful bravado, the odd duo bragged that they, in the words of Francis Crick—or at least in the memory of James Watson recalling the words of Francis Crick—"We have discovered the secret of life."

Indeed, they had. That very morning, the two men worked out the double helix structure of deoxyribonucleic acid, better known to every first-grader as DNA.

Mind you, they did not discover DNA. That scientific feat was actually accomplished in 1869 by Friedrich Miescher, a physiological chemist working in Basel, Switzerland. Miescher determined that DNA, a nucleic acid found in the cell's nucleus, was comprised of sugar, phosphoric acid, and several nitrogen containing bases. But for decades, no one quite knew much about its precise function.

In 1944, a trio of scientists, Oswald Avery, Colin Macleod, and Maclyn McCarty, determined that DNA was the "transforming principle," the substance that carries genetic information. Nevertheless, there remained many naysayers who felt that the

Literatim: Essays at the Intersections of Medicine and Culture. Howard Markel, Oxford University Press (2020).
© Oxford University Press.
DOI: 10.1093/oso/9780190087647.001.0001

chemical composition of DNA was far too simple to carry such complex data and, instead, argued that proteins must contain the true genetic material.

Proving how the simple brew of chemicals contained in DNA carried such an array of information required an elucidation of its actual structure, echoing a centuries' old concept in the history of medicine and science that continues to this very day: specifically, one must determine the form of a biological unit before one can begin to understand its function.

Watson and Crick worked with three-dimensional models to re-construct the DNA molecule, much as a college student uses those pesky sticks and balls to cram for an organic chemistry exam.

Only 50 miles away, however, a team of physicists at King's College in London was using a complex technique called X-ray crystallography to study DNA. One of them, Rosalind Franklin, succeeded in taking an X-ray diffraction pattern from a sample of DNA that showed a clearly recognizable cross or helical shape. Unbeknownst to Franklin, one of her colleagues at King's College, Maurice Wilkins, let Watson see the image a few days earlier.

Franklin's DNA picture experimentally confirmed the correctness of the theoretical double helical model Watson and Crick were developing. As Watson later reflected on the importance of Feb. 28, 1953: "The discovery was made on that day, not slowly over the course of the week. It was simple; instantly you could explain this idea to anyone. You did not have to be a high-powered scientist to see how the genetic material was copied."

They finished building their now-famous model on March 7, 1953.

Watson and Crick published their findings in the April 25, 1953, issue of *Nature*. It was a brief communication of less than 900 words that discussed the double helix of DNA and suggested that the two strands of DNA allowed it to create identical copies of itself. Regardless of the report's brevity, the announcement changed the world of medicine and science forever.

Tragically, in 1958 Rosalind Franklin died of ovarian cancer. She was 37 years old. Watson and Crick, along with Maurice Wilkins, won the Nobel Prize for Physiology or Medicine in 1962. But because the Nobel Prize rules prevent it from being awarded posthumously, Franklin did not receive the credit she so richly deserved until years after her death.

In the epilogue of his 1968 memoir, *The Double Helix*, James Watson discusses his less-than-gentlemanly rivalry with Rosalind Franklin as well the appreciation he later came to acquire for her brilliant work. Gallant, perhaps, but the credit was a dollar short and quite a few days too late.

Feb. 28, 1953, was a landmark day in human history, medicine and science as well as a transformative moment in the lives of Watson and Crick. Sadly, it was just another day in the laboratory for the unsung Rosalind Franklin.

CHAPTER 67

✦

The Surgeon General's Famous Report That Alerted Americans to the Deadly Dangers of Cigarettes

D ozens of distinguished physicians have served as the U.S. surgeon general in our nation's history. That said, we rarely remember their names, including the surgeon general who may have had the farthest-reaching influence on our collective health.

That man was Dr. Luther Terry. On January 11, 1964, he released an earthshaking, 150,000-word report entitled, *Smoking and Health*.

The study identified cigarette smoking as the chief cause of lung cancer in men (and later, as the gender gap between smokers narrowed, women too). Smoking was also named as the most important cause of chronic bronchitis in men and women and a major culprit for laryngeal cancer. Heading up a committee of 10 scientific experts, (which included five smokers and five non-smokers) Dr. Terry hammered a few more nails in the tobacco-lined coffin by declaring that smokers were 70 percent more likely to die of a fatal heart attack than nonsmokers, and that there was a strong association between cigarette smoking and cancer of the esophagus and bladder, emphysema, peptic ulcers, and premature babies.

His conclusion was clear and chilling in a country where at least 42 percent of all adults were smokers. "It is the judgment of the Committee that cigarette smoking contributes substantially to mortality from certain specific diseases and to the overall death rate," read the report.

Unfortunately, the public's health has long been stymied on this issue by the powerful tobacco industry, a business so ingrained in the American fabric that tobacco leaves are inscribed in stone on the façade of the U.S. Capitol Building.

Literatim: Essays at the Intersections of Medicine and Culture. Howard Markel, Oxford University Press (2020).
© Oxford University Press.
DOI: 10.1093/oso/9780190087647.001.0001

Nevertheless, the brave Dr. Terry orchestrated a 14-month review of more than 7,000 scientific and public health studies on the topic, or as he referred to it, "the most comprehensive analysis ever taken." Upon introducing this seminal document, he promised to "move promptly" in taking bold steps to "advise anyone to discontinue smoking" or, at least, recognize "the health hazard" of cigarettes. Although a number of roadblocks were put in his and his successors' way, he was responsible for one of the most famous warnings ever made in this history of medicine and public health:

"Caution: Cigarette smoking may be hazardous to your health."

The following year, Congress passed legislation requiring this warning to be prominently displayed on every package of cigarettes. On July 27, 1965, President Lyndon Johnson, a notorious smoker himself, signed the act into law. Sadly, it took another six years to fully implement. In 1971, cigarette manufacturers were finally banned from advertising on television. In each of these years, and up to the present, roughly half a million or more Americans died from the results of smoking.

Cigarette manufacturers did their best (or worst) to poke holes and discredit the 1964 study's scientific findings, which have only proved to be more ominous in the decades that followed. The tobacco industry also stepped up the marketing of their products not only to the millions of Americans who were already hooked on smoking, but also to women and minorities who had not previously taken up the habit. And they put millions of dollars into lobbying congressmen and senators to keep their products profitable and widely used. A few decades after the Terry report, the cigarette manufacturers tried to discredit subsequent scientific research on the dangers of second hand smoke and the addictive nature of nicotine. It was not until the 1980s, during the term of Surgeon General C. Everett Koop, that cigarette smoking finally began to be banned from airplanes, hospitals, restaurants and other public spaces.

Long after Dr. Terry stepped down from his federal government appointment, he continued to warn the American public about the dangers of smoking. In 1967, for example, in his role as chairman of the National Interagency Council on Smoking and Health, he said, "The period of uncertainty is over. There is no longer any doubt that cigarette smoking is a direct threat to the user's health. There was a time when we spoke of the smoking and health 'controversy.' To my mind, the days of argument are over . . . Today we are on the threshold of a new era, a time of action, a time for public and private agencies, community groups and individual citizens to work together to bring his hydra-headed monster under control."

That era came closer in the 1990s after a coalition of state attorneys general successfully sued the tobacco industry for the harm they had caused to so many addicted smokers.

And yet, we are nowhere near ending the profitable sales of these toxic and deadly products. According to the U.S. Centers for Disease Control and Prevention, cigarette smoking remains the leading cause of preventable disease and death in the United States; more than 480,000 deaths every year, or one of every five deaths, are attributed to smoking. In 2015, 15 out of every 100 American adults aged 18 years or older (15.1 percent) smoked cigarettes. This means that about 36.5 million adults in the United States currently smoke cigarettes. More than 16 million Americans live with a smoking-related disease.

We can take heart in the fact that current smoking has declined from nearly 21 of every 100 adults (20.9 percent) in 2005 to about 14 of every 100 adults (14.0 percent) in 2017. This means that roughly 34.3 million Americans currently smoke cigarettes and more than 16 million Americans live with a smoking-related illness. But even with the advent of electronic-cigarettes (which have already created a potent set of public health problems) and medical treatments to stop smoking, we still have a long way to go in ending this preventable scourge.

Take a tip from this aging doctor, if not from Surgeon General Terry: If you do smoke, get some help to kick the habit. If you have not yet picked up your first cigarette—DON'T! You will likely live longer as a result of this sound decision.

CHAPTER 68

∞

The Publication of *Alcoholics Anonymous*

One of the Most Influential Books in the History of Medicine and Public Health

April 10, 1939 marks the publication date of *Alcoholics Anonymous: The Story of How Many Thousands of Men and Women Have Recovered from Alcoholism*. One of the best-selling books of all time (it has sold more than 30 million copies), the volume is better known to millions of recovering alcoholics and addicts as "the Big Book." Its influence on the world's health and the treatment of alcoholism and other addictions is immeasurable. In 2011, *Time* Magazine placed the Big Book on its most 100 influential books written in English since 1923 (not coincidentally the year *Time* was founded). In 2012, the Library of Congress designated it as one of the 88 books that "shaped America".

The book's copyright application, filed April 19, 1939, lists William G. ("Bill") Wilson, the co-founder of Alcoholics Anonymous, as the sole author. In reality, the book was very much a group effort. Dozens of recovering alcoholics, many who attended the earliest AA meetings and who had an average sobriety time of 1 to 1.5 years, helped Bill Wilson with the writing of the book in 1938. Their express purpose was to spread the life-saving premises of Alcoholics Anonymous.

The heart of the Big Book can be found in the first 164 pages, which outlines the now famous 12-steps of recovery, chapters devoted to how the program works, advice to the alcoholic's spouse, family, and employer, as well as counsel for the agnostic who seeks the spirituality felt to be necessary for those seeking recovery but who has questions about the existence of a higher power. Equally compelling is the compendium of personal stories that follows these chapters and which was designed to give "experience, strength and hope" to those seeking recovery.

Literatim: Essays at the Intersections of Medicine and Culture. Howard Markel, Oxford University Press (2020).
© Oxford University Press.
DOI: 10.1093/oso/9780190087647.001.0001

As of 2018, the General Services Office of Alcoholics Anonymous estimated there are 125,352 AA groups in more than 180 nations with over 2,130,000 members. "The Big Book," now in its 4th edition, remains their basic, and most important, text.

One of the best-known stories about AA's origins concerns a business trip made by the newly recovering Bill Wilson in 1935 to Akron, Ohio. Stuck in the hotel lobby, between a bar and a phone booth with a registry of local churches, he began calling the various clergymen to inquire if they would recommend a suffering alcoholic he could work with in order to buttress his own sobriety. It took more than a few calls, but he was finally given the name of a once successful and now well-oiled surgeon named Bob Smith. Bill went over to Dr. Bob's house and history was made. The two initially recruited other suffering alcoholics both in New York and Akron. With time, support by many physicians, journalists, and the philanthropy of John D. Rockefeller, Jr., AA chapters sprung up across North America.

Less well known, however, was Bill Wilson's incredible "spiritual experience" while being treated for alcoholism in the Towns Hospital of New York City. Many historians argue it was this miraculous moment that really gave birth to Alcoholics Anonymous and the influential book it spawned.

By the early 1930s, Wilson was a full-blown alcoholic, consuming more than two quarts of whiskey a day. Between 1933 and 1934, Mr. Wilson was admitted to Towns Hospital four different times. Although Wilson made some progress in temporarily abstaining, he relapsed after each of the first three hospitalizations.

In early December of 1934, Wilson reunited with a drinking buddy named Ebby Thacher. Ebby told Bill that he had been able to quit alcohol thanks to the help of the Oxford Group, a church-based association devoted to living a sober life guided by Christianity. As a way of showing Bill Wilson his new way of life, Ebby Thacher took him to the Calvary Mission, where the most drunken of New York's Depression-era down-and-outers went to be fed and, it was hoped, "saved."

A few days later, a drunken Wilson staggered back into the Towns Hospital. His physician, William D. Silkworth, M.D. sedated him with chloral hydrate and paraldehyde, along with a regimen of pills, cathartics, and tincture of belladonna. The latter was thought to cure people of alcoholism even though it causes hallucinations when given in high and frequent doses.

On the third day of his treatment, Mr. Wilson had his now famous spiritual awakening. Earlier that evening, Mr. Thacher had visited and tried to persuade Mr. Wilson to turn himself over to the care of a Christian deity who would liberate him from the ravages of alcohol. Hours later, depressed and delirious, Mr. Wilson cried out: "I'll do anything! Anything at all! If there be a God, let him show himself!" He then witnessed a blinding light and felt an ecstatic sense of freedom and peace. When Mr. Wilson told Dr. Silkworth about the event, the physician responded: "Something has happened to you I don't understand. But you had better hang on to it."

Hang on to it he did. Indeed, this experience ultimately led Mr. Wilson to abstain from alcohol for the remaining 36 years of his life and to co-create the novel program whereby one alcoholic helps another through a commitment to absolute honesty and a belief that a higher power can help one achieve sobriety.

Skeptics have dismissed Bill Wilson's spiritual awakening, sobriety, and even the remarkably important book he helped write, as mere products of belladonna hallucinations; others have argued that it was the result of *delirium tremens* or the symptoms of alcohol withdrawal. Wiser men and women have accepted that something else happened to Bill Wilson on that long ago night, something that medical science simply cannot explain.

In the end, millions of people around the world who have benefited from Alcoholics Anonymous, and the life-changing book bearing its name, would say that such pharmacological, physical or spiritual parsing hardly matters. For them, the most important thing is that it works.

CHAPTER 69

∽

Presidents Get Sick and Die

What Happens Next Hasn't Always Been Clear

On July 18, 1947, President Harry Truman signed the Presidential Succession Act, a law designed to clarify the order of succession upon the death of a sitting president and/or vice president. At the time, the critical process of presidential succession was an issue left somewhat unsettled by the Founding Fathers when they wrote and ratified the Constitution in the late 18th century.

To be sure, in Article II, Section 1, Clause 6, the Constitution describes the legal transfer of presidential power to the vice president if the former resigns or dies while in office. But this guiding document does little to describe what happens if the president becomes seriously ill, or who has the legal authority to determine if a particular illness or condition is severe enough to prevent the president from fulfilling his or her job. One reason this issue might have been left unresolved was the state of medicine in the late 18th century; unlike today, people tended to die rather quickly of the most serious illnesses.

In 1791, the first U.S. Congress pondered what would happen if both the offices of president and vice president were left unfilled at the same time and several congressmen urged that the secretary of state be next in line. There was a festering political sore beneath this prescription: The secretary of state at the time was Thomas Jefferson, an ardent anti-Federalist who had many Federalist opponents in the Congress.

The following year, in 1792, the second U.S. Congress passed a law stating that in the event both the president and the vice-president were dead or disabled, first the Senate president *pro tempore* and then the speaker of the House would become the acting president until either the disability that prevented the sitting president

Literatim: Essays at the Intersections of Medicine and Culture. Howard Markel, Oxford University Press (2020).
© Oxford University Press.
DOI: 10.1093/oso/9780190087647.001.0001

or vice president from serving was resolved or, in the event of their deaths, a new election could be held.

Nevertheless, presidential succession remained a thorny issue throughout the 19th century and beyond.

In April of 1841, for example, William Henry Harrison died one month after beginning his presidency. His vice president, John Tyler, unilaterally insisted on taking the oath of president—as opposed to "acting president" as many of his colleagues suggested. Matters became complicated again when Abraham Lincoln was murdered in 1865. One of the issues debated in the aftermath of this tragedy was who should be third in line, either the president *pro tempore* of the Senate (the most senior, and often the oldest, senator in the chamber) or the secretary of state (an appointed rather than an elected official, but the most senior member of the presidential administration).

In 1866, it was agreed that the secretary of state, followed by cabinet officers in order of the tenure of their departments, would succeed the vacancies. But a special election was not yet required by law. The acting president would serve until the next presidential election was judged to be completed by the Electoral College. That said, there was still congressional hand-wringing when Andrew Johnson was impeached, but not removed, in 1868; when James Garfield was shot and left dying for months in 1881; and again, in 1886, when Grover Cleveland and members of Congress urged changes in the succession process after Cleveland's vice president Thomas Hendricks died in office. When William McKinley was assassinated in 1901, Teddy Roosevelt rose from vice president to president, but served the rest of that term without the benefit of a vice president.

Nearly half a century later, Harry Truman became president in 1945 after Franklin Roosevelt's death on April 12, one month into FDR's historic fourth term. Once sworn in, Truman lobbied for a return to the succession delineated in the 1792 act, with one key distinction. The speaker of the House would be third in line as acting president, followed by the president *pro tempore* of the Senate, and then cabinet officers based on the date their department was created (today, the secretary of state remains the most senior and the secretary of homeland security, a position which was created in 2002, is the most junior).

Some have argued that Truman wanted these changes because of his close relationship with then speaker of the House, Sam Rayburn. Truman instead claimed that because the speaker was the leader of "the elected representatives of the people," he or she should be next to ascend to the vacancy of vice president or president, if the situation arose. Just as important, Truman was acutely aware of the fragility of presidential health and learned first-hand the importance of having an unambiguous plan for presidential succession in place.

In 1967, the 25th Amendment of the Constitution was ratified and its four sections further address some (but not all) of the succession issues President Truman raised. The first two sections of the 25th Amendment deal with how presidential power is assumed in the event of a president's death or resignation and allows the president to nominate a vice president when that office becomes vacant. The third section delineates a president's voluntary resignation of power. The fourth section discusses the involuntary removal of a president, when he or she is deemed unable to perform the job, by members of the cabinet and of Congress—but this has never been acted upon in American history.

Ethicists and presidential historians insist there remain serious problems in terms of presidential succession, both in the 25th Amendment and in the 1947 Succession Act, particularly in terms of defining the disabilities, physical, or mental illnesses that might prevent the president or vice-president from fulfilling his or her duties.

To make matters worse, throughout the 20th century, candidates and elected officials have not always been fully forthcoming about their medical histories because of concerns that such disclosures might cost them votes or political support. Woodrow Wilson's concealment of his debilitating stroke and the role his wife, Edith Galt Wilson, played in both the "cover-up" and by secretly acting as president; FDR's lower body paralysis (as a result of his 1921 bout with poliomyelitis) and, later, his congestive heart failure, malignant hypertension, and related disabilities; Dwight D. Eisenhower's secrecy over his 1955 heart attack, 1956 intestinal obstruction, and 1957 stroke; John F. Kennedy's multiple health problems including Addison's disease and the many medications he took while negotiating sensitive geopolitical matters; Richard Nixon's mental health during the final months of his presidency; and Ronald Reagan's gunshot wounds, cancer surgeries, and the extent of his Alzheimer's disease are just a few examples of serious disabilities that can affect our chief executives. How have these disabilities affected world events? We will never quite know the answer to that query.

Today, poll after poll demonstrates that the American people want to know about the health of their elected officials, and especially their president. And while private citizens are certainly entitled to privacy with respect to their health, matters become decidedly different when running for or holding the highest office in the land. Some medical experts have suggested that the president undergo an annual physical and mental health examination (including evaluations for depression and Alzheimer's disease), which are made public upon completion in real time.

The obvious reality is that we all get sick and we are all going to die. No president—no matter how powerful, beloved, or despised—is immune to the slings and arrows of human disease. Fortunately, we live in an era when so many medical and mental health conditions can be successfully treated and individuals live healthy, normal lives despite having this or that illness. That said, this physician insists that the American voter deserves to know the medical and mental health histories of our nation's chief magistrate, from the moment they announce their candidacy to their last day in office.

Just as all voters need access to this critical health information as they execute the profound civic duty of electing the next president of the United States, every president should be able to rest easier with the knowledge that there exists a clear path of succession in place, in the event of illness, disability or death. As President Harry Truman once opined about presidential health and disability, "We ought not go on trusting to luck to see us through."

THE TWENTY-FIFTH AMENDMENT TO
THE U.S. CONSTITUTION

Section 1. In case of the removal of the president from office or of his death or resignation, the vice president shall become president.

Section 2. Whenever there is a vacancy in the office of the vice president, the president shall nominate a vice president who shall take office on confirmation by a majority vote of both houses of Congress.

Section 3. Whenever the president transmits to the president pro tempore of the Senate and the Speaker of the House of Representatives his written declaration that he is unable to discharge the powers and duties of his office, and until he transmits to them a written declaration to the contrary, such powers and duties shall be discharged by the vice president as acting president.

Section 4. Whenever the vice president and a majority of either the principal officers of the executive departments or of such other body as Congress may by law provide transmit to the president pro tempore of the Senate and the Speaker of the House of Representatives their written declaration that the president is unable to discharge the powers and duties of his office, the vice president shall immediately assume the powers and duties of the office as acting president.

Thereafter, when the president transmits to the president pro tempore of the Senate and the Speaker of the House of Representatives his written declaration that no inability exists, he shall resume the powers and duties of his office unless the vice president and a majority of either the principal officers of the executive department or of such other body as Congress may by law provide, transmit within 4 days to the president pro tempore of the Senate and the Speaker of the House of Representatives their written declaration that the president is unable to discharge the powers and duties of his office. Thereupon, Congress shall decide the issue, assembling within 48 hours for that purpose if not in session. If the Congress within 21 days after receipt of the latter written declaration, or, if Congress is not in session within 21 days after Congress is required to assemble, determines by two-thirds vote of both houses that the president is unable to discharge the powers and duties of his office, the vice president shall continue to discharge the same as acting president; otherwise, the president shall resume the powers and duties of his office.

CHAPTER 70

✧

December 14, 1799

The Excruciating Final Hours
of President George Washington

I t was a house call no physician would relish. On December 14, 1799, three doctors were summoned to Mount Vernon in Fairfax County, Va., to attend to a critically ill, 67-year-old man who happened to be known as "the father of our country."

On the afternoon of December 13, a little more than 30 months into his retirement, George Washington complained about a cough, a runny nose and a distinct hoarseness of voice. He had spent most of the day on horseback in the frigid rain, snow and hail, supervising activities on his estate. Late for dinner and proud of his punctuality, Washington remained in his damp clothes throughout the meal.

By 2 a.m. the following morning, Washington awoke clutching his chest with a profound shortness of breath. His wife Martha wanted to seek help but Washington was more concerned about her health as she had only recently recovered from a cold herself. Washington simply did not want her leaving the fire-warmed bedroom for the damp, cold outside. Nevertheless, Martha asked her husband's chief aide, Colonel Tobias Lear, to come into the room. Seeing how ill the general was, Colonel Tobias immediately sent for Dr. James Craik, who had been Washington's physician for more than 40 years, and the estate's overseer, George Rawlins, who was well practiced in the art of bloodletting.

Only a few hours later, 6 a.m., Washington developed a pronounced fever. His throat was raw with pain and his breathing became even more labored.

At 7:30 a.m., Rawlins removed 12 to 14 ounces of blood, after which Washington requested that he remove still more. Following the procedure, Colonel Lear gave the

Literatim: Essays at the Intersections of Medicine and Culture. Howard Markel, Oxford University Press (2020).
© Oxford University Press.
DOI: 10.1093/oso/9780190087647.001.0001

patient a tonic of molasses, butter and vinegar, which nearly choked Washington to death, so inflamed were the beefy-red tissues of his infected throat.

American history buffs know so much about George Washington's final illness because of a wealth of primary source documents as well as the herculean efforts of Dr. David Morens, an epidemiologist and the Senior Advisor to the Director of the National Institute for Allergy and Infectious Diseases. Dr. Morens wrote about these harrowing last hours for the *New England Journal of Medicine* in 1999. (1999; 341: 1845-1849). Another fascinating account of Washington's medical history can be found in a 1933 issue of the *Bulletin of the Institute of the History of Medicine* written by Dr. J.H. Mason Knox Jr. (1933; 1: 174-191). And even more intriguing is a long letter about Washington's last illness, written by Colonel Tobias as the events unfolded, and which copies exist both in the William Clements Library of the University of Michigan and at Rare Book Room of the University of Virginia.

Dr. Craik entered Washington's bedchamber at 9 a.m. After taking the medical history, he applied a painful "blister of cantharides," better known as "Spanish fly," to Washington's throat. The idea behind this tortuous treatment was based on a humoral notion of medicine dating back to antiquity called "counter-irritation." The blisters raised by this toxic stuff would supposedly draw out the deadly humors causing the General's throat inflammation.

At 9:30 a.m., another bloodletting of 18 ounces was performed followed by a similar withdrawal at 11 a.m. At noon, an enema was administered. Attempts at gargling with a sage tea, laced with vinegar were unsuccessful but Washington was still strong enough to walk about his bedroom for a bit and to sit upright in an easy chair for a few hours. His real challenge was breathing once he returned to lying flat on his back in bed.

Dr. Craik ordered another bleeding. This time, 32 ounces were removed even though Elisha Cullen Dick, the second physician to arrive at Mount Vernon, objected to such a heroic measure. A third doctor, Gustavus Richard Brown, made it to the mansion at 4 p.m. He suggested a dose of calomel (mercurous chloride) and a tartar emetic (antimony potassium tartrate), guaranteed to make the former president vomit with a vengeance.

After the fourth bloodletting, Washington appeared to rally somewhat. At 5 p.m., he was having an easier time swallowing and even had the energy to examine his last will and testament with Martha. Soon enough, he was again struggling for air. He told Dr. Craik: "Doctor, I die hard; but I am not afraid to go; I believed from my first attack that I should not survive it; my breath can not last long." Ever the gentleman, even *in extremis*, the General made a point of thanking all three doctors for their help.

By 8 p.m., blisters of cantharides were applied to his feet, arms and legs while wheat poultices were placed upon his throat with little improvement. At 10 p.m., Washington murmured some last words about burial instructions to Colonel Lear. Twenty minutes later, Lear's notes record, the former president settled back in his bed and calmly took his own pulse. At the very end, Washington's fingers dropped off from his wrist and the first president of our great Republic took his final breath. At the bedside were Martha Washington, his doctor, James Craik, Tobias Lear, his valet, Christopher Sheels, and three slave housemaids named Caroline, Molly and Charlotte.

Washington's physicians, as doctors are wont to do, argued heatedly over the precise cause of death. Dr. Craik insisted that it was "inflammatory quinsy," or peritonsillar abscess. Dr. Dick rejected such a possibility and offered three alternative diagnoses: *stridular suffocatis* (a blockage of the throat or larynx), *laryngea* (inflammation and suppuration of the larynx), or *cynanche trachealis*. The last arcane medical diagnosis (from the Latin, for "dog strangulation"), which prevailed as the accepted cause of Washington's death for some time, referred to an inflammation and swelling of the glottis, larynx and upper trachea severe enough to obstruct the airway.

Back in 1799, Washington's physicians justified the removal of more than 80 ounces of his blood (2.365 liters or 40 percent of his total blood volume) over a 12-hour period in order to reduce the massive inflammation of his windpipe and constrict the blood vessels in the region. Theories of humoralism and inflammation aside, this massive blood loss—along with the accompanying dehydration, electrolyte imbalance, and viscous blood flow—could not have helped the president's dire condition.

A fourth physician, William Thornton (who also designed the U.S. Capitol Building), arrived after Washington succumbed. Thornton had expertise in the tracheotomy procedure, an extremely rare operation at the time that was performed only in emergencies and with occasional success. Dr. Dick, too, advocated this procedure—rather than the massive bloodletting—but given the primitive nature of surgical science in 1799, it is doubtful it would have helped much.

In the more than 215 years since Washington died, several retrospective diagnoses have been offered ranging from croup, quinsy, Ludwig's angina, Vincent's angina, diphtheria, and streptococcal throat infection to acute pneumonia. But Dr. Morens's suggestion of acute bacterial epiglottitis seems most likely. In the end, we will never really know, which constitutes half of the fun enjoyed by doctors who argue over the final illnesses of historical figures.

At this late date, it is all too easy to criticize Washington's doctors. Indeed, even in real time and for decades thereafter, critics complained that the physicians bled Washington to death. But the truth of the matter is that they did the best they could, against a pathologically implacable foe, using now antiquated and discredited theories of medical practice.

The president's last hours must have been agonizing to watch and, of course, to experience. Like any human being, General Washington hoped his physicians would help him to an easy death. Between the massive bloodletting, the painful blistering treatments, and the awful sensation of suffocation, this was not at all possible.

Excruciating though his death was, George Washington's life continues to teach us valuable lessons of citizenship, leadership and devotion to duty. In an era when there are so few heroes in public life, it remains inspiring to recall Henry ("Light-Horse Harry") Lee Jr.'s famous phrase from the eulogy of Washington he delivered to the U.S. Congress on December 26, 1799: "First in war, first in peace, and first in the hearts of his countrymen."

CHAPTER 71

∿

The Dirty, Painful Death of President James A. Garfield

On September 19, 1881, James Abram Garfield, the 20th president of the United States, died. His final weeks were an agonizing march towards oblivion that began on July 2, while preparing to leave Washington for a family vacation to the New Jersey seashore.

A man of great energy, eloquence and charm, Garfield was in a superlative mood that morning. At the breakfast table, he horsed around with his two teenaged sons while singing a few patter songs written by the musical kings of his day, Gilbert and Sullivan.

A few hours later, the president was strolling through the Baltimore and Potomac train station. Before he reached the platform, a mentally disturbed lawyer and writer named Charles Guiteau broke through the crowd and entered the history books. He shot Garfield twice. The first bullet grazed his arm but the second passed the first lumbar vertebra of his spine and lodged in his abdomen. Fully conscious, in awful pain, and unable to stand, President Garfield cried out, "My God, what is this?"

A battery of Washington doctors rushed to the scene. One of them, an expert in gunshot wounds named Doctor (no joke, that was his first name!) Willard Bliss, ultimately became Garfield's chief physician.

Focused on finding and removing the bullet, Bliss and the other doctors stuck their unwashed fingers in the wound and probed around, all for naught and without applying the numbing power of ether anesthetic. In late 19th century America, such a grimy search was a common medical practice for treating gunshot wounds. A key principle behind the probing was to remove the bullet, because it was thought that leaving buckshot in a person's body led to problems ranging from

Literatim: Essays at the Intersections of Medicine and Culture. Howard Markel, Oxford University Press (2020).
© Oxford University Press.
DOI: 10.1093/oso/9780190087647.001.0001

"morbid poisoning" to nerve and organ damage. Indeed, this was the same method the doctors pursued in 1865 after John Wilkes Booth shot Abraham Lincoln in the head.

President Garfield was taken back to the White House where the medical treatment truly became brutal. Still hellbent on finding and removing the bullet, the doctors argued whether it damaged the spinal cord (Garfield complained of numbness in his legs and feet) or one of the many organs in the abdomen. Dr. Bliss even recruited Alexander Graham Bell to apply his newly invented metal detector device to find the errant bullet.

As the summer waned, Garfield was suffering from a scorching fever, relentless chills, and increasing confusion. The doctors tortured the president with more digital probing and many surgical attempts to widen the three-inch deep wound into a 20-inch-long incision, beginning at his ribs and extending to his groin. It soon became a super-infected, pus-ridden, gash of human flesh.

This assault and its aftercare probably led to an overwhelming infection known as sepsis, from the Greek verb, "to rot." It is a total body inflammatory response to an overwhelming infection that almost always ends badly—the organs of the body simply quit working. The doctors' dirty hands and fingers are often blamed as the vehicle that imported the infection into the body. But given that Garfield was a surgical and gunshot-wound patient in the germ-ridden, dirty Gilded Age, a period when many doctors still laughed at germ theory, there might have been many other sources of infection as well.

During his last 80 days of life, Garfield wasted away from a plump 210 pounds to a bony 130 pounds. On September 6, a special train transported him to his seashore cottage at Long Branch, New Jersey. The president's final breaths were inspired on the evening of September 19. Clutching his chest and wailing, "This pain, this pain," he died. Without the aid of a stethoscope, Dr. Doctor W. Bliss raised his head from the president's chest at 10:35 pm and announced to Mrs. Garfield and the medical retinue, "It is over." The assigned causes of death include a fatal heart attack, the rupture of the splenic artery, which resulted in a massive hemorrhage, and, more broadly, septic blood poisoning.

Guiteau was later found guilty of murder and sentenced to death, even though he was one of first high-profile cases in American history to plead not guilty by reason of insanity. He was hanged on June 20, 1882, in Washington D.C.

In recent years, a wave of revisionist historians has taken Garfield's doctors to task for not applying sterile technique, and, thus, saving the President's life.

There is, indeed, a grain of truth to the assassin Guiteau's claim "the doctors killed Garfield, I just shot him." But this odd and disgusting medical history requires a more nuanced clarification.

To be sure, in 1881, when Garfield was shot, Louis Pasteur and Robert Koch were at work scientifically demonstrating the germ theory of disease to great public acclaim. Beginning in the late 1860s, the surgeon Joseph Lister beseeched his colleagues to apply these discoveries and adopt "anti-sepsis" in their operating rooms. This technique required surgeons and nurses to thoroughly wash their hands and instruments in anti-septic chemicals, such as carbolic acid or phenol, before touching the patient.

The number of surgeons who actually followed Lister's edicts of cleanliness as late as 1881, however, was hardly universal. From the distance of more than a century, it is tempting to imagine that germ theorists, or "contagionists," overtook "anti-contagionist" medical practices with the speed of light. In real time, however, many mainstream physicians and surgeons did not fully adopt anti-septic techniques until into the mid-to-late 1890s, and for some, as late as the early 1900s.

Blaming his doctors may be a tantalizing literary trope but President Garfield had an excellent chance of dying from the ordeal no matter who treated him during his awful, last summer. Nevertheless, Bliss and his colleagues certainly cannot be credited with helping Mr. Garfield all that much either.

In the final, post-mortem analysis, the president desperately needed a modern medical miracle long before his doctors were equipped to produce one.

CHAPTER 72

∿

When a "Secret President" Ran the Country

Woodrow Wilson may have been one of our hardest-working chief executives and, by the fall of 1919, he looked it.

For most of the six months between late December 1918 and June 1919, our 28th president was in Europe negotiating the Treaty of Versailles and planning for the nascent League of Nations, efforts for which he was awarded the 1919 Nobel Peace Prize (an award he did not officially receive until 1920). Back home, however, the ratification of the treaty met with mixed public support and strong opposition from Republican senators, led by Henry Cabot Lodge (R-Mass.), as well as Irish Catholic Democrats. As the summer progressed, President Wilson worried that defeat was in the air.

Bone-tired but determined to wage peace, on September 3, 1919, Woodrow Wilson embarked on a national speaking tour across the United States so that he could make his case directly to the American people. For the next three and a half weeks, the president, his wife Edith Bolling Galt Wilson, assorted aides, servants, cooks, Secret Service men and members of the press rode the rails. The presidential train car, quaintly named the *Mayflower*, served as a rolling White House. Also joining the party was the president's personal physician, Cary T. Grayson, who had grave concerns over his patient's health.

Not that Woodrow Wilson was the picture of health before beginning this grueling crusade.

When Wilson took office, the famed physician and part-time novelist Silas Weir Mitchell ominously predicted that the president would never complete his first term. Dr. Weir was wrong on that prognosis even though Dr. Grayson did fret aloud and often about Wilson's tendency to overwork.

Literatim: Essays at the Intersections of Medicine and Culture. Howard Markel, Oxford University Press (2020).
© Oxford University Press.
DOI: 10.1093/oso/9780190087647.001.0001

For example, while negotiating with European leaders on arriving at an equitable peace to end "the Great War," Wilson worked incessantly, eliminating all the exercise, entertainment and relaxation sessions from his schedule. In early April of 1919, like tens of millions of other people during the worst pandemic in human history, the American president succumbed to a terrible case of influenza.

All during September of 1919, as the presidential train traveled across the Midwest, into the Great Plains states, over the Rockies into the Pacific Northwest and then down the West Coast before turning back East, the president became thinner, paler and ever frailer. He lost his appetite, his asthma grew worse and he complained of unrelenting headaches.

Unfortunately, Woodrow Wilson refused to listen to his body.

He had too much important work to do. Combining his considerable skills as a professor, scholar of history, political science and government, orator and politician, he threw himself into the task of convincing the skeptics and preaching to the choir on the importance of ratifying the treaty and joining the League of Nations. At many of the "whistle stops," vociferous critics heckled and shouted down his proposals. In the Senate, his political opponents criticized Wilson's diplomacy, complained that the treaty reduced the Congress's power to declare war, and ultimately voted the treaty down.

Late on the evening of September 25, 1919, after speaking in Pueblo, Colorado, Edith discovered Woodrow in a profound state of illness; his facial muscles were twitching uncontrollably and he was experiencing severe nausea. Earlier in the day, he complained of a splitting headache.

Six weeks after the event, Dr. Grayson told a journalist that he had noted a "curious drag or looseness at the left side of [Wilson's] mouth—a sign of danger that could no longer be obscured." In retrospect, this event may have been a transient ischemic attack (T.I.A.), the medical term for a brief loss of blood flow to the brain, or "mini-stroke," which can be a harbinger for a much worse cerebrovascular event to follow—in other words, a full-fledged stroke.

On September 26, the president's private secretary, Joseph Tumulty, announced that the rest of the speaking tour had been canceled because the president was suffering from "a nervous reaction in his digestive organs." The *Mayflower* sped directly back to Washington's Union Station. Upon arrival, on September 28, the president appeared ill but was able to walk on his own accord through the station. He tipped his hat to awaiting crowd, shook the hands of a few of the people along the track's platform, and was whisked away to the White House for an enforced period of rest and examination by a battery of doctors.

Everything changed on the morning of October 2, 1919. According to some accounts, the president awoke to find his left hand numb to sensation before falling into unconsciousness. In other versions, Wilson had his stroke on the way to the bathroom and fell to the floor with Edith dragging him back into bed. However those events transpired, immediately after the president's collapse, Mrs. Wilson discretely phoned down to the White House chief usher, Ike Hoover and told him to "please get Dr. Grayson, the president is very sick."

Grayson quickly arrived. Ten minutes later, he emerged from the presidential bedroom and the doctor's diagnosis was terrible: "My God, the president is paralyzed," Grayson declared.

What would surprise most Americans today is how the entire affair, including Wilson's extended illness and long-term disability, was shrouded in secrecy. The recent discovery of the presidential physicians' clinical notes at the time of the illness confirm that the president's stroke left him severely paralyzed on his left side and partially blind in his right eye, along with the emotional maelstroms that accompany any serious, life-threatening illness, but especially one that attacks the brain. Only a few weeks after his stroke, Wilson suffered a urinary tract infection that threatened to kill him. Fortunately, the president's body was strong enough to fight that infection off but he also experienced another attack of influenza in January of 1920, which further damaged his health.

Protective of both her husband's reputation and power, Edith shielded Woodrow from interlopers and embarked on a bedside government that essentially excluded Wilson's staff, the Cabinet and the Congress. During a perfunctory meeting the president held with Senators Gilbert Hitchcock (D-Neb.) and Albert Fall (R-NM) on December 5, he and Edith even tried to hide the extent of his paralysis by keeping his left side covered with a blanket. Senator Fall, who was one of the president's most formidable political foes told Wilson, "I hope you will consider me sincere. I have been praying for you, Sir." Edith later recalled that Woodrow was, at least, well enough to jest, "Which way, Senator?" A great story, perhaps, but Wilson's biographer, John Milton Cooper, Jr. doubts its veracity and notes that neither Edith nor Dr. Grayson recorded such a clever rejoinder in their written memoranda from that day.

By February of 1920, news of the president's stroke began to be reported in the press. Nevertheless, the full details of Woodrow Wilson's disability, and his wife's management of his affairs, were not entirely apparent to the American public at the time.

What remained problematic was that in 1919 there did not yet exist clear constitutional guidelines of what to do, in terms of the transfer of presidential power, when severe illness struck the chief executive. What the U.S. Constitution's Article II, Section 1, Clause 6 on presidential succession does state is as follows:

> In Case of the Removal of the President from Office, or of his Death, Resignation, or Inability to discharge the Powers and Duties of the said Office, the Same shall devolve on the Vice President, and the Congress may by Law provide for the Case of Removal, Death, Resignation or Inability, both of the President and Vice President, declaring what Officer shall then act as President, and such Officer shall act accordingly, until the Disability be removed, or a President shall be elected.

But Wilson, of course, was not dead and not willing to resign because of inability. As a result, Vice President Thomas Marshall refused to assume the presidency unless the Congress passed a resolution that the office was, in fact, vacant, and only after Mrs. Wilson and Dr. Grayson certified in writing, using the language spelled out by the Constitution, of the president's "inability to discharge the powers and duties of the said office." Such resolutions never came.

In fact, it was not until 1967 that the 25th Amendment to the Constitution was ratified, which provides a more specific means of transfer of power when a president dies or is disabled. Parenthetically, many presidential health scholars continue to argue that even the 25th Amendment is not clear enough in terms of presidential succession and needs revision, especially in the face of 21st century medicine and the increased chances of surviving major illnesses with severe and impairing disabilities.

For the remainder of her life, Edith Wilson steadfastly insisted that her husband performed all of his presidential duties after his stroke. As she later declared in her 1938 autobiography, *My Memoir*:

> So began my stewardship, I studied every paper, sent from the different Secretaries or Senators, and tried to digest and present in tabloid form the things that, despite my vigilance, had to go to the President. I, myself, never made a single decision regarding the disposition of public affairs. The only decision that was mine was what was important and what was not, and the very important decision of when to present matters to my husband.

Over the last century, historians have continued to dig into the proceedings of the Wilson administration and it has become clear that Edith Wilson acted as much more than a mere "steward." She was, essentially, the nation's chief executive until her husband's second term concluded in March of 1921. Nearly three years later, Woodrow Wilson died in his Washington, D.C., home, at 2340 S Street, NW, at 11:15 AM on Sunday, February 3, 1924.

According to the February 4, 1924 issue of *The New York Times*, the former president uttered his last sentence on Friday, February 1: "I am a broken piece of machinery. When the machinery is broken—I am ready." And on Saturday, February 2, he spoke his last word: *Edith*.

As we look forward to future presidential campaigns it seems appropriate to recall that October 2, 1919 may well mark the first time in American history a woman became *de facto* president of the United States, even if Edith Wilson never officially held the elected position. Indeed, the prolonged blockage of blood flow to his brain changed more than the course of Woodrow Wilson's life; it changed the course of history.

CHAPTER 73

∾

The "Strange" Death
of Warren G. Harding

At 7:20 p.m. on the evening of August 2, 1923, a terrible event of national importance occurred in the presidential suite of San Francisco's Palace Hotel. President Warren G. Harding's wife, Florence, was reading the latest issue of the *Saturday Evening Post* to him. The article in question was about Mr. Harding and appeared to please him because he was last heard to utter, "That's good, go on." Immediately thereafter, he shuddered and dropped dead onto his bed.

Recently ill with cramps, indigestion, fever and a distressing shortness of breath, the president chalked up his feeling so poorly to a week after succumbing to "food poisoning" and the stresses of his being on a 15,000-mile, cross-country speaking tour, including the territory of Alaska, the first time a U.S. President had visited that part of the nation. His aides, already planning a re-election campaign, labeled the trip, "The Voyage of Understanding."

As the week progressed, Harding seemed to be improving somewhat but that was merely illusory. The 29th president of the United States and the 6th chief magistrate to die in office was never a healthy man. (Since Harding's death, two more presidents sadly have joined that list, Franklin D. Roosevelt and John F. Kennedy).

Harding had long suffered from an overly nervous condition then known as neurasthenia. Some of his doctors warned Harding, while he was still in the U.S. Senate, that his multiple amorous affairs might physically injure his delicate and enlarged heart. Since at least 1918, Harding suffered from shortness of breath, bouts of chest pain, and difficulty sleeping unless his head was propped up on several pillows, all signs of congestive heart disease.

Mr. and Mrs. Harding's favorite doctor was an odd and charismatic homeopathic physician from Ohio named Charles Sawyer, who the president appointed as a Brigadier General in the U.S. Army and the chairman of the Federal Hospitalization

Literatim: Essays at the Intersections of Medicine and Culture. Howard Markel, Oxford University Press (2020).
© Oxford University Press.
DOI: 10.1093/oso/9780190087647.001.0001

Board. Harding's other physician was the far better trained Joel T. Boone, a U.S. naval officer and Medal of Honor winner. Dr. Sawyer was given to dosing the ailing president with purgatives, laxatives and injections of heart stimulants, including the once commonly prescribed arsenic, which did not always sit well with Dr. Boone. Medical disagreements notwithstanding, President Harding's doctors arranged for him to be examined while he was in San Francisco, by Ray Lyman Wilbur, the president of Stanford University, a president of the American Medical Association, and a leading heart specialist. (Wilbur later became Herbert Hoover's Secretary of the Interior, from 1929-1933).

The nurses present on the scene instructed the Secret Service agent on duty to find Dr. Sawyer, who was down the hall, and Dr. Boone, who was out dining with General John J. "Black Jack" Pershing. The first official to reach the death scene was the Secretary of Commerce, Herbert Hoover. By the time the president's doctors arrived, around 7:30 p.m., Harding was already dead. The vice president, Calvin Coolidge, was sworn into office at 2:43 a.m. Eastern time, at his home in Plymouth, Vermont.

Mrs. Harding refused all entreaties to allow the doctors to conduct an autopsy and instead ordered that her husband be embalmed shortly after his death. Dr. Wilbur was especially frustrated by this refusal because the press and a bereaved public blamed the president's doctors for incompetence, malpractice and even plots of poisoning the president. "We were accused of being abysmally ignorant, stupid and incompetent," Dr. Wilbur griped in later years.

In 1930, Gaston Means, an embittered, former Harding Administration official, published a book entitled *The Strange Death of President Harding*. In addition to his short stint with the Department of Justice's Bureau of Investigation, he was also a notorious confidence man and bootlegger who died in Leavenworth Prison in 1938, after being convicted for a con he tried to pull related to the Charles Lindbergh Jr. kidnapping.

In his 1930 book, Means falsely claimed that Florence Harding poisoned her husband. He also gathered together tall tales and scandals within the Harding administration, including "Teapot Dome" and Prohibition violations, as well as Harding's clandestine love affairs—one of which may, or may not, have led to the birth of an illegitimate child. Mr. Means' ghostwriter, May Dixon, later exposed the book as a pack of lies. Beyond the published falsehoods he asked her to record, her anger stemmed from the fact that Means failed to pay her any of the royalties owed to her.

Nevertheless, rumors are powerful things and they continue to swirl about Harding's memory to the present day.

On the evening of the president's death, Herbert Hoover sent out the official news that the president had died of "a stroke of cerebral apoplexy." But it was most likely a sudden myocardial infarction, or heart attack, that ended Harding's life at the age of 58, two years more than the average life span for an American male in 1923 (56.1 years).

In the end, President Harding's death was hardly strange at all, merely premature by 21st century standards.

CHAPTER 74

ojo

Franklin D. Roosevelt's Painfully
Eloquent Final Words

At 1:00 in the afternoon of April 12, 1945, Franklin Delano Roosevelt was sitting in a chair near the fireplace of his cottage, which was perched atop Pine
Mountain in Warm Springs, Georgia. Over the previous 12 years, reporters came to
refer to the president's quaint lodge of respite as "the Little White House."

The president was in high spirits despite a long period of poor health and, a few
weeks earlier, a bout of arduous negotiating at the Yalta conference, which mapped
out the end of World War II. Also present at the Little White House were his
cousins Daisy Suckley and Laura "Polly" Delano, his secretary Grace Tully, some
military aides and medical attendants, an artist named Elizabeth Shoumatoff, who
was making some sketches in preparation for a presidential portrait, and, perhaps
most relevant for FDR's improved mood, his mistress, Lucy Mercer Rutherfurd.

Lucy, it may be recalled, was Eleanor's social secretary while Franklin was
Woodrow Wilson's assistant secretary of the Navy. Eleanor found out about his affair
with the beautiful socialite just after Franklin returned from Europe in September
of 1918 with a galloping case of the Spanish influenza. While unpacking his things,
Mrs. Roosevelt found a packet of love letters from Lucy. Eleanor vowed to divorce
FDR if the relationship did not end *pronto*, and Sara Roosevelt, FDR's mother,
threatened to write him out of the family's money. These two blows would have
effectively ended his political career. The affair re-heated during FDR's presidency.
During the war, his daughter Anna arranged for visits with Lucy when Eleanor was
out of town.

After traveling some 14,000 miles to Yalta and back, Franklin Roosevelt arrived
to Warm Springs on March 30, 1945, looking haggard and gaunt, with dark circles
under his eyes, obvious weight loss, and an overall aura of fatigue. This was decidedly not the picture of health and optimism that the jaunty FDR famously exhibited

Literatim: Essays at the Intersections of Medicine and Culture. Howard Markel, Oxford University Press (2020).
© Oxford University Press.
DOI: 10.1093/oso/9780190087647.001.0001

in years past. The president hoped that a few weeks of rest and recreation in the warm mineral waters of Georgia would do the trick before traveling west to San Francisco for the United Nations conference on international organization to be held on April 25.

There was more to the president's poor appearance than mere overwork. He had long suffered the effects of poorly controlled hypertension, (high blood pressure) in an era when one of the only medications available to lower it a bit was the soporific phenobarbital. The president also suffered from hypertension's most common aftermaths: atherosclerosis, arteriosclerosis, and congestive heart failure.

On the morning of the 12th, Roosevelt woke up at 9:20 a.m. and had a light breakfast. He complained of a mild headache and some neck stiffness but the latter seemed to resolve with mild massage. Despite the warm and humid clime, FDR felt a chill and asked for a warm cape to be draped on his shoulders. As the president casually read the newspapers and composed a few letters at a card table that served as his make-shift desk, the artist Shoumatoff set up her easel and painted away. At 1:00 pm, the president said, "We have about 15 minutes more to work."

At that point, Daisy thought Franklin had dropped one of his ever-present cigarettes because his head drooped forward and he seemed unable to raise it. She asked her cousin what was wrong. He raised his left hand to the rear of his head and said in a soft whisper, "I have a terrific pain in the back of my head." Those were Franklin Roosevelt's final words.

Despite the ministrations of his doctors, he was declared dead at 3:35 pm. Only an hour before his demise, Lucy Rutherfurd and Elizabeth Shoumatoff hurriedly left the Little White House and drove their way to Aiken, South Carolina.

Franklin Roosevelt, the nation's longest serving president and, perhaps its most successful commander-in-chief, died 83 days into his fourth term. He was 63 years old. The immediate cause was a massive cerebral hemorrhage.

A number of physicians and conspiracy theorists have long debated that FDR was not of sound mind and body during his last months of office. This is an argument Roosevelt's own physicians, close friends and relatives have heatedly denied. One of the great shibboleths in this debate concerns his last address to Congress on March 1, 1945, which he made from his wheelchair rather than gripping onto a lectern.

"I hope that you will pardon me for this unusual posture of sitting down," the president began his speech, "but I know you will realize that it makes it a lot easier for me not to have to carry about 10 pounds of steel around on the bottom of my legs." On the radio, many listeners noted an occasional hesitance or loss for words, something rarely, if ever, heard in an FDR speech. When asked about it later by reporters, Roosevelt laughed it off and explained how he had gone "off book" from his prepared remarks and then encountered difficulties finding his place when returning to the printed speech.

In the years since Roosevelt's death, some retrospective diagnoses have included a series of mini-strokes before his final "cerebrovascular accident," all the way to poisoning by enemies of the state, and a malignant melanoma that spread into his brain, causing his cerebral hemorrhage. Alas, an autopsy was not performed at Eleanor's request.

In the end, FDR's health—once threatened so severely by his bout of poliomyelitis in 1921 and the resultant paralysis of his lower body—finally gave out after years of carrying the weight of the United States, and ultimately the free world, on his muscular shoulders.

Ten years to the day of the president's death, on April 12, 1955, representatives of his foundation, the National Foundation for Infantile Paralysis (the March of Dimes) announced Dr. Jonas Salk's effective and safe vaccine to prevent polio. A more fitting memorial for one of our greatest American presidents is difficult to imagine.

CHAPTER 75

cW∂

How Florence Nightingale Cleaned up "Hell on Earth" Hospitals and Became an International Hero

In all of medical history, few names have been sung more brightly than Florence Nightingale. She was born on May 12, 1820. Credited with founding the first modern, secular nursing school in 1860 (at St. Thomas's Hospital in London, and currently part of King's College, University of London), Florence's birthday has been designated International Nursing Day.

Nicknamed "the Lady of the Lamp" by an intrepid journalist for the *London Times*, and subsequently immortalized by Henry Wadsworth Longfellow in his 1857 poem *Santa Filomena*, Florence Nightingale first came to prominence during the Crimean War.

In 1855, she organized and trained a group of nurses to help the soldiers injured during that conflict. Appalled by the primitive hospital facilities, the lack of beds, bandages, and bathing facilities, all wrapped into a decidedly filthy, vermin-ridden environment, Nightingale later wrote, "the British high command had succeeded in creating the nearest thing to hell on earth." Initially, her nurses were not allowed to see the suffering soldiers and, instead, ordered to clean the hospital floors. As the casualties mounted and the physicians became overwhelmed, Nightingale's nurses were finally enlisted to help.

Nightingale's poetic moniker was the result of her late evening rounds visiting the wounded soldiers while carrying a lamp for illumination. When the war ended and she returned home to London, she was lauded as a national hero and showered with awards and medals including a jewel from Queen Victoria.

Ever busy advancing the profession of nursing, Nightingale worked extraordinarily hard to counter the prevalent (and negative) view of nurses, such as that

Literatim: Essays at the Intersections of Medicine and Culture. Howard Markel, Oxford University Press (2020).
© Oxford University Press.
DOI: 10.1093/oso/9780190087647.001.0001

described by Charles Dickens in his 1842-1843 novel, *Martin Chuzzlewit*. One of the minor characters in this delightful tome is an incompetent, poorly trained and negligent nurse named Sarah Gamp is best recalled as an alcoholic, far more interested in her next glass of gin than the needs of her patients.

Nightingale's 1859 book, *Notes on Nursing*, on the other hand, sheds a far better light on the profession and soon became a standard textbook for training nurses around the globe.

Florence was also consumed with advancing the cause of cleanliness in the hospital setting and beyond by using the newly developed mathematical methods of statistics to prove that such interventions made a difference.

Beginning with her war work, Nightingale noted that 10 times more soldiers died of the so-called filth diseases, such as cholera, dysentery, typhoid and typhus, than those who succumbed to bullets and cannon balls. She determined the cause to be related to the overcrowding of soldiers, paltry latrine and sewer facilities and, in an era when "poisonous miasmas" were still thought to the source of many infectious diseases, poor ventilation in the hospital wards. Indeed, her insistence on adequate ventilation led to a worldwide trend of building hospitals with large windows and cross-ventilation schemes, a design one can still see in the few late-19th century hospital buildings that remain in various American and European cities.

Working with the pioneering British statistician William Farr and public health and urban poverty expert Edwin Chadwick, she compiled, analyzed and presented understandable and detailed information on the living conditions of England's poorest citizens, as well as the living conditions, public health, and medical care of those living in India. Florence Nightingale pioneered in the graphical representation of the numbers she crunched. She was an early adopter of the "pie chart" and developed her own "rose diagram," which is a circular histogram of data she called the "coxcomb" and used to describe seasonal changes in patient mortality, first in various military theaters and, subsequently, among Britain's poor.

This work led to the passage of England's Public Health Acts of 1874 and 1875, which required property owners to connect their sewage lines to main drain pipes, as a means of controlling the dumping of huge amounts of human waste onto city streets, and giving control of public health problems to local authorities who saw the unhealthy conditions first hand, rather than the previous system of granting those powers to centralized government officials in a faraway office. Both these reforms are credited with playing a vital role in extending the lifespan of British subjects (as well as citizens in other industrialized, western nations) by 20 years, between 1891 and the mid-1930s, when there were not yet the advantages of antibiotics, intravenous fluids or other modern medical conveniences.

A deeply religious woman, Florence was the advantaged child of a wealthy family. She managed to use those advantages, as well as surmount the disadvantages of being an ambitious, professional woman in Victorian England. Florence was truly committed to helping the neediest and most vulnerable, both to the ravages of poverty and disease.

Every May 12, on International Nurse's Day, we celebrate Florence's many accomplishments and the work of dedicated nurses around the world who continue to make a huge difference in caring for the ill.

When reflecting on the life of this extraordinary woman, the doctor in me is forced to recall a lesson he learned the hard way as an intern: if you want to know what is really going on with a patient, make sure you ask his or her nurse first.

CHAPTER 76

∽

Celebrating Rebecca Lee Crumpler, First African American Woman Physician

Rebecca Lee Crumpler (1831–1895 is best remembered as the first African-American woman physician in the United States. Born Rebecca Davis in Delaware on February 8, 1831, she grew up in Pennsylvania, where her aunt provided care for the ill.

A bright girl, Rebecca attended a prestigious private school, the West Newton English and Classical School in Massachusetts, as a "special student." In 1852, she moved to Charlestown, Massachusetts, and worked as a nurse. In 1860, she took the bold step of applying to medical school and was accepted into the New England Female Medical College.

The New England Female Medical College was based in Boston and attached to the New England Hospital for Women and Children. It was founded by Drs. Israel Tisdale Talbot and Samuel Gregory in 1848. The school accepted its first class of 12 women in 1850. From its inception, many male physicians derided the institution, complaining that women lacked the physical strength to practice medicine; others insisted that not only were women incapable of mastering a medical curriculum and that many of the topics taught were inappropriate for their "sensitive and delicate nature."

Fortunately, Drs. Talbot and Gregory ignored such false claims and organized a school that required "a good English education," a "thesis on some medical subject," and a set of courses on the theory and practice of medicine, *materia medica*, chemistry and therapeutics, anatomy, medical jurisprudence, obstetrics and diseases of women and children, and physiology and hygiene. The coursework was 17 weeks in length (30 or more hours per week) during the first year of instruction. Following this was a two-year preceptorship, or apprenticeship, under an established physician's supervision.

Literatim: Essays at the Intersections of Medicine and Culture. Howard Markel, Oxford University Press (2020).
© Oxford University Press.
DOI: 10.1093/oso/9780190087647.001.0001

In 1864, Rebecca became the New England Female Medical College's only African-American graduate (the school closed its doors in 1873.) A few statistics help put her remarkable achievement in perspective. In 1860, there were only 300 women doctors out of the 54,543 physicians then practicing in the United States and none of them were African-American. Some historians have wondered if Rebecca even knew of her status as "the first" given that for many decades in the 20th century that credit was awarded to Dr. Rebecca Cole, an African-American woman who received her medical degree from the Woman's Medical College of Pennsylvania in 1867. The first "historically black" medical school in the U.S., Howard University College of Medicine, would not open until 1868. As late as 1920, there were only 65 African-American women doctors in the United States.

Around the time of her graduation, Rebecca married for the second time. (Her first marriage to Wyatt Lee, from 1852 to 1863, ended with his death in 1863.) In 1864, she married Arthur Crumpler. Rebecca began a medical practice in Boston.

After the end of the Civil War in 1865, the Crumplers moved to Richmond, Virginia, where, to use her own words, she found "the proper field for real missionary work, and one that would present ample opportunities to become acquainted with the diseases of women and children." Rebecca worked under the aegis of General Orlando Brown, the Assistant Commissioner of the Freedman's Bureau for the State of Virginia. The Freedman's Bureau was the federal agency charged with helping more than 4,000,000 slaves make the arduous transition from bondage to freedom. In Richmond, Rebecca valiantly ignored daily episodes of racism, rude behavior, and sexism from her colleagues, pharmacists, and many others, in order to treat, as she later wrote, "a very large number of the indigent, and others of different classes, in a population of over 30,000 colored."

In 1869, the Crumplers returned to Boston and they settled in a predominantly African-American neighborhood on Beacon Hill. She practiced medicine there, as well. In 1880, she and her husband moved, once again, this time to Hyde Park, New York. Although there exists little evidence that she practiced much medicine after this point, she did write a fine book, *A Book of Medical Discourses in Two Parts*, which was published by Cashman, Keating and Co., of Boston, in 1883.

The book is divided, as the title implies, into two sections. The first part focuses on "treating the cause, prevention, and cure of infantile bowel complaints, from birth to the close of the teething period, or after the fifth year." The second section contains "miscellaneous information concerning the life and growth of beings; the beginning of womanhood; also, the cause, prevention, and cure of many of the most distressing complaints of women, and youth of both sexes." The volume, which may well be the first medical text by an African-American author, is dedicated "to mothers, nurses, and all who may desire to mitigate the afflictions of the human race."

Rebecca Davis Lee Crumpler died on March 9, 1895, in Hyde Park. She is an inspiration to all who face adversity, seek diversity, and forge the difficult path forward. Her passion "to mitigate the afflictions of the human race" was Rebecca's gift and historic legacy.

CHAPTER 77

༄

How Elizabeth Blackwell Became the First Female Doctor in the United States

It was a cold, wintry day in upstate, western New York when a 28-year-old Elizabeth Blackwell received her diploma from the Geneva Medical College of New York. As she accepted her sheepskin, Charles Lee, the medical school's dean, stood up from his chair and made a courtly bow in her direction.

Only two years earlier, in October of 1847, her medical future was not so certain. Already rejected from medical schools in Charleston, Philadelphia and New York City, matriculating into Geneva represented her only chance of becoming a medical doctor.

Dean Lee and his all male faculty were more than hesitant to make such a bold move as accepting a woman student. Consequently, Dr. Lee decided to put the matter up to a vote among the 150 men who made up the medical school's student body. If one student voted "No," Lee explained, Miss Blackwell would be barred from admission.

Apparently, the students thought the request was little more than a silly joke and voted unanimously to let her in; they were surprised, to say the least, when Elizabeth Blackwell arrived at the school ready to learn how to heal.

Geneva Medical College required only a year and a half of formal lectures, and young Elizabeth found her new home to be somewhat daunting. Too shy to ask questions of her fellow classmates or even her teachers, she figured out on her own where to purchase her books and how to study the rather arcane language of 19th century medicine.

Most male medical students of this era were raucous and rude; it was not uncommon for crude jokes and jeers to be hurled at the lecturer, no matter what

Literatim: Essays at the Intersections of Medicine and Culture. Howard Markel, Oxford University Press (2020).
© Oxford University Press.
DOI: 10.1093/oso/9780190087647.001.0001

the subject. But with Miss Blackwell in the room, as the legend goes, her male classmates quieted down and immediately became more studious than those the Geneva faculty had taught in the past.

One of her greatest hurdles was the class in reproductive anatomy. The professor, James Webster, felt that the topic would be too "unrefined" for a woman's "delicate sensibilities" and asked her to step out of the lecture hall. An impassioned Blackwell disagreed and somehow convinced Webster to let her stay, much to the support of her fellow students.

Nevertheless, medical school and her summer clinical experiences at the Blockley Almshouse in Philadelphia were hardly a bed of roses. Few male patients were eager to let her examine them, and not a few of her male colleagues there treated her with great animosity.

Undaunted, Elizabeth persevered and gained a great deal of clinical expertise, especially in the treatment of one of the most notorious infectious diseases of the poor: typhus fever, which became the subject of her doctoral thesis.

In April of 1849, Dr. Blackwell crossed the Atlantic to study in the medical meccas of Paris and London. In June, she began her postgraduate work at the famed Parisian maternity hospital, La Maternité, and was acclaimed by her teachers as a superb obstetrician.

Only few months later, on November 4, 1849, Dr. Blackwell was treating a baby with a bacterial infection of the eyes, most likely gonorrhea contracted from the infant's mother while passing through the birth canal. During her examination, Elizabeth contaminated her left eye and eventually lost sight in it. This injury prevented her from becoming a surgeon.

She subsequently studied at St. Bartholomew's Hospital in London. Ironically, she was permitted to practice all the branches of medicine except for gynecology and pediatrics—the two fields in which she was to garner her greatest fame.

When Dr. Blackwell returned to the United States in 1850, she began practice in New York City but found it tough going, and the patients in her waiting room were few and far between. In 1853, she established a dispensary for the urban poor near Manhattan's Tompkins Square.

By 1857, she had expanded the dispensary into the New York Infirmary for Women and Children. One of her colleagues there was her younger sister Emily, who was the third woman in the U.S. to be granted a medical degree.

Dr. Blackwell traveled widely across Europe and became increasingly interested in social reform movements dedicated to women's rights, family planning, hygiene, eugenics, medical education, sexual purity and Christian socialism.

She was also an avid writer whose by-line attracted many readers on a wide range of subjects, including advice to young girls and new parents, household health, medical education, medical sociology and sexual physiology.

Dr. Blackwell returned to London a number of times during the 1860s and 1870s. Between 1874 and 1875, she helped establish a medical school for women, the London School of Medicine for Women. She remained a professor of gynecology there until 1907, when she suffered serious injuries after falling down a flight of stairs.

Dr. Blackwell died only a few years later, in 1910, after suffering a paralytic stroke at her home in Hastings, East Sussex, England. Her ashes were buried at St. Munn's Parish Church in Kilmun, Argyllshire, Scotland.

Most often remembered as the first American woman to receive an M.D. degree, Dr. Blackwell worked tirelessly to secure equality for all members of the medical profession. Many might argue we still have a long way to go.

CHAPTER 78

ᐛ

Clara Barton's Crusade to Bring the Red Cross to America

May 21, 1881 marks the founding of the American Red Cross. Over its long and distinguished history, the Red Cross has provided a wide menu of services to help the needy, disaster victims, military personnel and their families. The American Red Cross is also a major participant in the collection, processing and distribution of blood and blood products, the development of educational programs on health, preparedness and safety, and, in partnership with other affiliate organizations of the International Federation of Red Cross and Red Crescent Societies, relief and development efforts all over the world.

The American Red Cross's Washington headquarters, right near the White House, is both a monument to "the women who died in the Civil War" and a National Historic Landmark. The organization is governed by volunteers and supported by both generous contributions from the public and income generated from health and safety training and from blood products.

One could write volumes about the American Red Cross's distinguished history and positive impact on the nation and the world. But for historical purposes, it seems wise to begin with a profile of its founder, the remarkable nurse, health activist, teacher and humanitarian Clara Barton (1821-1912).

In 1855, Barton obtained a prestigious post as a clerk in the U.S. Patent Office in Washington, D.C. She briefly enjoyed the rare distinction of earning the same salary as a man. Sadly, the times did not allow for this situation to last long and her position was initially reduced to copyist and, in 1856, eliminated entirely. After Abraham Lincoln was elected president, Barton returned to the U.S. Patent Office as a "temporary copyist" with the goal of paving the way for more women to engage in government service.

Literatim: Essays at the Intersections of Medicine and Culture. Howard Markel, Oxford University Press (2020).
© Oxford University Press.
DOI: 10.1093/oso/9780190087647.001.0001

Her second stint in Washington coincided with the onslaught of the Civil War. The capital was in a state of mass confusion because of the arrival of thousands of newly recruited soldiers all requiring uniforms, food, housing and preparation for the rigors of the battlefield. Barton immediately jumped into the fore, working to provide both assistance for the new recruits and, as the war progressed, relief for the injured. Her greatest contribution to the messy business of war (and, subsequently, natural disasters) was to organize a system of distributing medical care and supplies for the injured and providing information for the families of those injured or killed.

Barton soon realized she and her peers were most needed on the battlefields. She demonstrated extraordinary bravery at bloody locales such as Antietam by ordering the drivers of Red Cross supply wagons to follow the fighting men, often ahead of other military units. She and her associates provided nursing, comfort and meals to the wounded in the midst of danger and death.

Barton also organized an Office of Correspondence with Friends of the Missing Men of the United States Army, which she operated out of her apartment for four years. It was an operation that drew the praise of President Lincoln. Her group responded to more than 63,000 letters and identified more than 22,000 missing men.

In 1869, Barton traveled to Europe, ostensibly in search of rest. During her travels, she was introduced to the Red Cross in Geneva, which was part of the global Red Cross network of service organizations founded by Henry Durant and codified by the "Red Cross Treaty" or Geneva Convention. A major focus of treaty, which was endorsed by 12 European nations in 1864, was the humanitarian protection for those not participating in a conflict or battle, such as prisoners of war, soldiers wounded on the battlefield, and doctors, nurses and hospital units displaying the Red Cross emblem (literally, a red cross on a white background).

In 1877, Barton lobbied President Rutherford B. Hayes to endorse the Geneva Convention of 1864. Hayes initially expressed interest but worried that the treaty would be seen as a "possible entangling alliance" with European nations and ultimately rejected her petition.

Undaunted, Barton established the American Red Cross and held the first meeting in her Washington apartment on May 21, 1881. She also founded a local branch in Livingston County, New York, on August 22, 1881, where she had a country home. Around this time, Barton approached President James Garfield about ratifying the Geneva treaty. He appeared to be supportive but his death from an assassin's bullet prevented him from taking a definitive role. His successor, Chester A. Arthur, however, did agree to sign the treaty and on May 16, 1882, the U.S. Senate ratified it.

The U.S. Congress awarded the American Red Cross its first federal charter in 1900 and again in 1905. In 1904, at the age of 83, Clara Barton resigned as president of the organization.

In the years since, the American Red Cross has become one of the premier medical aid organizations in the world. Whenever and wherever a disaster has occurred on American soil, the Red Cross has been there to help and comfort the afflicted. It has also conducted major humanitarian efforts in war zones and disasters, ranging from the natural to the man-made, around the world.

It is difficult to fathom how our nation would survive crises ranging from hurricanes and earthquakes to the terrorist attacks of 9/11 and beyond, without the essential presence of the American Red Cross. Fortunately, thanks to the hundreds of thousands of women and men who have generously worked—and continue to work—under its banner and, especially, to the visionary Clara Barton, this is a question that need not be answered.

CHAPTER 79

∽

Happy Birthday to the Woman Who Revolutionized Endocrinology

July 19, 1921 marks the birthdate of the second woman to receive the Nobel Prize for Physiology or Medicine. Her name was Rosalyn Yalow and she received this great honor in 1977. (The first woman to receive the Nobel Prize for Physiology or Medicine, incidentally, was Gerty Theresa Cori, in 1947. Eight women have won the physiology or medicine award since).

Dr. Yalow was a medical physicist who co-discovered the radioimmunoassay, an exquisitely sensitive means of using "radioactive tracers" to measure hormones in the bloodstream, such as insulin, thyroid, reproductive and growth hormones, as well as levels of vitamins, viruses and many other substances in the body.

A sample size of only a few drops of blood is required to make these critical determinations, which not only saved lives and guided medical care but was also used, for example, to prevent mental retardation for thyroid hormone deficient babies still in the womb. For decades it has been a major tool in clinical medicine and medical research. Indeed, her work revolutionized the field of endocrinology, the study of diseases of hormonal systems.

Yalow's origins were humble and she conducted her entire life and career with humility and grace. She was born in the Bronx, to an immigrant mother and a father from New York's Lower East Side, neither of whom completed high school. In 1941, at age 19, Yalow graduated *magna cum laude* from Hunter College, the all-women's college of the tuition-free City University of New York, majoring in physics. Initially fascinated by chemistry, she became attracted to physics after reading Eve Curie's 1937 biography of her famous mother, Madame Marie Curie, who studied the effects of radioactivity and won the Nobel twice (for physics in 1903 and chemistry in 1911).

Literatim: Essays at the Intersections of Medicine and Culture. Howard Markel, Oxford University Press (2020).
© Oxford University Press.
DOI: 10.1093/oso/9780190087647.001.0001

Gaining acceptance into graduate school, however, was no easy task. As the *New York Times* reported in Yalow's obituary on June 1, 2011, when one of her Hunter professors recommended her for a graduate assistant's position in physics at Purdue University, a skeptical physicist wrote back, "She is from New York. She is Jewish. She is a woman. If you can guarantee her a job afterward, we'll give her an assistantship."

There was no guaranteed job and the position at Purdue fell through. That now-forgotten physicist at Purdue had no clue regarding the mettle of this courageous woman. Yalow subsequently won a job as a secretary at the Columbia University College of Physicians and Surgeons, taking additional courses in physics. Once World War II began, however, opportunities for women to assume roles tradition-ally held by men began to open up a bit. As a result, she was offered a teaching assis-tantship at the University of Illinois College of Engineering in Champagne-Urbana. With glee and excitement of pursuing her dreams, she tore up her stenographer's pads and moved to the Midwest.

Once there, Yalow learned that she was the only woman in a group of 400 teaching fellows and professors. After receiving an "A minus" in a lab course, the chairman of the physics department taunted her with the observation that women did not do well with laboratory work. She proved him wrong in ways she could not even have dreamed in 1945, when she received her Ph.D.

Moving back to New York, she again had trouble finding a job and taught at Hunter College as well as doing "volunteer" (read: unpaid) medical research at Columbia, where she was introduced to the nascent fields of radiation medicine and radiotherapy. In 1947, she moved to the Bronx Veterans Affairs Medical Center and in 1950 she joined its staff, full-time, where she worked for the remainder of her professional career.

It was at this point in time that she met her long-time collaborator, a brilliant young internist named Solomon A. Berson. They taught each other medicine and physics and then developed and perfected the radioimmunoassay, beginning in 1959. Because Berson died in 1972 and the Nobel Prize is not awarded post-humously, he did not share in the award. To commemorate his work, however, Dr. Yalow named her laboratory after Dr. Berson, so that every paper she subse-quently wrote would carry his name. Dr. Yalow was also elected to the National Academy of Sciences in 1975 and won the prestigious Lasker Award in 1976.

Yalow was known for her single-minded devotion to her research and her family. She met her husband Aaron Yalow in 1943, while both were physics grad-uate students at the University of Illinois. He, too, was a medical physicist and worked at the Montefiore Hospital in the Bronx. They had two children and two grandchildren, lived in Riverdale, New York, less than a mile from her laboratory, and were married for nearly 50 years before Aaron died in 1992.

In 1982, Dr. Yalow gave an informal speech to a group of schoolchildren about the joys and tribulations of a career as a scientist. Enthralling the youngsters with her dedication, brilliance and modesty, Dr. Yalow told the kids, "Initially, new ideas are rejected. Later they become dogma. And if you're really lucky, you can publish your rejections as part of your Nobel presentation."

Dr. Yalow may have been "lucky," but she really made her own luck by being incredibly smart, determined and talented.

CHAPTER 80

cᴧɔ

The Quarantine of "Typhoid Mary" Malone

North Brother Island is a 16.5-acre bump of land jutting out of the East River, 1,500 feet east of 140th Street in the South Bronx and 2,500 feet west of Riker's Island. Once the site of New York City's lazaretto, or quarantine hospital, it is now a favorite nesting point for herons and egrets. In its long career as an agent of quarantine, however, North Brother Island deserves mention as the enforced residence of New York City cook Mary Malone, or as she was better known, "Typhoid Mary."

In 1884, Mallon emigrated from Tyrone County in Ireland to the United States. She was only 15. Mary earned her income as a domestic and a cook in the New York City area. Between 1900 and 1907, she infected many people with *Salmonella typhosa*—then the name for the causative organism of typhoid fever. Less understood to doctors of the time—and explicated so nicely through Mary Malone's case–was that *Salmonella* carriers can be completely asymptomatic while still spreading the germ, which tends to harbor in a person's gall bladder. Modern bacteriology has explained how the Salmonella microbe sheds in feces and urine, thus demanding excellent hand washing, especially before preparing food, to cut down on the spread.

An intrepid New York City Health Department epidemiologist named George Soper tracked down a spate of typhoid cases that began in a Park Avenue penthouse where Mary Malone worked. Dr. Soper demanded she turn over urine and stool samples, but Mary refused. As his investigation continued, Soper discovered that of eight families Mary had previously worked for as a cook, seven of them had experienced bouts of typhoid fever. Soper made many more entreaties to Malone, all for naught. Once when she was hospitalized he even promised to write a book about her and give her all the royalties. Still, Mary refused to cooperate, insisted that she

Literatim: Essays at the Intersections of Medicine and Culture. Howard Markel, Oxford University Press (2020).
© Oxford University Press.
DOI: 10.1093/oso/9780190087647.001.0001

had done nothing wrong, and complained that she was being persecuted by the City of New York. In 1907, city officials arrested her in the name of the public's health. More than one newspaper reported she was "crawling with typhoid bugs." But it was the *Journal of the American Medical Association,* in a 1908 issue, that is credited with coining the now infamous epithet, "Typhoid Mary."

The New York City health department physicians gave her an ultimatum: submit to an operation to remove her gall bladder or be imprisoned on the lazaretto. Abdominal surgery of that era was fraught with deadly complications and infections and Mary understandably rejected such a choice. The officials then, literally, sent her up the river to North Brother Island, where, under sections 1169 and 1170 of the Greater New York City Charter, she lived in a tiny brick bungalow until she was released in 1910.

One of the conditions of her freedom was a promise that she would no longer earn her income working as a cook. Initially Mary worked as a laundress. But soon enough, to make ends meet, she took on kitchen jobs against doctor's orders. The result were still more outbreaks of the deadly typhoid.

On March 27, 1915, the New York City Sanitary Police tracked her down, this time on a Long Island estate. Mary Malone was confined to North Brother Island, never to return to a normal or free life. She resided there until her death, at age 69, in 1938. One of her "jobs" there was to wash the bottles and glassware used in the quarantine hospital's laboratory. Upon her autopsy, the pathologist diagnosed evidence of live typhoid bacilli in her gall bladder.

"Typhoid Mary" lives on in the popular culture because the very name conjures the personification of someone spreading an epidemic or contagious crisis. Perhaps more important, Mary's case history introduced physicians to the concept of a carrier state, whereby seemingly healthy people can spread an infectious disease as they harbor the disease-producing microbe in their bodies without apparent harm to themselves.

As reflect on Mary Malone's sentence to a life in quarantine, it is worth recalling how harshly public health officials once handled those deemed a contagious threat to others. And what a terrible life sentence it must have been. A little less than century later, standing on the rocky shoals of the island, peering into the distance, the city seems remote and inaccessible. From Mary's perspective of forced isolation for more than 25 years, it must have been truly painful.

CHAPTER 81

∽

How Nellie Bly Went Undercover
to Expose Abuse of the Mentally Ill

May 5, 1864 is the birthday of Elizabeth Cochrane Seaman. Better known by her *nom de plume* Nellie Bly (taken and misspelled from the title of a Stephen Foster tune, *Nelly Bly*), she was the pioneering, if not the very first, American investigative journalist.

Bly was born in Cochran's Mills, Pennsylvania, just outside of Pittsburgh. In 1889, she made a famous, widely reported and intrepid 72-day trip around the globe. It was the fastest journey of her era and one that shattered the fictional record of Jules Verne's wanderer, Phineas Fogg, in his novel *Around the World in 80 Days*. It was a journey she made traveling by herself rather than with a chaperone.

Medical historians and patient advocates, however, rightly revere Bly for her infamous exposé of the New York City Lunatic Asylum on Blackwell's (now Roosevelt) Island in the East River.

First reported in October 1887 on the pages of Joseph Pulitzer's flagship newspaper, the *New York World*, Bly subsequently published her daring dispatches as a book, *Ten Days in a Mad-House*. It is a slim volume that remains a classic in the annals of psychiatry and a cogent warning against inhumane treatment of the mentally ill. The book proved so embarrassing to the city aldermen that they appropriated an extra "$1,000,000 per annum" to correct many of the abuses Bly exposed.

The fascinating question to answer, of course, is how did she do it?

Bly began her journalistic career in 1880 at the age of 16, writing "women's columns" on home, hearth, gardening, society and childrearing for the *Pittsburgh Dispatch*. Soon enough, she convinced her editor to investigate such vanguard topics as how divorce affected women. Too impatient to be restricted only to domestic matters, she spent six months in Mexico as a special correspondent. Soon

Literatim: Essays at the Intersections of Medicine and Culture. Howard Markel, Oxford University Press (2020).
© Oxford University Press.
DOI: 10.1093/oso/9780190087647.001.0001

after her return, she flew the constraining coop of Pittsburgh, leaving behind a note, "I am off for New York. Look out for me. —Bly"

After talking her way into the city room of the *New York World*, she impressed the editors there enough to leave with a plum assignment: "I was asked by the *World* if I could have myself committed to one of the asylums for the insane in New York, with a view to writing a plain and unvarnished narrative of the treatment of the patients therein."

Getting committed proved rather easy, even if neither Bly nor her editors had a clear plan of getting her released once the story was secured. She took a room at a cheap boarding house, "Temporary Home for Females, No. 84 Second Avenue," under the name Bly Brown and began questioning and imitating the women who seemed most insane to her. Soon enough, it was Bly who was deemed "crazy." The matron of the house enlisted a few cops to escort Bly to the Essex Market Police Courtroom, where an impatient judge named Duffy pronounced her insane and ordered her to be confined at Bellevue Hospital, the city's largest charitable hospital. A few days later, she boarded a ferry boat filled stem to stern with unwashed and uncomprehending women for Blackwell's Island, "an insane place," one ambulance driver told her, "where you'll never get out of."

Taking careful notes of both her own experiences and those of her fellow inmates, Bly painted a dire picture in which 16 doctors were assigned to the care of some 1,600 inmates. "Excepting two," she recorded, "I have never seen them pay any attention to the patients." She questioned the judge's ability to pronounce a woman insane "by merely bidding her good morning and refusing to hear her pleas of release? Even the sick ones know it is useless to say anything for the answer will be that it is their imagination." She also reported on the cultural insensitivity and language barriers experienced by immigrant women who spoke little or no English and a host of hostile and abusive treatments, from mandatory cold baths to confinement in small, damp, vermin-infested, locked rooms.

After a few days on Blackwell's Island, Bly dropped her act of appearing insane and tried to present herself in a more fit mental state. Such efforts were all for naught until the *New York World* sent an attorney to arrange for her release. Two days later, on Sunday, Oct. 9, 1887, the *World* ran the first installment of her story, titled *Behind Asylum Bars*, and Bly became an overnight sensation. The psychiatrists who had erroneously diagnosed her as insane offered profuse apologies, even as the remaining stories were widely syndicated across the nation.

Not only did the New York City municipal government appropriate more money to the care of the mentally ill on Blackwell's Island, a grand jury was impaneled to investigate the abuses and poor treatments Bly uncovered at the asylum. Approximately one month after her articles ran in print, many of the most glaring problems she reported had improved: better living and sanitary conditions were instituted, more nourishing meals were provided, translators were hired for the foreign born who were not necessarily mentally ill but simply could not understand their keepers, and the most abusive nurses and physicians were fired and replaced.

Bly sailed from one journalistic triumph to the next, including a series of dispatches from the Eastern Front during World War I, and reports on the women's suffrage movement. In 1895, at age 31, she married the 73-year-old millionaire Robert Seaman, who ran the Iron Clad Manufacturing Company, which made steel milk cans, stacking garbage cans and boilers. Due to her husband's failing health (he died in 1904), she retired from journalism and took over the reins of the company.

Bly died of pneumonia at the age of 57 in 1922. One can only speculate what further triumphs and good deeds this remarkable woman might have achieved if only she lived a few years longer.

At the very least, she helped create the field of investigative journalism. She also led the charge to change the plights of the mentally ill in America—a problem, sadly, that still requires our collective attention and concern to this very day.

ACKNOWLEDGMENTS

I should begin this page of acknowledgements by thanking my students over the past three decades at the University of Michigan Medical School and the University of Michigan College of Literature, Science and the Arts and its Department of English Literature and Language. These energetic, ambitious, and book-hungry young scholars inspired me to think, read, and write about a wide variety of topics, many of which are included in this volume.

I am also grateful to my colleague Michael S. Schoenfeldt, Professor of English at the University of Michigan, who has co-taught my Literature and Medicine course over the past several years, so that we can provide two perspectives to our teaching; one from a historian of medicine and a physician, the other, a literary critic and Shakespeare scholar. I learn far more from him than the reverse and so do the students!

I am fortunate to direct and work at the University of Michigan Center for the History of Medicine, where my scholarship is advanced daily thanks to my colleagues Heidi Mueller and Dr. J. Alexander Navarro. I would also like to formally thank my cousin, Dr. Sheldon F. Markel, who first urged me to collect these essays in book form, and my former professors at Michigan, Bert G. Hornback, Arthur J. Vander, the late George R. DeMuth, and the late Horace W. Davenport; and at Johns Hopkins, the late Frank A. Oski and the late Barton Childs.

Debbie Malina, who edits the "Perspectives" section for the *New England Journal of Medicine*, worked diligently to enrich the essays I wrote for that august journal. I am also grateful to her colleagues, Jeffrey Drazen, Steven Morrissey, and Edward Campion.

At the *Journal of the American Medical Association*, I long wrote a column called "Literatim." Many of those essays appear in this book and they were edited and improved by Drs. Catherine DeAngelis, Phil Fontanarosa, and John Zeller, Annette Flanigan, and Dr. Howard Bauchner.

Since 2012, I have contributed a monthly essay on medical history for the *PBS NewsHour*. There, I have, or had, the joy of working with Jason Kane, Molly Finnegan, Erica Hendry, Jenny Marder, Travis Daub, Margaret Myers, Murrey Jacobsen, and Sara Just. At WUOM/Michigan Radio, the National Public Radio affiliate for the University of Michigan, I have had the pleasure of converting many of these PBS essays into conversations with the incomparable Cynthia Canty and her superb producers, Alexandra Billings and Mike Blank.

I would be remiss if I did not thank my long-time editor at the *New York Times*, the late Barbara Strauch, who taught me the value of explaining complex ideas in 800 words, or less, and on deadline. She was a gem of a newspaperwoman.

I would also like to thank the editorial staff at Oxford University Press, my superb editor Chad Zimmerman and Chloe Layman.

For the time writing these essays on weekends took away from my two daughters, Bess and Samantha Markel, while they were growing up, I apologize. On the other hand, both of them have matured into bright, able young women who are devoted readers with curious minds. So, perhaps, my digging about in books, papers, and journals during their most impressionable years had a hand in their developing those fine traits. At any rate, I love them both dearly. They are the lights of my life.

INDEX

Tables, figures, and boxes are indicated by *t, f,* and *b* following the page number.

For the benefit of digital users, indexed terms that span two pages (e.g., 52–53) may, on occasion, appear on only one of those pages.